Clinical Handbook of Psychotropic Drugs

Twelfth Revised Edition

Kalyna Z. Bezchlibnyk-Butler, BScPhm

Principal Editor

J. Joel Jeffries, MB, FRCPC[A]

Co-Editor

The Editors Wish to Acknowledge Contributions from

Roger S. McIntyre, MD, FRCPC[A]

(Antidepressants, Anticonvulsants)

Gary J. Remington, MD, PhD, FRCPC[A]

(Antipsychotics)

Barry A. Martin, MD, FRCPC[A]

(Electroconvulsive Therapy)

Umesh Jain, MD, FRCPC, DAPBN[A]

(Psychostimulants)

Andrius Baskys, MD, PhD[B]

(Cognition Enhancers)

Robert Dickey, MD, FRCPC[A]

(Sex-Drive Depressants)

[A]Centre for Addiction and Mental Health and Department of Psychiatry, University of Toronto, Toronto, Canada

[B]Department of Psychiatry and Human Behavior, University of California, Irvine, CA, USA

Hogrefe & Huber Publishers

Seattle • Toronto • Göttingen • Bern

Library of Congress Cataloging-in-Publication Data

Clinical handbook of psychotropic drugs/Kalyna Z. Bezchlibnyk-Butler, principal editor; J. Joel Jeffries, co-editor
p. cm
Bibliography: p.
ISBN 0-88937-258-6
1. Psychotropic drugs –Handbooks, manuals, etc. I. Bezchlibnyk-Butler, Kalyna Z., 1947– . II. Jeffries, J. Joel, 1939– .
RM315.C547 2002 88-21704
615'.788--dc19 CIP

Canadian Cataloguing in Publication Data

Main entry under title:

Clinical handbook of psychotropic drugs
12th rev. ed.
Includes bibliographical references and index

ISBN 0-88937-258-6

1. Psychotropic drugs – Handbooks, manuals, etc.
I. Bezchlibnyk-Butler, Kalyna Z., 1947– .
II. Jeffries, J. Joel, 1939– .

RM315.C55 2002 615'.788 C93-094102-0

12th completely revised edition

ISBN 0-88937-258-6
Hogrefe & Huber Publishers **Seattle • Toronto • Göttingen • Bern**

INTRODUCTION

The *Clinical Handbook* is a user-friendly and very practical resource guide on the use of psychotropic drugs. Its content is based on published literature (including basic science data, controlled clinical trials, and anecdotal case reports) as well as clinical experience, and is continually updated. New sections, periodically added, reflect changes in therapy and in current practice.

Charts and tables of comparisons are employed whenever possible to enable the reader to have quick access to information.

Both Canadian and American trade names are used throughout the text. Though plasma levels are given in SI units, conversion rates to Imperial U.S. units are available in the text.

Dose comparisons and plasma levels are based on scientific data. However, it is important to note that some patients will respond to doses outside the reported ranges. Age, sex, and the medical condition of the patient must always be taken into consideration when prescribing any psychotropic agent.

Patient Information Sheets have been included for all drug categories, to facilitate education/counselling of patients receiving these medications.

As the *Clinical Handbook* is intended to be a clinical summary of current information, the authors welcome input from readers as to the content or format. Please write to

Mrs K.Z. Butler
E-mail: kalyna@sympatico.ca

Information on how to obtain future editions of this handbook is given at the end.

Table of Contents

ANTIDEPRESSANTS

GENERAL COMMENTS

- Antidepressants can be classified as follows:

Chemical Class[A]	Agent	Page
Cyclic Antidepressants		
Selective Serotonin Reuptake Inhibitors (SSRI)	Example: Citalopram	See p. 3
Norepinephrine Dopamine Reuptake Inhibitor (NDRI)	Bupropion	See p. 14
Selective Serotonin-Norepinephrine Reuptake Inhibitor (SNRI)	Venlafaxine	See p. 19
Serotonin-2 Antagonists/Reuptake Inhibitors (SARI)	Example: Nefazodone	See p. 22
Noradrenergic/Specific Serotonergic Agent (NaSSA)	Mirtazapine	See p. 28
Non-Selective Cyclic Agents (Mixed Reuptake Inhibitor/Receptor Blockers)		See p. 31
NE-Reuptake Inhibitors	Example: Desipramine	See p. 31
Mixed NE/5-HT reuptake inhibitors	Example: Amitriptyline	See p. 31
Serotonin Reuptake Inhibitors	Example: Clomipramine	See p. 31
Monoamine Oxidase Inhibitors		
Reversible MAO-A Inhibitor (RIMA)	Moclobemide	See p. 44
Irreversible MAO-A-B Inhibitors (MAOIs)	Example: Phenelzine	See p. 48

[A] Antidepressants are currently classified on the basis of their specificity on the reuptake of brain neurotransmitters. This specificity confers a pharmacologic profile on the drugs that determines their spectrum of activity and adverse effects (see Table p. 39).

- Antidepressants increase psychomotor activity before affecting the depression; as energy increases, suicide is an ongoing risk
- Certain non-selective cyclic and MAOI antidepressants are toxic in overdose; limited quantities should be prescribed to patients with suicidal propensities
- Different classes of antidepressants can be combined for additive efficacy in refractory cases, but caution must be exercised – see Interactions
- Prophylaxis of depression is most effective if the therapeutic dose is maintained
- Patients with resistant depression may receive augmentation therapy (see Augmentation Strategies p. 58)

THERAPEUTIC EFFECTS

- Elevation of mood, improved appetite and sleep patterns, increased physical activity, improved clarity of thinking, better memory; decreased feelings of guilt, worthlessness, helplessness, inadequacy, decrease in delusional preoccupation and ambivalence

Selective Serotonin Reuptake Inhibitors (SSRI)

PRODUCT AVAILABILITY

Chemical Class	Generic Name	Trade Name[A]	Dosage Forms and Strengths
Phthalane derivative	Citalopram	Celexa	Tablets: 20 mg, 40 mg Oral solution[B]: 10 mg/5 ml
Bicyclic	Fluoxetine	Prozac	Capsules: 10 mg, 20 mg Enteric-coated tablets: 90 mg Delayed release pellets 90 mg[B] Oral solution: 20 mg/5 ml
Monocyclic	Fluvoxamine	Luvox	Tablets: 50 mg, 100 mg
Phenylpiperidine	Paroxetine	Paxil Paxil CR[B]	Tablets: 10 mg, 20 mg, 30 mg, 40 mg[B] Oral suspension[B]: 10 mg/5 ml Controlled-release tablets[B]: 12.5 mg, 25 mg
Tetrahydronaphthylmethylamine	Sertraline	Zoloft	Oral solution: 20 mg/ml[B] Capsules/Tablets: 25 mg, 50 mg, 100 mg

[A] Generic preparations may be available, [B] Not marketed in Canada

INDICATIONS*

- ▲ Major depression
- ▲ Prophylaxis of recurrent major depressive disorder (unipolar affective disorder)
- ▲ Treatment of secondary depression in other mental illnesses, e.g., schizophrenia, dementia
- ▲ Depressed phase of bipolar affective disorder (see Precautions)
- ▲ Bulimia nervosa (approved for fluoxetine and sertraline)
- ▲ Obsessive compulsive disorder (OCD) (approved for fluvoxamine, fluoxetine, paroxetine and sertraline)
- ▲ Panic disorder with or without agoraphobia (paroxetine, sertraline)
- ▲ Social phobia (paroxetine)
- ▲ Posttraumatic stress disorder (sertraline, paroxetine)
- ▲ Premenstrual dysphoric disorder (fluoxetine – USA)
- Dysthymia
- Atypical depression
- Generalized anxiety disorder (paroxetine)
- Major depressive disorder in patients with comorbid medical disorder (i.e., poststroke depression, myocardial infarction) or Alzheimer's disease
- Double-blind study suggests efficacy of fluvoxamine in binge-eating disorder
- Aggression, impulsive behavior, behavior disturbances of dementia and borderline personality disorder
- May aid in smoking cessation, and withdrawal from drugs, including alcohol – variable response reported
- Benefit reported in chronic fatigue syndrome, body dysmorphic disorder
- Preliminary data suggest efficacy in pervasive developmental disorder (autism) and elective mutism
- Pain management (e. g., diabetic neuropathy, arthritis), phantom limb pain (fluoxetine, sertraline), Raynaud's phenomenon (fluoxetine), fibrositis and fibromyalgia (fluoxetine) – data conflicting as to efficacy

* ▲ Approved indications

Selective Serotonin Reuptake Inhibitors (SSRI) (cont.)

- May reduce episodes of cataplexy
- Premature ejaculation
- Early data suggest a role in the treatment of functional enuresis
- Preliminary data suggests a role in reducing hot flashes
- Overview of studies and clinical experience is contradictory in terms of efficacy of SSRIs in the treament of paraphilias and paraphilia-related disorders. Use of these agents in high-risk patients should be approached with caution

PHARMACOLOGY

- Exact mechanism of antidepressant action unknown; SSRIs, through inhibition of serotonin uptake (and with paroxetine, potent NE reuptake inhibition), cause a down-regulation of receptors (e.g., 5-HT_2) while influencing other neurotransmitter systems as well, e.g., dopamine, norepinephrine

GENERAL COMMENTS

- SSRIs may be less effective than tricyclic antidepressants for severe refractory melancholic depression
- Suggested that women may respond better to SSRIs (and less well to tricyclics) than men; premenopausal women show better response

DOSING

- See p. 55
- SSRIs have flat dose-response curves, i.e., approximately 75 % of patients respond to the initial (low) dose. Do not increase the dose till steady state is reached (4 weeks for fluoxetine and 1 week for other drugs); "therapeutic window" of response is suggested for fluoxetine
- Dosage should be decreased (by 50%) in patients with hepatic impairment as plasma levels can increase up to 3-fold; no dosage reduction required in kidney impairment with most SSRIs (sertraline levels may increase 1.5-fold)
- Higher doses may be required in the treatment of OCD
- Lower starting dose may be required in panic disorder due to patient sensitivity to stimulating effects
- Dosing interval of every 2 to 7 days has been used with fluoxetine in prophylaxis of depression; once weekly dosing used in the maintenance treatment of panic disorder
- Intermittent dosing (during luteal phase of menstrual cycle) found effective for the treatment of premenstrual dysphoric disorder

PHARMACOKINETICS

- Rapidly absorbed; undergo little first-pass effect
- Highly bound to plasma protein; all SSRIs (least – citalopram and fluvoxamine) will displace other drugs from protein binding and elevate their plasma level (see Interactions, p. 9)
- Metabolized primarily by the liver; all SSRIs affect cytochrome P-450 metabolizing enzyme (least – citalopram) and will affect the metabolism of other drugs metabolized by this system (see Interactions, p. 9). Fluoxetine and paroxetine have been shown to decrease their own metabolism over time
- Peak plasma level of sertraline is 30% higher when drug taken with food, as first-pass metabolism is reduced
- Fluoxetine as well as its active metabolite, norfluoxetine, have the longest half-lives (up to 70 h and 330 h, respectively); this has implications for reaching steady-state drug levels as well as for drug withdrawal
- Once weekly dose of enteric-coated fluoxetine 90 mg results in mean steady state plasma concentration of fluoxetine and norfluoxetine, achieved with a daily dose of 10–20 mg; peak to trough differences vary (enteric coating used to reduce GI effects)
- Clearance of fluoxetine, sertraline and fluvoxamine reduced in patients with liver cirrhosis; clearance of citalopram reduced in elderly females

ONSET AND DURATION OF ACTION

- SSRIs are long-acting drugs and can be given in a single daily dose, usually in the morning; fluvoxamine may cause sedation and can be prescribed at night
- Therapeutic effect seen after 7–28 days; most patients with depression respond to the initial (low) dose; increasing the dose too

rapidly due to absence of therapeutic effect or adverse effects can ultimately result in an overshoot of the therapeutic range

- Tolerance to effects seen in some patients after months of treatment ("poop-out syndrome") [Check compliance with therapy; dosage adjustment may help; switching to an alternate antidepressant (p. 57) or augmentation strategies (p. 58) have also been tried]

ADVERSE EFFECTS

- The pharmacological and side effect profile of SSRIs is dependent on their *in vivo* affinity for and activity on neurotransmitters/receptors (see Table p. 40)
- See accompanying chart (p. 43) for incidence of adverse effects at therapeutic doses
- Incidence may be greater in early days of treatment; patients adapt to many side effects over time
- Rule out withdrawal symptoms of previous antidepressant – can be misattributed to side effects of current drug

1. CNS Effects

- A result of antagonism at histamine H_1-receptors and α_1-adrenoreceptors
- Headache common, worsening of migraines [Management: analgesics prn]
- Seizures reported, primarily in patients with underlying seizure disorder (risk low)

a) Cognitive Effects

- Both activation and sedation can occur early in treatment
- Activation, excitement, impulse dyscontrol, agitation, and restlessness; more frequent at higher doses [may respond to lorazepam]
- Decreased REM sleep, insomnia, and increased awakenings with all SSRIs; increased dreaming, nightmares, sexual dreams and obsessions reported with fluoxetine [may respond to clonazepam or cyproheptadine 2–4 mg]
- Drowsiness – more common with fluvoxamine; prescribe bulk of dose at bedtime; sedation with fluoxetine may be related to high concentration of metabolite norfluoxetine
- Precipitation of hypomania or mania (up to 30% of patients with a history of BAD – less frequent if patient receiving lithium)
- Psychosis, panic reactions, anxiety, or euphoria may occur; isolated reports of antidepressants causing agitation, motor activation, aggression, impulsivity, and suicidal urges
- Lethargy, apathy or amotivational syndrome (asthenia) reported – may be dose-related [prescribe bulk of dose at bedtime; bromocriptine 2.5–20 mg/day (rarely up to 60 mg/day), bupropion, buspirone or psychostimulant (e.g., methyphenidate 5–20 mg bid) may be helpful]
- Case reports of cognitive impairment, decreased attention and short-term memory [early data suggest donepezil 2.5–10 mg/day may be of benefit]

b) Neurological Effects

- Fine tremor [may respond to dose reduction or to propranolol]
- Akathisia [may respond to dose reduction, to propranolol or to a benzodiazepine]
- Dystonia, dyskinesia, parkinsonism or tics; more likely in older patients
- Tinnitus
- Myoclonus (e.g., periodic leg movements during sleep) [may respond to lamotrigine, gabapentin or bromocriptine]; may increase spasticity; recurrence of restless legs syndrome (paroxetine)
- Dysphasia, stuttering
- May induce or worsen extrapyramidal effects when given with antipsychotics (see Interactions, page 9)
- Increased extrapyramidal symptoms reported in patients with Parkinson's disease
- Case reports of tardive dyskinesia following chronic fluoxetine, sertraline and paroxetine use; more likely in older patients
- Nocturnal bruxism reported – may result in morning headache or may lead to damage to teeth or bridgework [may respond to buspirone up to 50 mg/day]
- Paresthesias; may be caused by pyridoxine deficiency [Management: pyridoxine 50–150 mg/day]
- Joint pain

2. Cardiovascular Effects

- Rare reports of tachycardia, palpitations, hypertension, and atrial fibrillation
- Bradycardia occurs more frequently
- Dizziness and impaired balance reported, especially in the elderly
- May cause coronary vasoconstriction; caution in patients with angina/ischemic heart disease

Selective Serotonin Reuptake Inhibitors (SSRI) (cont.)

- Slowing of sinus node reported with fluoxetine; caution in sinus node disease and in patients with serious left ventricular impairment

3. GI Effects

- A result of inhibition of 5-HT reuptake (activation of 5-HT_3 receptors)
- Nausea; vomiting – generally decreases over time due to gradual desensitization of 5-HT_3 receptors [may respond to taking drug with meals; cyproheptadine 2 mg or lactobacillus acidophilus (e.g., yogurt)]; diarrhea, bloating – usually transient and dose-related
- Anorexia and weight loss frequently reported during early treatment – more pronounced in overweight patients and those with carbohydrate cravings
- Reports of upper GI bleeding
- Weight gain reported: 5–10% of individuals gain more than 7% of body weight with chronic use (more common with paroxetine); citalopram associated with phasic craving for carbohydrate
- Case reports of stomatitis with fluoxetine

4. Sexual Side Effects

- A result of altered dopamine (D_2) activity, acetylcholine (ACh) blockade, inhibition of serotonin (5-HT) reuptake, and reduced nitric oxide levels – appears to be dose-related
- Decreased libido, impotence, ejaculatory disturbances occur relatively frequently [Management: amantadine (100–400 mg prn), bethanechol (10 mg tid or 10–50 mg prn), cyproheptadine (4–16 mg prn – loss of antidepressant response reported occasionally), neostigmine (7.5–15 mg prn), yohimbine (5.4–16.2 mg prn or 5.4 mg tid), buspirone (15–60 mg od or prn), bupropion 100–300 mg/day; sildenafil (25–100 mg prn), granisetron (1–2 mg prn), or "drug holidays"]
- Genital anesthesia (fluoxetine, sertraline) [Management: ginkgo biloba 240–900 mg]
- Anorgasmia or delayed orgasm [Management: amantadine (100–400 mg prn); cyproheptadine (4–16 mg prn) [loss of antidepressant response reported occasionally with cyproheptadine], buspirone (15–60 mg od or prn), bupropion (75–150 mg od), mirtazapine (15–45 mg od), nefazodone (50–150 mg prn), yohimbine (5.4–10.8 mg od or prn), methylphenidate (5–40 mg od), dextroamphetamine (5–40 mg od), ginseng, ginkgo biloba (180–900 mg), granisetron (1–2 mg prn), sildenafil (25–100 mg prn)]
- Spontaneous orgasm with yawning
- Cases of clitoral priapism with citalopram

5. Endocrine Effects

- Can induce SIADH (syndrome of inappropriate secretion of antidiuretic hormone) with hyponatremia; risk increases with age (up to 28% incidence), female sex, smoking and concomitant diuretic use
- Elevated prolactin; cases of galactorrhea reported
- Up to 30% decrease in fasting blood glucose has been reported
- Breast enlargement

6. Allergic Reactions

- Rare
- Jaundice, hepatitis, rash, urticaria, psoriasis, pruritis, edema
- Rare blood dyscrasias including neutropenia and aplastic anemia
- Serum sickness
- Bleeding disorders including petechiae, purpura (1% risk with fluoxetine); epistaxis, thrombocytopenia with fluoxetine; bruising reported with all SSRI drugs (rare) [suggested that ascorbic acid 500 mg may ameliorate bleeding]

7. Other Adverse Effects

- Case reports of alopecia
- Rhinitis common
- Sweating [Management: daily showering, talcum powder; in severe cases: Drysol solution, terazosin: 1–10 mg daily, oxybutynin up to 5 mg bid, clonidine 0.1 mg bid, guanfacine 2 mg hs, benztropine 0.5 mg hs; drug may need to be changed]
- Case reports of urinary retention, urgency, incontinence or cystitis
- Case reports of photosensitivity/photoallergic reactions
- Case report of acute angle-closure with paroxetine in patient with narrow angle glaucoma

- Case reports of exacerbation of Raynaud's syndrome
- Several cases of decreased thyroid indices reported with sertraline

WITHDRAWAL

- Abrupt withdrawal from high doses may cause a syndrome consisting of *somatic symptoms:* dizziness (exacerbated by movement), lethargy, nausea, headache, fever, sweating, chills, malaise, incoordination, insomnia, vivid dreams; *neurological symptoms:* myalgia, paresthesias, dyskinesias, "electric-shock-like" sensations, visual discoordination; *psychological symptoms:* anxiety, agitation, crying, irritability, confusion, slowed thinking, disorientation; rarely aggression, impulsivity, hypomania, mania and depersonalization.
- Most likely to occur 24–48 h after withdrawal
- Incidence (of 2–40%) is related to half-life of antidepressant – reported most frequently with paroxetine, least with fluoxetine

☞ **THEREFORE THESE MEDICATIONS SHOULD BE WITHDRAWN GRADUALLY AFTER PROLONGED USE**

Management

- Re-institute drug and taper more slowly
- Report that ginger can mitigate nausea and disequilibrium effects; substitution with one dose of fluoxetine (10–20 mg) also recommended to help in the withdrawal process

PRECAUTIONS

- May impair the mental and physical ability to perform hazardous tasks (e.g., driving a car or operating machinery); may potentiate the effects of alcohol
- May induce manic reactions in up to 20% of patients with bipolar affective disorders (BAD) – reported more frequently with fluoxetine; because of risk of increased cycling, BAD is a relative contraindication

☞ Use of SSRIs with other serotonergic agents may result in a hypermetabolic **Serotonin Syndrome – usually occurs within 24 hours of medication initiation, overdose or change in dose. Symptoms include: nausea, diarrhea, chills, sweating, dizziness, elevated temperature, elevated blood pressure, palpitations, increased muscle tone with twitching, tremor, myoclonic jerks, hyperreflexia, unsteady gait, restlessness, agitation, excitation, disorientation, confusion and delirium; may progress to rhabdomyolysis, coma and death (see Interactions) [Treatment: stop medication and administer supportive care, cyproheptadine 4–16 mg may reduce duration of symptoms]**

- Fluoxetine, paroxetine and sertraline will displace drugs from protein binding and elevate their plasma levels
- Fluoxetine, fluvoxamine, and paroxetine affect cytochrome P-450 and will inhibit the metabolism (and elevate the levels) of drugs metabolized by this system; sertraline will inhibit metabolism in higher doses (over 100 mg/day) (see Interactions, p. 9)
- Combination of SSRIs with other cyclic antidepressants can lead to increased plasma level of other antidepressant. Combination therapy has been used in the treatment of resistant patients. Caution when switching from fluoxetine to another antidepressant (see Interactions). Caution when switching from one SSRI to another
- Lower doses should be used in patients with renal or hepatic disease

TOXICITY

- SSRIs have a low probability of causing dose-related toxicity (one fatality reported with dose of 6000 mg of fluoxetine; seizure reported in adolescent after ingestion of 1880 mg); fatal outcome in 6 patients with citalopram 840–3920 mg (5 had also taken other sedative drugs or alcohol); fatalities reported with overdoses of citalopram and moclobemide
- Symptoms include: nausea, vomiting, tremor, myoclonus, irritability; ECG changes and seizures rarely reported with citalopram
- Case of serotonin syndrome reported after overdose of 8 g of sertraline

Treatment

- Treatment: symptomatic and supportive

PEDIATRIC CONSIDERATIONS

- SSRIs have been used in the treatment of depression, dysthymia, social phobia, anxiety, panic disorder, bulimia, OCD, autism, selective mutism, Gilles de la Tourette syndrome, and attention deficit hyperactivity disorder (ADHD); preliminary data suggest efficacy in some children with pervasive developmental disorders (autism) and elective mutism
- SSRIs are absorbed and metabolized more quickly in children than in adults; dosage requirements may be relatively higher (e.g., up to 80 mg daily of fluoxetine has been used)
- Children are more prone to behavioral adverse effects including: agitation, restlessness (32–46%), activation, hypomania (up to 13%), insomnia (up to 21%), irritability and social disinhibition (up to 25%)
- Nausea (up to 21%), dyspepsia (6–21%) reported; minimize by starting with a low dose (e.g., 5 mg fluoxetine) and give with food; anorexia (up to 12%)

Selective Serotonin Reuptake Inhibitors (SSRI) (cont.)

- Increased risk of headache (21%)
- Amotivational syndrome reported to emerge after several months of treatment (suggestive of frontal lobe dysfunction) – rule out subthreshold depression and hypothyroidism
- Efficacy of SSRIs for treatment of severe PMS in adolescent girls remains unclear

GERIATRIC CONSIDERATIONS

- SSRIs considered safe in the elderly due to a low risk of CNS, anticholinergic, and cardiovascular effects
- Initiate dose lower and increase more slowly; higher doses of fluoxetine have been associated with delirium
- Elderly patients may take longer to respond and may need trials of at least 12 weeks before treatment response noted
- Half-life of paroxetine increased by 170% in the elderly; clearance of sertraline decreased
- Monitor for drug-drug interactions
- Both weight gain and weight loss reported; monitor for excessive weight loss in debilitated patients
- Neurological side effects more likely in elderly persons
- Improvement in cognitive functioning in elderly depressed patients has been noted
- Impaired balance and falls reported; more likely with higher doses
- Monitor serum electrolytes; hyponatremia can present with confusion, somnolence, fatigue, delirium, hallucinations, urinary incontinence, hypotension and vomiting

USE IN PREGNANCY

- SSRIs have not been demonstrated to have teratogenic effects in humans; possible increased risk of miscarriage
- If possible, avoid during first trimester; when stopping the SSRI, taper the dose gradually to minimize adverse fetal outcome; with fluoxetine be aware of long half-life of metabolite, norfluoxetine
- Reports of an increase in premature births and poor neonatal adaptation when drug taken in the third trimester
- Withdrawal effects reported in neonate include jitteriness, restlessness, irritability, tremors (with fluoxetine is related to blood level of fluoxetine and norfluoxetine)

Breast milk

- Fluoxetine and citalopram appear in breast milk in therapeutic levels; caution: infant can receive up to 17% of maternal dose of fluoxetine and up to 9% of dose of citalopram
- Sertraline, paroxetine and fluvoxamine are present in very low concentrations in plasma of breast-fed infants
- The American Academy of Pediatrics considers SSRIs as "drugs whose effect on nursing infants is unknown but may be of concern."

NURSING IMPLICATIONS

- Psychotherapy and education are also important in the treatment of depression
- Monitor therapy by watching for adverse effects, mood and activity level changes
- Be aware that the medication reduces the degree of depression and may increase psychomotor activity; this may create concern about suicidal behavior
- Excessive ingestion of caffeinated foods, drugs, or beverages may increase anxiety and agitation and confuse the diagnosis
- Fluvoxamine tablets should be swallowed whole, with water, without chewing
- Sertraline should be given with food

PATIENT INSTRUCTIONS

For detailed patient instructions on SSRI antidepressants, see the Patient Information Sheet on p. 236.

- Avoid driving a car or operating hazardous machinery until response to drug has been determined
- Alcohol or other CNS depressants may cause an increase in sleepiness
- Do not stop these drugs suddenly, unless advised to do so by your physician, as withdrawal reactions can occur
- Avoid exposure to extreme cold, heat, and humidity as these drugs may affect the body's ability to regulate temperature
- Check with your doctor before taking other medication, including over-the-counter drugs, such as cold remedies, cough syrups
- These drugs may interact with medication used by a dentist, so let him/her know the name of the drug you are taking
- Avoid ingestion of grapefruit juice while taking fluvoxamine and sertraline, as the blood level of the antidepressant may rise

DRUG INTERACTIONS • Clinically significant interactions are listed below

Class of Drug	Example	Interaction Effects
Anorexiant	Fenfluramine, dexfenfluramine Phentermine	Increased serotonergic effects – data conflicting Case reports of mania and psychosis in combination
Antiarrhythmic	Propafenone, flecainide, mexiletine	Increased plasma level of antiarrhythmic with fluoxetine and paroxetine due to inhibited metabolism via CYP2D6
Antibiotic	Clarithromycin Erythromycin	Case of delirium with fluoxetine; case of serotonin syndrome with citalopram Increased plasma level of citalopram due to inhibited metabolism via CYP3A4 is possible but not confirmed
Anticoagulant	Warfarin	Loss of anticoagulant control with fluoxetine – data contradictory 65% increase in plasma level of warfarin with fluvoxamine and paroxetine; increased bleeding Increased prothrombin ratio or INR response with paroxetine and sertraline
Anticonvulsant	Barbiturates	Barbiturate metabolism inhibited by fluoxetine; reduced plasma level of SSRIs due to enzyme induction
	Carbamazepine, phenytoin, phenobarbital	Decreased plasma level of SSRIs; half-life of paroxetine decreased by 28% Increased plasma level of carbamazepine or phenytoin due to inhibition of metabolism with fluoxetine and fluvoxamine; elevated phenytoin level with sertraline and paroxetine
	Valproate, valproic acid, divalproex	Increased nausea with fluvoxamine and carbamazepine Increased plasma level of valproate (up to 50%) with fluoxetine Valproate may increase plasma level of fluoxetine
	Topiramate	Two case reports of angle-closure glaucoma in females on combination
Antidepressant Cyclic (non-selective)	Amitriptyline, desipramine, imipramine	Elevated plasma level of cyclic antidepressant with fluoxetine, fluvoxamine and paroxetine due to release from protein binding and inhibition of oxidative metabolism; can occur with higher doses of sertraline Increased desipramine level (by 50%) with citalopram
	Clomipramine	Additive antidepressant effect in treatment-resistant patients Increased serotonergic effects
Irreversible MAOI	Phenelzine, tranylcypromine	Hypermetabolic syndrome ("serotonin syndrome" – see p. 7) and death reported with combined use. Suggest waiting 5 weeks when switching from fluoxetine to MAOI and vice versa. Increased plasma level of tranylcypromine (by 15%) reported with paroxetine
RIMA	Moclobemide	Combined therapy may have additive antidepressant effect in treatment-resistant patients; use caution and monitor for serotonergic effects
NDRI	Bupropion	Additive antidepressant effect in refractory patients. Bupropion may reverse SSRI-induced sexual dysfunction Cases of anxiety, panic, delirium, tremor, myoclonus and seizure reported with fluoxetine due to inhibited metabolism of bupropion (via CYP3A4 and 2D6), competition for protein binding, and additive pharmacological effects

Selective Serotonin Reuptake Inhibitors (SSRI) (cont.)

Class of Drug	Example	Interaction Effects
NaSSA	Mirtazapine	Combination reported to alleviate insomnia and augment antidepressant response May mitigate SSRI-induced sexual dysfunction and "poop-out" syndrome through $5HT_3$ blockade Increased serotonergic effects possible Increased sedation and weight gain reported with combination
SARI	Nefazodone, trazodone	Additive antidepressant effect Elevated plasma level of SARI; increased serotonergic effects (case report of serotonin syndrome with fluoxetine and nefazodone) Nefazodone may reverse SSRI-induced sexual dysfunction and enhance REM sleep Increased level of MCPP metabolite of trazodone and nefazodone, with paroxetine (via inhibition of CYP2D6) resulting in increased anxiogenic potential
Antifungal	Ketoconazole, itraconazole	Increased plasma level of citalopram due to inhibited metabolism via CYP3A4 is possible but not confirmed
Antihistamine	Terfenadine, astemizole	Case reports of cardiovascular symptoms including intermittent sinus tachycardia, premature atrial contractions and couplets, shortness of breath and orthostatic hypotension, with fluoxetine and fluvoxamine; felt to be due to inhibition of metabolism of the antihistamine leading to accumulation of parent compound and resultant cardiac effects (loratidine, cetirizine and fexofenadine considered safe)
Antipsychotic	Chlorpromazine, fluphenazine, haloperidol, perphenazine, pimozide, clozapine, risperidone, olanzapine, thioridazine, mesoridazine	Increased serum level of neuroleptic (up to 100% increase reported with haloperidol and fluvoxamine or fluoxetine) (2- to 7-fold increase with clozapine and fluvoxamine, 76% increase with fluoxetine, and 40–45% increase with paroxetine and sertraline) (up to 21-fold increase in peak plasma level of perphenazine with paroxetine) (increased AUC by 119% and decreased clearance (by 50%) of olanzapine with fluvoxamine) (3-fold increase in thioridazine and mesoridazine levels with fluvoxamine). DO NOT COMBINE fluvoxamine, fluoxetine or paroxetine with mesoridazine or thioridazine due to risk of conduction disturbances May worsen extrapyramidal effects and akathisia, especially if antidepressant added early in the course of neuroleptic therapy May be useful for negative symptoms of schizophrenia Additive effect in treatment of OCD
Anxiolytic		
Benzodiazepine	Alprazolam, diazepam, bromazepam	Increased plasma level of alprazolam (by 100%), bromazepam, triazolam, midazolam and diazepam with fluvoxamine and fluoxetine, due to inhibited metabolism; small (13%) decrease in clearance of diazepam reported with sertraline Increased sedation, psychomotor and memory impairment
Buspirone		May potentiate anti-obsessional effects Anxiolytic effects of buspirone may be antagonized Increased plasma level of buspirone (3-fold) with fluvoxamine May mitigate SSRI-induced sexual dysfunction

Class of Drug	Example	Interaction Effects
β-Blockers	Propranolol, metoprolol	Decreased heart rate and syncope (additive effect) reported Increased side effects, lethargy, and bradycardia with fluoxetine and fluvoxamine due to decreased metabolism of the β-blocker (five-fold increase in propranolol level reported with fluvoxamine) Increased metoprolol level (100%) with citalopram
	Pindolol	Increased concentration of serotonin at post-synaptic sites; increased onset of therapeutic response Increased half-life of pindolol (by 28%) with fluoxetine; increased plasma level with paroxetine due to inhibited metabolism via CYP2D6
Benztropine		Increased plasma level of benztropine with paroxetine
Caffeine		Increased caffeine levels with fluvoxamine due to inhibited metabolism via CYP1A2; half-life increased from 5 to 31 h Increased jitteriness and insomnia
Ca-channel blocker	Nifedipine, verapamil	Increased side effects (headache, flushing, edema) due to inhibited clearance of Ca-channel blocker with fluoxetine
	Diltiazem	Bradycardia in combination with fluvoxamine
Cimetidine		Inhibited metabolism and increased plasma level of sertraline (by 25%) and paroxetine (by 50%)
CNS depressant	Alcohol, antihistamines	Potentiation of CNS effects; low risk Rate of fluvoxamine absorption increased by ethanol
	Chloral hydrate	Increased sedation and side effects with fluoxetine due to inhibited metabolism of chloral hydrate
Cyclobenzaprine		Increased side effects of cyclobenzaprine with fluoxetine, due to inhibited metabolism; observe for QT prolongation
Cyclosporin		Decreased clearance of cyclosporin with sertraline due to competition for metabolism via CYP3A4
Cyproheptadine		Report of reversal of antidepressant and antibulimic effects of fluoxetine and paroxetine
Digoxin		Decreased level (area under curve) of digoxin by 18% reported with paroxetine
Ergot alkaloid	Dihydroergotamine	Increased serotonergic effects with intravenous use – **AVOID**. Oral, rectal and subcutaneous routes can be used, with monitoring
	Ergotamine	Elevated ergotamine levels possible due to inhibited metabolism, via CYP3A4, with fluoxetine and fluvoxamine
Ginkgo biloba		Possible increased risk of petechiae and bleeding due to combined anti-hemostatic effects
Grapefruit juice		Decreased metabolism of fluvoxamine and sertraline resulting in increased plasma levels
Insulin		Increased insulin sensitivity reported

Selective Serotonin Reuptake Inhibitors (SSRI) (cont.)

Class of Drug	Example	Interaction Effects
Lithium		Increased serotonergic effects Changes in lithium level and clearance reported Caution with fluoxetine and fluvoxamine; neurotoxicity and seizures reported Increased tremor and nausea reported with sertraline and paroxetine Additive antidepressant effect in treatment-resistant patients
L-Tryptophan		May result in central and peripheral toxicity, hypermetabolic syndrome ("serotonin syndrome" – see p. 7)
MAO-B inhibitor	Selegiline (L-deprenyl)	Case reports of serotonin syndrome, hypertension, and mania when combined with fluoxetine
Narcotic	Codeine, oxycodone, hydrocodone	Decreased analgesic effect with fluoxetine and paroxetine due to inhibited metabolism to active moiety – morphine, oxymorphone and hydromorphone, respectively (interaction may be beneficial in the treatment of dependence by decreasing morphine and analog formation and opiate reinforcing properties)
	Pentazocine, tramadol	Report of excitatory toxicity (serotonergic) with fluoxetine and pentazocine; and with paroxetine, sertraline and tramadol
	Dextromethorphan	Visual hallucinations reported with fluoxetine
	Methadone	Elevated plasma level of methadone by 10–100% reported with fluvoxamine
	Morphine , fentanyl	Enhanced analgesia
NSAIDS		Early data suggest increased risk of upper GI bleed with combined use
Omeprazole		Increased plasma level of citalopram due to inhibited metabolism via CYP2C19
Procyclidine		Increased plasma level of procyclidine with paroxetine (by 40%)
Proguanil		Increased plasma level of proquanil with fluvoxamine due to inhibited metabolism via CYP2C19
Protease inhibitor	Ritonavir	Increased plasma level of sertraline due to competition for metabolism; moderate increase in level of fluoxetine and paroxetine. Serotonin syndrome reported in combination with high dose of fluoxetine Cardiac and neurological side effects reported with fluoxetine, due to elevated ritonavir level (19% increase AUC)
Sibutramine		Increased serotonergic effects possible
Sildenafil		Possible enhanced hypotension due to inhibited metabolism of sildenafil via CYP3A4 with fluoxetine and fluvoxamine
Smoking – cigarettes		Increased metabolism of fluvoxamine by 25% via CYP1A2
St. John's Wort		May augment serotonergic effects – several reports of serotonin syndrome
Stimulant	Amphetamine, methylphenidate, pemoline	Potentiated effect in depression, dysthymia, and OCD, in patients with comorbid ADHD; may improve response in treatment-refractory paraphilias and paraphilia-related disorders Plasma level of antidepressant may be increased
	Fenfluramine, dexfenfluramine	Possible risk of serotonergic reaction

Class of Drug	Example	Interaction Effects
Sulfonylurea antidiabetic agent	Glyburide, tolbutamide	Increased hypoglycemia reported in diabetics Increased plasma level of tolbutamide due to reduced clearance (up to 16%) with sertraline
Tacrine		Increased plasma level of tacrine with fluvoxamine; peak plasma level increased 5-fold and clearance decreased by 88% due to inhibited metabolism via CYP1A2
Theophylline		Increased plasma level of theophylline with fluvoxamine due to decreased metabolism via CYP1A2
Thyroid drug	Triiodothyronine (T_3-liothyronine)	Antidepressant effect potentiated Elevated serum thyrotropin (and reduced free thyroxine concentration) reported with sertraline
Tolterodine		Decreased oral clearance of tolterodine by up to 93% with fluoxetine
Triptan	Sumatriptan, rizatriptan, zolmitriptan	Increased serotonergic effects possible (rare); exacerbation of migraine headache reported with combination
Zolpidem		Case reports of hallucinations and delirium when combined with sertraline, fluoxetine and paroxetine Chronic (5-night) administration of sertraline resulted in faster onset of action and increase in peak plasma concentration of zolpidem

Norepinephrine Dopamine Reuptake Inhibitor (NDRI)

PRODUCT AVAILABILITY

Chemical Class	Generic Name	Trade Name[A]	Dosage Forms and Strengths
Monocyclic agent (aminoketone)	Bupropion (amfebutamone)	Wellbutrin[B] Wellbutrin-SR, Zyban[D]	Tablets[B]: 75 mg, 100 mg Sustained-release tablets: 100 mg, 150 mg

[A] Generic preparations may be available, [B] Not marketed in Canada, [D] Marketed as aid in smoking cessation

INDICATIONS*

- ▲ Major depression
- ▲ Prophylaxis of recurrent major depression
- ▲ Depressed phase of bipolar affective disorder
- ▲ Aid in smoking cessation (Zyban)
- May play a role in the treatment of addictive disorders (e.g., cocaine)
- Efficacy reported in seasonal affective disorder, dysthymia and chronic fatigue syndrome; case reports of efficacy in social phobia
- Controlled studies suggest benefit in ADHD in adults and children
- Early data suggest efficacy in alleviating hyperarousal and depressive symptoms in PTSD; intrusive symptoms less responsive
- Reports of efficacy in alleviating sexual dysfunction (anorgasmia, erectile problems) induced by SSRIs and SNRI
- May promote weight loss
- Early data suggest bupropion reduces movements in depressed patients with periodic limb movement disorder
- Case reports and open-label studies suggest benefit in neuropathic pain

PHARMACOLOGY

- Inhibits the re-uptake of primarily norepinephrine (and dopamine to a lesser extent) into presynaptic neurons
- Antidepressant activity is mediated primarily through noradrenergic and/or dopaminergic pathways

GENERAL COMMENTS

- May have a lower switch rate (to hypomania or mania) than other antidepressants

DOSING

- See p. 55
- Drug should be prescribed in divided doses, with a maximum of 150 mg per dose
- In adults with ADHD: begin at 150 mg/day and titrate dose gradually to a maximum of 450 mg/day in divided doses; up to 4 weeks may be required for maximum drug effect

PHARMACOKINETICS

- Rapid absorption with peak concentration occurring within 3 h (mean = 1.5 h); peak plasma concentration of sustained-release preparation is 50–85% of the immediate-release tablets after single dosing, and 25% after chronic dosing
- Highly bound to plasma protein (80–85%)
- Metabolized predominantly by the liver primarily via CYP2B6 and to a lesser extent by other isoenzymes – 6 metabolites; 3 are active
- Bupropion and hydroxybupropion inhibit CYP2D6 isoenzyme
- Elimination half-life: 11–14 h; with chronic dosing: 21 h (mean); increased half-life of bupropion and its metabolites and decreased clearance reported in the elderly
- Weak inducer of its own metabolism, as well as that of other drugs
- Use cautiously in patients with hepatic impairment – reduce dose or frequency of administration

* ▲ Approved indications

ONSET AND DURATION

- Therapeutic effect seen after 7–28 days

ADVERSE EFFECTS

- See chart on p. 43 for incidence of adverse effects

1. CNS Effects

- A result of antagonism at histamine H_1-receptors and α_1-adrenoreceptors

a) Cognitive

- Insomnia; vivid dreams and nightmares reported; decreased REM latency and increased REM sleep
- Agitation, anxiety, irritability, dysphoria, aggression
- Precipitation of hypomania or mania felt to be less likely than with other cyclic antidepressants
- Can exacerbate psychotic symptoms
- Very high doses can result in CNS toxicity including confusion, impaired concentration, hallucinations, delusions, delirium, EPS and seizures
- Reported to exacerbate symptoms of obsessive compulsive disorder
- Short-term memory loss reported

a) Neurological

- Seizures can occur after abrupt dose increases, or use of daily doses above 450 mg; use divided doses (maximum single dose no greater than 150 mg) – bulimic patients may be at higher risk. Risk of seizures at doses of 100–300 mg = 0.1%; at 300–450 mg = 0.4%; above 450 mg risk increases 10-fold; risk with SR preparation = 0.15% (doses up to 300 mg)
- Disturbance in gait, fine tremor, myoclonus
- Headache, arthralgia (4%), neuralgias (5%), myalgia [Management: analgesics prn]
- Tinnitus reported
- Reversible dyskinesia reported; may aggravate neuroleptic-induced tardive dyskinesia

2. Anticholinergic Effects

- Occur rarely
- Dry mouth, sweating

3. Cardiovascular Effects

- Modest sustained increases in blood pressure reported in adults and children (more likely in patients with pre-existing hypertension)
- Orthostatic hypotension, dizziness occurs occasionally – caution in the elderly
- Palpitations
- Case of transient ischemic attacks reported
- Cases of myocarditis, myocardial infarction and cardiac death

4. Endocrine Effects

- Menstrual irregularities reported (up to 9% risk)
- Cases of hypoglycemia reported

5. Other Adverse Effects

- Urticarial or pruritic rashes have been reported; rare cases of erythema multiforme and Stevens-Johnson syndrome
- Reports of serum sickness
- Clitoral priapism reported
- Urinary frequency
- Anorexia
- Alopecia
- Case report of rhabdomyolysis in a patient with hepatic dysfunction
- Anaphylactoid reactions with pruritis, urticaria, angioedema, and dyspnea (up to 0.3%)
- Case reports of liver failure
- Delayed hypersensitivity reactions with arthralgia, myalgia, fever and rash

WITHDRAWAL

- None known

SPECIAL CONSIDERATIONS

- Bupropion does not potentiate the sedative effects of alcohol
- Rarely impairs sexual functioning or behavior; some improvement noted
- There is no evidence of increased abuse potential (considering bupropion is related to the sympathomimetic drug diethylpropion)

Norepinephrine Dopamine Reuptake Inhibitor (NDRI) (cont.)

PRECAUTIONS

- May lower the seizure threshold; therefore administer cautiously to patients with a history of convulsive disorders, organic brain disease and when combining with other drugs that may lower the seizure threshold. To minimize seizures, do not exceed a dose increase of 100 mg in a 3-day period. No single dose should exceed 150 mg for the immediate-release or the sustained-release preparation
- Contraindicated in patients with history of bulimia, undergoing alcohol or benzodiazepine withdrawal, or with other conditions predisposing to seizures
- Use with caution (i.e., use lower dose and monitor regularly in patients with hepatic impairment)
- Zyban, marketed for smoking cessation, contains bupropion – DO NOT COMBINE with Wellbutrin

TOXICITY

- Rare reports of death following massive overdose, preceded by uncontrolled seizures, bradycardia, cardiac failure and cardiac arrest

Management

- Induce vomiting
- Activated charcoal given every 6 h to 12 h
- Supportive treatment
- Monitor ECG and EEG

PEDIATRIC CONSIDERATIONS

- Exacerbation of tics reported in ADHD and Tourette's syndrome
- Dosage in children: initiate at 1 mg/kg/day, in divided doses, and increase gradually to a maximum of 6 mg/kg/day (divided doses)
- Rash reported in up to 17% of youths

GERIATRIC CONSIDERATIONS

- The elderly are at risk for accumulation of bupropion and its metabolites due to decreased clearance
- Orthostatic hypotension or dizziness may predispose to falls
- Prior to prescribing bupropion, screen for factors that may predispose an elderly patient to seizures

USE IN PREGNANCY

- No harm to fetus reported in animal studies; no data on effects in humans

Breast milk

- Bupropion and metabolites are secreted in breast milk; infant can receive up to 2.7% of maternal dose – effects on infant unknown

NURSING IMPLICATIONS

- Risk of seizures increases if any single dose exceeds 150 mg (immediate-release or sustained-release), or if total daily dose exceeds 300 mg
- Crushing or chewing the sustained-release preparation destroys the slow-release activity of the product; cutting or splitting the SR preparation in half will increase the rate of drug release in the first 15 minutes
- Bupropion degrades rapidly on exposure to moisture, therefore tablets should not be stored in an area of high humidity
- If the patient has difficulty sleeping, ensure that the last dose of bupropion is no later than 1500 h

PATIENT INSTRUCTIONS

For detailed patient instructions on bupropion, see the Patient Information Sheet on p. 238.

- Do not chew or crush bupropion-SR as this will negate the sustained-release action of the product
- If you have been advised by your doctor to break bupropion SR tablets in half, do so just prior to taking your medication and discard the other half unless used within 24 h
- Doses above 150 mg should be taken in divided doses, preferably 8 h apart
- Inform your doctor if you are taking any medication for smoking cessation treatment
- Store tablets away from high humidity (e.g., washroom medicine cabinet)

DRUG INTERACTIONS

- Clinically significant interactions are listed below

Class of Drug	Example	Interaction Effects
Amantadine		Case reports of neurotoxicity in elderly patients; delirium
Antiarrhythmics (Type 1c)	Propafenone, flecainide	Increased plasma level of antiarrhythmic due to inhibited metabolism via CYP2D6
Antibiotics – Quinolone	Ciprofloxacin	Seizure threshold may be reduced
Anticholinergic	Antiparkinsonian agents, antihistamines, etc. Orphenadrine	Increased anticholinergic effect Altered levels of either drug due to competition for metabolism via CYP2B6
Anticonvulsant	Carbamazepine, phenytoin, phenobarbital Valproate	Decreased plasma level of bupropion and increased level of its metabolite hydroxybupropion due to increased metabolism by the anticonvulsant Increased level of hydroxybupropion due to inhibited metabolism; level of bupropion not affected
Antidepressant Cyclic (non-selective) Irreversible MAOI SSRI	 Imipramine, desipramine, nortriptyline Phenelzine Fluoxetine	 Elevated imipramine level (by 57%) and nortriptyline level (by 200%) with combination; desipramine peak plasma level and half-life increased 2-fold due to increased metabolism (via CYP2D6) Seizure threshold may be reduced Additive antidepressant effect in treatment-refractory patients DO NOT COMBINE – dopamine metabolism inhibited Case of delirium, anxiety, panic and myoclonus with fluoxetine due to inhibited metabolism of bupropion (via CYP3A2 and 2D6), competition for protein binding and additive pharmacological effects Additive antidepressant effect in treatment-refractory patients; bupropion may mitigate SSRI-induced sexual dysfunction
Antimalarial		Seizure threshold may be reduced
Antipsychotic	Thioridazine Chlorpromazine	Increased plasma level of thioridazine due to decreased metabolism via CYP2D6; increased risk of thioridazine-related ventricular arrhythmias and sudden death. DO NOT COMBINE Seizure threshold may be reduced
Beta-blocker	Metoprolol	Increased plasma level of β-blocker possible due to inhibited metabolism via CYP2D6
Corticosteroid (systemic)		Seizure threshold may be reduced
Insulin		Seizure threshold may be reduced
L-Dopa		Increased side effects, including excitement, restlessness, nausea, vomiting and tremor due to increased dopamine availability
Lithium		Additive antidepressant effect
Nicotine transdermal		Combination reported to promote higher rates of smoking cessation than either drug alone Increased risk of hypertension with combination

Norepinephrine Dopamine Reuptake Inhibitor (NDRI) (cont.)

Class of Drug	Example	Interaction Effects
Nitrogen mustard analogues	Cyclophosphamide, ifosfamide	Altered levels of either drug due to competition for metabolism via CYP2B6
Protease inhibitor	Ritonavir, nelfinavir, efavirenz	Increased plasma level of bupropion due to decreased metabolism via CYP2B6; risk of seizure
Stimulant	Methylphenidate, dextroamphetamine	Additive effect in ADHD
Sympathomimetic	Pseudoephedrine	Report of manic-like reaction with pseudoephedrine Seizure threshold may be reduced
Theophylline		Seizure threshold may be reduced
Tramadol		Seizure threshold may be reduced

Selective Serotonin Norepinephrine Reuptake Inhibitor (SNRI)

PRODUCT AVAILABILITY

Chemical Class	Generic Name	Trade Name[(A)]	Dosage Forms and Strengths
Bicyclic agent (phenethylamine)	Venlafaxine	Effexor Effexor XR	Tablets: 25 mg[(B)], 37.5 mg, 50 mg[(B)], 75 mg, 100 mg[(B)] Sustained-release tablets: 37.5 mg, 75 mg, 150 mg

[(A)] Generic preparations may be available, [(B)] Not marketed in Canada

INDICATIONS*

- ▲ Major depressive disorder (MDD)
- ▲ Generalized anxiety disorder (GAD)
- Depressed phase of bipolar affective disorder
- Preliminary data suggest efficacy in treatment-resistant depression, dysthymia, postpartum depression and melancholic depression
- Preliminary studies suggest efficacy in obsessive compulsive disorder, panic disorder, social phobia, premenstrual dysphoria, borderline personality disorder, fibromyalgia, and in children and adults with ADHD
- Anecdotal reports of efficacy in alleviating sexual dysfunction induced by SSRIs
- Preliminary data suggest a role in reducing hot flashes
- Early data suggest a possible role in management of migraine and tension headaches, and for chronic pain associated with diabetic neuropathy

PHARMACOLOGY

- Potent inhibitor of serotonin at low doses; at moderate doses norepinephrine reuptake occurs; inhibition of dopamine reuptake occurs at high doses
- Rapid down-regulation of β-receptors; may slow early onset of clinical activity

GENERAL COMMENTS

- Dosing is similar for MDD and GAD; some patients with GAD, however, may require a slower titration
- Early data suggest that postmenopausal females show better response to venlafaxine than to SSRIs

DOSING

- See p. 55
- Initiate drug at 37.5–75 mg (once daily for XR preparation and twice daily for regular preparation), and increase after 1 week in increments no greater than 75 mg q 4 days, up to 225 mg/day (in divided doses); some patients may require up to 375 mg/day (in divided doses)
- Dosage adjustment in healthy elderly patients is not required
- Decrease dose by 50% in hepatic disease and by 25–50% in renal disease

PHARMACOKINETICS

- Well absorbed from GI tract: food has no effect on absorption; absorption of XR formulation is slow (15 ± 6 h)
- Less than 35% bound to plasma protein
- Peak plasma level reached by parent drug in 1–3 h and by active metabolite (O-desmethylvenlafaxine, ODV) in 2–6 h; with XR formulation peak plasma level reached by parent drug in 6 h and metabolite in 8.8 h (mean)
- Steady-state of parent and metabolite reached in about 3 days
- Elimination half life of oral tablet: parent = 3–7 h and metabolite = 9–13 h; XR elimination half-life is dependent on absorption half-life (15 h mean)
- Major elimination is via the urine; clearance decreased by 24% in renal disease and by 50% in hepatic disease
- Parent drug metabolized by CYP2D6 and is also a weak inhibitor of this enzyme; ODV metabolite is metabolized by CYP3A3/4

* ▲ Approved indications

Selective Serotonin Norepinephrine Reuptake Inhibitor (SNRI)

ONSET AND DURATION

- Therapeutic effect seen after 7–28 days

ADVERSE EFFECTS

- Generally dose-related; see chart p. 43 for incidence of adverse effects

1. CNS Effects

- Both sedation and insomnia reported; disruption of sleep cycle, decreased REM sleep, vivid nightmares
- Headache
- Nervousness, agitation, asthenia
- Risk of hypomania/mania estimated to be 0.5%
- 10–30% of patients who improve initially can have breakthrough depression after several months ("poop-out syndrome") – an increase in dosage or augmentation therapy may be of benefit
- Seizures reported rarely (0.3%)
- Case reports of restless legs syndrome

2. Anticholinergic Effects

- May be mediated through NE-reuptake inhibition
- Dry mouth
- Sweating
- Urinary retention
- Constipation
- Cases of elevated ocular pressure in patients with narrow angle glaucoma

3. Cardiovascular Effects

- Modest, sustained increase in blood pressure can occur, usually within two months of dose stabilization; seen in over 3% of individuals on less than 100 mg/day and about 13% of individuals on doses above 300 mg/day; caution in patients with history of hypertension; recommended that patients on doses above 225 mg/day have BP monitored for 2 months at each dose level
- Tachycardia; increase by 4 beats/min in about 2% of individuals
- Dizziness, hypotension occasionally reported

4. GI Effects

- Nausea occurs frequently at start of therapy and tends to decrease after 1–2 weeks; less frequent with XR formulation
- No weight gain reported

5. Sexual Side Effects

- Sexual side effects reported in over 30% of patients [see SSRIs p. 6 for suggested treatments]

6. Other

- Mean increase in serum cholesterol of 3 mg/dL reported
- Case report of breast engorgement and pain
- Case reports of hyponatremia

WITHDRAWAL

- Abrupt withdrawal, even after several weeks' therapy can occur within 8–16 h of discontinuation and can last for 8 days
- Symptoms include: asthenia (2%), dizziness (3%), headache (3%), insomnia (3%), tinnitus, nausea (6%), nervousness (2%), confusion, nightmares, auditory hallucinations, "electric-shock" sensations, chills, cramps and diarrhea
- Cases of inter-dose withdrawal reported with regular-release tablet; withdrawal reactions also reported with XR product

☞ **THEREFORE THIS MEDICATION SHOULD BE WITHDRAWN GRADUALLY AFTER PROLONGED USE**

Management

- Suggested to taper slowly over a two-week period (some suggest over 6 weeks)
- Substituting one dose of fluoxetine (10 or 20 mg) near the end of the taper may help in the withdrawal process; ondansetron 8–12 mg/day over 10 days suggested to be helpful during the taper

PRECAUTIONS

- Use cautiously in patients with hypertension, as venlafaxine can cause modest, sustained increases in blood pressure

- May induce manic reaction in patients with BAD and rarely in unipolar depression

TOXICITY

- Symptoms of toxicity include somnolence, mild tachycardia, increase in QTc interval, seizures – no deaths reported due to overdose

PEDIATRIC CONSIDERATIONS

- Preliminary data suggest efficacy in ADHD
- Children may metabolize venlafaxine more rapidly than adults
- May cause behavior activation and aggravate symptoms of hyperactivity

GERIATRIC CONSIDERATIONS

- Dosage adjustments in healthy elderly patients are not required

USE IN PREGNANCY

- Animal studies show a decrease in offspring weight, as well as stillbirths with high doses
- No teratogenic effects reported in humans, to date; may be a trend toward higher rates of spontaneous abortion

Breast milk

- Unknown if secreted into breast milk

NURSING IMPLICATIONS

- A gradual titration of dosage at start of therapy will minimize nausea
- Psychotherapy and education are also important in the treatment of depression
- Monitor therapy by watching for adverse effects as well as mood and activity level changes; keep physician informed
- Be aware that the medication may increase psychomotor activity; this may create concern about suicidal behavior
- Excessive ingestion of caffeinated foods, drugs, or beverages may increase anxiety and agitation and confuse the diagnosis

PATIENT INSTRUCTIONS

For detailed patient instructions on venlafaxine, see the Patient Information Sheet on p. 240.

- Do not chew or crush the sustained-release tablet (Effexor XR), but swallow it whole
- If a dose is missed, do not attempt to make it up; continue with regular daily schedule (divided doses)

DRUG INTERACTIONS

- Clinically significant interactions are listed below

Class of Drug	Example	Interaction Effects
Anticholinergic	Antiparkinsonian agents, antipsychotics, etc.	Increased anticholinergic effects
Antidepressant		
Irreversible MAOI	Phenelzine	**AVOID**; possible hypertensive crisis and serotonergic reaction
RIMA	Moclobemide	Enhanced effects of norepinephrine and serotonin; caution – no data on safety with combined use
Antipsychotic	Haloperidol	Increased peak plasma level and AUC of haloperidol; no change in half-life
Cimetidine		Increased plasma level of venlafaxine due to decreased clearance by 43%; peak concentration increased by 60%
MAO-B inhibitor	Selegiline	Case report of serotonergic reaction
Protease inhibitor	Ritonavir	Moderate decrease in clearance of venlafaxine with ritonavir
	Indinavir	Both increases (by 13%) and decreases (by 60%) in total concentration (AUC) of indinavir reported
Zolpidem		Case report of delirium and hallucinations with combination

Serotonin-2 Antagonists/Reuptake Inhibitors (SARI)

PRODUCT AVAILABILITY

Chemical Class	Generic Name	Trade Name[(A)]	Dosage Forms and Strengths
Phenylpiperidine	Nefazodone	Serzone	Tablets: 50 mg, 100 mg, 150 mg, 200 mg, 250 mg[(B)]
Triazolopyridine	Trazodone	Desyrel	Tablets: 50 mg, 100 mg, 150 mg, 300 mg[(B)]

[(A)] Generic preparations may be available, [(B)] Not marketed in Canada

INDICATIONS*

- ▲ Major depressive disorder
- ▲ Prophylaxis of recurrent major depression (unipolar affective disorder)
- ▲ Depressed phase of bipolar affective disorder (see Precautions)
- Treatment of secondary depression in other mental illnesses, e.g., schizophrenia, dementia
- Chronic depression (nefazodone)
- Agoraphobia associated with panic disorder
- Efficacy in dysthymia reported
- Bulimia nervosa
- Early data reports benefit in social phobia (nefazodone)
- Efficacy against intrusive symptoms of posttraumatic stress disorder reported (nefazodone)
- Insomnia (trazodone)
- Premenstrual syndrome (nefazodone)
- Preliminary data suggest benefit in generalized anxiety disorder (nefazodone)
- Erectile impotence (trazodone), anorgasmia (nefazodone)
- Trazodone reported to decrease disturbed behavior in patients with dementia and improve delirium (case reports); open trials suggest efficacy in treatment of aggression in children
- Preliminary data suggest nefazodone decreases nonparaphilic compulsive sexual behavior
- Open trials suggest nefazodone improves fatigue, sleep disturbances and mood in patients with chronic fatigue syndrome

PHARMACOLOGY

- Exact mechanism of action unknown; equilibrate the effects of biogenic amines through various mechanisms; cause downregulation of β-adrenergic receptors

GENERAL COMMENTS

- Studies demonstrate improved outcomes in chronic depression with combination of nefazodone and psychotherapy

DOSING

- See p. 55
- Initiate drug at a low dose and increase dose every 3 to 5 days to a maximum tolerated dose based on side effects; there is a wide variation in dosage requirements
- Trazodone should be taken on an empty stomach as food delays absorption and decreases drug effect
- Regular ingestion of grapefruit juice while on nefazodone may affect the antidepressant plasma level (see Interactions)
- Prophylaxis is most effective if therapeutic dose is maintained

* ▲ Approved indications

PHARMACOKINETICS

- Completely absorbed from the gastrointestinal tract; food significantly delays and decreases peak plasma effect of trazodone
- Large percentage metabolized by first-pass effect
- Highly bound to plasma protein
- Metabolized primarily by the liver
- Elimination half-life, see p. 55; steady state reached in about 5 days
- Half-life of nefazodone is dose-dependent

ONSET AND DURATION OF ACTION

- Therapeutic effect is seen after 7–28 days
- Sedative effects are seen within a few hours of oral administration; decreased sleep disturbance reported after a few days

ADVERSE EFFECTS

- The pharmacological and side effect profile of SARI antidepressants is dependent on their affinity for and activity on neurotransmitters/receptors (see table p. 40)
- See chart p. 43 for incidence of adverse effects at therapeutic doses; incidence of adverse effects may be greater in early days of treatment; patients adapt to many side effects over time

1. CNS Effects

- A result of antagonism at histamine H_1-receptors and α_1-adrenoreceptors
- Occur frequently

a) Cognitive Effects

- Drowsiness (most common adverse effect) [Management: prescribe bulk of dose at bedtime]
- Weakness, lethargy, fatigue
- Conversely, excitement, agitation and restlessness have occurred
- Confusion, disturbed concentration, disorientation
- Nefazodone increases REM sleep and sleep quality
- Improved psychomotor and complex memory performance reported with nefazodone after single doses; dose-related impairment noted after repeated doses
- Precipitation of hypomania or mania, psychosis, panic reactions, anxiety, or euphoria may occur

b) Neurological Effects

- Fine tremor
- Akathisia (rare – check serum iron for deficiency)
- Seizures rarely can occur following abrupt drug increase or after drug withdrawal; risk increases with high plasma levels
- Tinnitus
- Paresthesias reported with nefazodone (approximate risk 4%)
- Myoclonus; includes muscle jerks of lower extremities, jaw, and arms, and nocturnal myoclonus – may be severe in up to 9% of patients [If severe, clonazepam, valproate or carbamazepine may be of benefit]
- Dysphasia, stuttering
- Disturbance in gait, parkinsonism, dystonia
- Headache; worsening of migraine reported with nefazodone and trazodone

2. Anticholinergic Effects

- A result of antagonism at muscarinic receptors (ACh)
- Uncommon; occur more frequently in elderly patients
- Include dry eyes, blurred vision, constipation, dry mouth [see Cyclic Antidepressants p. 33 for treatment suggestions]

3. Cardiovascular Effects

- A result of antagonism at α_1-adrenoreceptors, muscarinic, 5-HT_2 and H_1-receptors and inhibition of sodium fast channels
- More common in elderly
- Risk increases with high plasma levels
- Bradycardia seen with nefazodone
- Orthostatic hypotension [Management: sodium chloride tablets, caffeine, fludrocortisone (0.1–0.5 mg), midodrine (2.5–10 mg tid), use of support stockings]
- Prolonged conduction time; contraindicated in heart block or post-myocardial infarction

Serotonin-2 Antagonists/Reuptake Inhibitors (SARI) (cont.)

4. GI Effects

- A result of inhibition of 5-HT uptake and ACh antagonism
- Weight gain reported with trazodone; rare with nefazodone
- Peculiar taste, "black tongue," glossitis
- Reports of upper GI bleeding wtih trazodone

5. Sexual Side Effects

- A result of altered dopamine (D_2) activity, 5-HT_2 blockade, inhibition of 5-HT reuptake, α_1-blockade, and ACh blockade
- Occur rarely
- Testicular swelling, painful ejaculation, retrograde ejaculation, increased libido and priapism (with trazodone; not seen with nefazodone); spontaneous orgasm with yawning (trazodone)

6. Endocrine Effects

- Decreases in blood sugar levels reported (nefazodone)
- Can induce syndrome of SIADH with hyponatremia; risk increased with age

7. Allergic Reactions

- Rare
- Rash, urticaria, pruritis, edema, blood dyscrasias
- Jaundice, hepatitis, hepatic necrosis and hepatic failure reported with therapeutic doses of nefazodone (laboratory evidence includes: increased levels of ALT, AST, GGT, bilirubin and increased prothrombin time) – Cases of liver failure and death reported. Recommend baseline and periodic liver function tests with nefazodone. Monitor for signs of hepatotoxicity

8. Other Adverse Effects

- Rare reports of alopecia with nefazodone
- Cases of palinopsia with both trazodone and nefazodone
- Case reports of burning sensations, in various parts of the body, with nefazodone

WITHDRAWAL

- Reported incidence 20–80% – likely due to cholinergic and adrenergic rebound
- Abrupt withdrawal from high doses may occasionally cause a "flu-like" syndrome consisting of fever, fatigue, sweating, coryza, malaise, myalgia, headache; psychological symptoms: anxiety, dizziness, nausea, vomiting, akathisia, dyskinesia, insomnia, nightmares, panic and priapism (trazodone)
- Most likely to occur 24–48 h after withdrawal, or after a large dosage decrease
- Rebound depression can occur (even in individuals not previously depressed – such as patients with obsessive compulsive disorders)
- Paradoxical mood changes reported on abrupt withdrawal, including hypomania or mania

☞ **THEREFORE THESE MEDICATIONS SHOULD BE WITHDRAWN GRADUALLY AFTER PROLONGED USE**

Management

- Reinstitute the drug at a lower dose and taper gradually over several days

PRECAUTIONS

- Use cautiously in patients in whom excess anticholinergic activity could be harmful (e.g., prostatic hypertrophy, urinary retention, narrow-angle glaucoma)
- Use with caution in patients with respiratory difficulties, since antidepressants can dry up bronchial secretions and make breathing more difficult
- May lower the seizure threshold; therefore, administer cautiously to patients with a history of convulsive disorders, organic brain disease, or a predisposition to convulsions (e.g., alcohol withdrawal)
- May impair the mental and physical ability to perform hazardous tasks (e.g., driving a car or operating machinery); will potentiate the effects of alcohol
- May induce manic reactions in patients with bipolar affective disorder and rarely in unipolar depression; because of risk of increased cycling, bipolar affective disorder is a relative contraindication
- Use caution in prescribing nefazodone for patients with a history of alcoholism or liver disorder. Monitor liver function tests periodically, and for clinical signs of liver dysfunction

- Combination of SARI antidepressants with SSRIs can lead to increased plasma level of the SARI antidepressant. Combination therapy has been used in the treatment of resistant patients; use caution and monitor for serotonergic reaction
- Use caution when switching from a SARI antidepressant to fluoxetine and vice versa (see Interactions, p. 26, and Switching Antidepressants, p. 57)

TOXICITY

- SARI antidepressants have a low probability of causing dose-related toxicity (e.g., nausea, vomiting and sedation reported after 11.2 g nefazodone); no seizures or cardiovascular effects reported

PEDIATRIC CONSIDERATIONS

- SARI antidepressants are used in major depressive disorder and behavior disturbances in children (agitation, aggression)
- Trazodone used in acute and chronic treatment of insomnia and night terrors
- Start drug at a low dose (10–25 mg) and increase gradually by 10–25 mg every 4–5 days
- Plasma levels of nefazodone and its metabolites reported to be higher in children than adolescents

GERIATRIC CONSIDERATIONS

- Initiate dose lower and slower than in younger patients; elderly patients may take longer to respond and may require trials of up to 12 weeks before response is noted
- Monitor for excessive CNS and anticholinergic effects
- Caution when combining with other drugs with CNS and anticholinergic properties; additive effects can result in confusion, disorientation, and delirium; elderly are sensitive to anticholinergic effects
- Caution regarding cardiovascular side effects: orthostatic hypotension (can lead to falls)
- Cognitive impairment can occur

USE IN PREGNANCY

- Trazodone in high doses was found to be teratogenic and toxic to the fetus in some animal species; data in humans is unclear
- If possible, avoid during first trimester

Breast milk

- SARI antidepressants are excreted into breast milk
- The American Academy of Pediatrics classifies SARI antidepressants as drugs "whose effects on nursing infants are unknown but may be of concern."

NURSING IMPLICATIONS

- Psychotherapy and education are also important in the treatment of depression
- Monitor therapy by watching for adverse side effects, mood and activity level changes; keep physician informed
- Be aware that the medication may increase psychomotor activity; this may create concern about suicidal behavior
- Expect a lag time of 7–28 days before antidepressant effects will be noticed
- Reassure patient that drowsiness and dizziness usually subside after first few weeks; if dizzy, patient should get up from lying or sitting position slowly, and dangle legs over edge of bed before getting up
- Excessive use of caffeinated foods, drugs, or beverages may increase anxiety and agitation and confuse the diagnosis

PATIENT INSTRUCTIONS

For detailed patient instructions on SARI, see the Patient Information Sheet on p. 242.

- Avoid driving a car or operating hazardous machinery until response to drug has been determined
- Alcohol or other CNS depressants will cause an increase in sleepiness, dizziness, and lightheadedness
- Check with your doctor before taking other medication, including over-the-counter drugs, such as cold remedies
- Avoid ingestion of grapefruit juice while taking nefazodone, as the blood level of the antidepressant may increase

Serotonin-2 Antagonists/Reuptake Inhibitors (SARI) (cont.)

DRUG INTERACTIONS

- Clinically significant interactions are listed below

Class of Drug	Example	Interaction Effects
Alcohol		Short-term or acute use reduces first-pass metabolism of antidepressant and increases its plasma level; chronic use induces metabolizing enzymes and decreases its plasma level
Anticholinergic	Antiparkinsonian agents, antihistamines	Increased anticholinergic effect; may increase risk of hyperthermia, confusion, urinary retention, etc.
Anticonvulsant	Carbamazepine, phenytoin	Increased plasma level of carbamazepine or phenytoin due to inhibition of metabolism with trazodone Increased plasma level of carbamazepine with nefazodone due to inhibited metabolism via CYP3A4
	Carbamazepine, barbiturates, phenytoin	Decreased plasma level of trazodone and nefazodone due to enzyme induction via CYP3A4
Anticoagulant	Warfarin	Decreased prothrombin time with trazodone
Antidepressant		
Irreversible MAOI	Phenelzine, tranylcypromine	Low doses of trazodone (25–50 mg) used to treat antidepressant-induced insomnia Combined SARI and MAOI therapy has additive antidepressant effects; monitor for serotonergic effects
RIMA	Moclobemide	Additive antidepressant effect in treatment-resistant patients; monitor for serotonergic effects
NDRI	Bupropion	Additive antidepressant effect in treatment-resistant patients
SSRI	Fluoxetine, fluvoxamine, paroxetine, sertraline	Elevated SARI plasma level (due to release from protein binding and inhibition of oxidative metabolism); monitor plasma level and for signs of toxicity Nefazodone metabolite (mCPP) level increased 4-fold with fluoxetine; case report of serotonin syndrome with combination Additive antidepressant effect in treatment-resistant patients; nefazodone may reverse SSRI-induced sexual dysfunction and may enhance sleep
Antihistamine	Terfenadine, astemizole, loratadine	Inhibited metabolism of antihistamine by nefazodone (via CYP3A4) leading to accumulation of parent compound and resultant adverse cardiac effects; potentiation of QT prolongation (cetirizine and fexofenadine levels elevated, but considered safe)
Antihypertensive	Bethanidine, clonidine, debrisoquin, methyldopa, guanethidine, reserpine	Decreased antihypertensive effect due to inhibition of α-adrenergic receptors
	Acetazolamide, thiazide diuretics	Hypotension augmented

Class of Drug	Example	Interaction Effects
Antipsychotic	Chlorpromazine, haloperidol, perphenazine Clozapine	Increased plasma level of either agent Potentiation of hypotension with trazodone Increased plasma level of clozapine and norclozapine with nefazodone due to inhibited metabolism via CYP3A4
Anxiolytic	Alprazolam, triazolam, midazolam, bromazepam, diazepam	Increased plasma level of benzodiazepines metabolized by oxidation (via CYP3A4) with nefazodone; triazolam by 500%, alprazolam by 200% and desmethyldiazepam by 87%
Ca-channel blocker	Amlodipine	Elevated amlodipine level due to inhibited metabolism by nefazodone, via CYP3A4
CNS depressant	Hypnotics, antihistamines, benzodiazepines	Increased sedation, CNS depression
Cholestyramine		Decreased absorption of antidepressant, if given together
Digoxin		Increased digoxin plasma level, with possible toxicity, with trazodone and nefazodone
Ergot alkaloid	Ergotamine	Elevated ergotamine levels possible due to inhibited metabolism by nefazodone via CYP3A4
Ginkgo Biloba		Case report of coma with trazodone (postulated to be due to excess stimulation of GABA receptors)
Grapefruit juice		Decreased metabolism of trazodone and nefazodone via CYP3A4
Immunosuppressant	Cyclosporin, tacrolimus	Increased plasma level of cyclosporin (by approx. 70%) and tacrolimus (5-fold) with nefazodone due to inhibition of CYP3A4
Insulin		Hypoglycemia reported with nefazodone
Lithium		Additive antidepressant effect
L-Tryptophan		Additive antidepressant effect; monitor for serotonergic effects
MAO-B inhibitor	L-deprenyl (selegiline)	Reports of serotonergic reactions
Protease inhibitor	Ritonavir	Increased plasma levels of trazodone and nefazodone due to decreased metabolism
Sildenafil		Possible enhanced hypotension due to inhibited metabolism of sildenafil by nefazodone via CYP3A4
Statins	Simvastatin, pravastatin, atorvastatin	Inhibited metabolism of statins by nefazodone (via CYP3A4); increased plasma level and adverse effects – myositis and rhabdomyolysis reported
St. John's Wort		May augment serotonergic effects – case reports of serotonergic reactions
Sulfonylurea	Tolbutamide	Increased hypoglycemia
Thyroid drug	Triiodothyronine (T_3-liothyronine), L-thyroxine (T_4)	Additive antidepressant effect in treatment-resistant patients

Noradrenergic/Specific Serotonergic Antidepressants (NaSSA)

PRODUCT AVAILABILITY

Chemical Class	Generic Name	Trade Name(A)	Dosage Forms and Strengths
Tetracyclic agent	Mirtazapine	Remeron Remeron SolTab(B)	Tablets: 15 mg(B), 30 mg(B), 45 mg(B) Oral disintegrating tablets: 15 mg, 30 mg, 45 mg

(A) Generic preparations may be available, (B) Not marketed in Canada

INDICATIONS*

- ▲ Major depression
- Early data suggest mirtazapine may mitigate SSRI-induced sexual dysfunction and "poop-out" syndrome
- Preliminary reports of efficacy in panic disorder, generalized anxiety disorder, OCD, PTSD, dysthymia and premenstrual dysphoric disorder
- Early data suggest mirtazapine may benefit negative symptoms of schizophrenia and psychotic depression

PHARMACOLOGY

- Selective antagonist at α_2-adrenergic auto- and heteroreceptors which are involved in regulation of neuronal release of norepinephrine and serotonin (increases noradrenergic and serotonergic transmission via blockade of α-adrenoreceptors; increases the release of norepinephrine and serotonin, and blocks 5-HT_{2A+C} and 5-HT_3 receptors)

GENERAL COMMENTS

- Reduces sleep latency and prolongs sleep duration due to H_1 and 5-HT_{2A+C} blockade
- Early data suggest mirtazapine may have a faster onset of antidepressant action than some other classes of antidepressants (e.g., most SSRIs) – may be secondary to early restoration of sleep and decrease of anxiety

DOSING

- See p. 55
- Initiate at 15–30 mg daily for 4 days; increase to 30 mg and maintain for at least 10 days; if ineffective, can increase to 60 mg daily

PHARMACOKINETICS

- Bioavailability is approximately 50% because of gut wall and hepatic first-pass metabolism; food decreases rate of absorption to a small degree
- Remeron SolTabs dissolve on the tongue within 30 seconds; can be swallowed with or without water, chewed, or allowed to dissolve
- Peak plasma level achieved in 2 h
- Protein binding of 85%
- Females and the elderly show higher plasma concentrations than males and young adults
- Extensively metabolized via CYP1A2, 2D6 and 3A4; desmethyl metabolite has some clinical activity
- Half-life: 20–40 h – half-life significantly longer in females than in males
- Hepatic clearance decreased by 40% in patients with cirrhosis
- Clearance reduced by 30–50% in patients with renal impairment

ONSET AND DURATION OF ACTION

- Therapeutic effects seen after 7–28 days

ADVERSE EFFECTS

- See p. 43

1. CNS Effects

- Sedation in over 30% of patients; fatigue, insomnia, agitation, restlessness and nervousness reported occasionally; less sedation at doses above 15 mg due to increased effect on α_2-receptors and increased release of NE
- Decreases REM sleep; vivid dreams reported
- Rarely delirium, psychosis
- Seizures (very rare – 0.04%)

* ▲ Approved indications

2. Anticholinergic Effects

- Dry mouth frequent; constipation [for treatment suggestions see Non-selective Cyclic Antidepressants, p. 33)]
- Increased sweating, blurred vision and urinary retention reported rarely

3. Cardiovascular Effects

- Hypotension, hypertension, vertigo, tachycardia and palpitations reported rarely
- Edema 1–2%
- No significant ECG changes reported

4. GI Effects

- Rare reports of bitter taste, dyspepsia, nausea, vomiting and diarrhea
- Increased appetite and weight gain (of over 4 kg) reported in approximately 16% of patients (due to potent antihistaminic properties); occur primarily in the first 4 weeks of treatment and may be dose-related
- Decreased appetite and weight loss occasionally reported

5. Other Adverse Effects

- Case reports of erotic dream-related ejaculation in elderly patients
- Rare reports of tremor, hot flashes
- Transient elevation of ALT reported in about 2% of patients
- Neutropenia (1.5% risk) and agranulocytosis (0.1%) reported; monitor WBC if patient develops signs of infection [some recommend doing baseline and annual CBC]
- Increases in plasma cholesterol, to over 20% above the upper limit of normal, seen in 15% of patients; increases in non-fasting triglyceride levels (7%)
- Cases of joint pain or worsening of arthritis reported
- Myalgia and flu-like symptoms in 2–5% of patients
- Case of palinopsia reported

WITHDRAWAL

- Case report of dizziness, nausea, anxiety, insomnia and paresthesia following abrupt withdrawal
- Case report of hypomania

☞ **THEREFORE THESE MEDICATIONS SHOULD BE WITHDRAWN GRADUALLY AFER PROLONGED USE**

Management

- Reinstitute drug at a lower dose and taper gradually over several days

PRECAUTIONS

- Caution in patients with compromised liver function or renal impairment
- Monitor WBC if patient develops signs of infection; a low WBC requires discontinuation of therapy
- May induce manic reactions in patients with BAD and rarely in unipolar depression

TOXICITY

- Low liability for toxicity in overdose if taken alone; no changes in vital signs, with dose of 900 mg, reported
- No fatalities when drug used alone

PEDIATRIC CONSIDERATIONS

- Safety not established

GERIATRIC CONSIDERATIONS

- Clearance reduced in elderly males by up to 40%, and in elderly females by up to 10%
- Dosing: start at 7.5 mg hs and increase to 15 mg after 1–2 weeks, depending on response and side effects; monitor for sedation, hypotension and anticholinergic effects

USE IN PREGNANCY

- Data not available

Breast milk

- Data not available

NURSING IMPLICATIONS

- Psychotherapy and education are also important in the treatment of depression
- Monitor therapy by watching for adverse effects, mood and activity level changes

Noradrenergic/Specific Serotonergic Antidepressants (NaSSA) (cont.)

PATIENT INSTRUCTIONS

- For detailed patient instructions on mirtazapine, see Patient Information Sheet on p. 244
- Should you develop signs and symptoms of infections (e.g., sore throat, fever, mouth sores, elevated temperature), this should be reported, as soon as possible, to the physician

DRUG INTERACTIONS

- Clinically significant interactions are listed below

Class of Drug	Example	Interaction Effects
Anticonvulsant	Carbamazepine	Decreased plasma level of mirtazapine by 60% due to induction of metabolism via CYP3A4
Antidepressant		
Irreversible MAOI	Phenelzine, tranylcypromine	Possible serotonergic reaction; DO NOT COMBINE
SSRI		Combination reported to alleviate insomnia and augment antidepressant response; may have activating effects May mitigate SSRI-induced sexual dysfunction and "poop-out" syndrome Increased serotonergic effects possible Increased sedation and weight gain reported with combination
CNS depressant	Alcohol, benzodiazepines	Impaired cognition and motor performance
Stimulant	Phentermine, dextroamphetamine, methylphenidate	May increase agitation and risk of mania, especially in patients with bipolar disorder

Non-Selective Cyclic Antidepressants

PRODUCT AVAILABILITY

Chemical Class[D]	Generic Name	Trade Name[A]	Dosage Forms and Strengths
Tricyclic antidepressant (TCA)	Amitriptyline	Elavil, Endep[B]	Tablets: 10 mg, 25 mg, 50 mg, 75 mg, 100 mg[B], 150 mg[B] Oral suspension: 10 mg/5ml Injection[B]: 10 mg/ml
	Clomipramine	Anafranil	Tablets: 10 mg, 25 mg, 50 mg, 75 mg[B]
	Desipramine	Norpramin	Tablets: 10 mg, 25 mg, 50 mg, 75 mg, 100 mg, 150 mg[B]
	Doxepin	Sinequan, Adapin[B]	Capsules: 10 mg, 25 mg, 50 mg, 75 mg, 100 mg, 150 mg
	Imipramine	Tofranil	Tablets: 10 mg, 25 mg, 50 mg, 75 mg[C] Capsules[B]: 75 mg, 100 mg, 125 mg, 150 mg Injection[B]: 12.5 mg/ml
	Nortriptyline	Aventyl[C], Pamelor[B]	Capsules: 10 mg, 25 mg, 50 mg[B], 75 mg[B] Syrup[B]: 10 mg/5ml
	Protriptyline	Triptil[C], Vivactil[B]	Tablets: 5 mg[B], 10 mg
	Trimipramine	Surmontil	Tablets: 12.5 mg[C], 25 mg, 50 mg, 100 mg Capsules: 75 mg
Dibenzoxazepine	Amoxapine	Asendin	Tablets: 25 mg, 50 mg, 100 mg, 150 mg[B]
Tetracyclic	Maprotiline	Ludiomil	Tablets: 10 mg[C], 25 mg, 50 mg, 75 mg

[A] Generic preparations may be available, [B] Not marketed in Canada, [C] Not marketed in USA, [D] Include: NE-reuptake inhibitors, Mixed 5 HT/NE reuptake inhibitors, Serotonin reuptake inhibitors

INDICATIONS*

- ▲ • Major depressive disorder
- ▲ • Prophylaxis of recurrent major depression (unipolar affective disorder)
- ▲ • Treatment of secondary depression in other mental illnesses, e.g., schizophrenia, dementia
- ▲ • Depressed phase of bipolar affective disorder (see Precautions)
- ▲ • Obsessive-compulsive disorder (clomipramine)
- ▲ • Treatment of enuresis (imipramine)
- • Panic disorder prophylaxis (imipramine, desipramine)
- • Agoraphobia associated with panic disorder
- • Efficacy in dysthymia reported (imipramine, desipramine)
- • Bulimia
- • Efficacy against intrusive symptoms of posttraumatic stress disorder reported

* ▲ Approved indications

Non-Selective Cyclic Antidepressants (cont.)

- Attention deficit hyperactivity disorder not responsive to psychostimulants
- Used in autism for ritualistic behavior and aggression (clomipramine) or hyperactivity (desipramine)
- Premenstrual syndrome (clomipramine, nortriptyline)
- Cataplexy (protriptyline)
- Premature ejaculation (clomipramine)
- Sialorrhea induced by clozapine (amitriptyline)
- Anti-ulcer effect (doxepin)
- Pain management, including migraine headache, diabetic neuropathy, postherpetic neuralgia, chronic oral-facial pain
- Antipsychotic effect reported with low dose amoxapine
- Aid in smoking cessation (nortriptyline)

PHARMACOLOGY

- Exact mechanism of action unknown; equilibrate the effects of biogenic amines through various mechanisms; cause downregulation of β-adrenergic receptors
- The action in the treatment of enuresis may involve inhibition of urination due to the anticholinergic effect and CNS stimulation, resulting in easier arousal by the stimulus of a full bladder

GENERAL COMMENTS

- Suggested that men respond better to tricyclics (and less well to SSRIs) than women
- Studies suggest improved outcomes in panic disorder with combination of imipramine and psychotherapy

DOSING

- Initiate drug at a low dose and increase dose every 3 to 5 days to a maximum tolerated dose based on side effects
- There is a wide variation in dosage requirements (partially dependent on plasma levels) (see pp. 55–56)
- Once steady-state is reached, give drug as a single bedtime dose; use divided doses if patient develops nightmares
- Prophylaxis is most effective if therapeutic dose is maintained

Dosing route

- Usual route of administration is oral – IM injection has no advantage except with patients unwilling or unable to receive drug orally
- Clomipramine IV up to 300 mg daily for treatment of obsessive-compulsive disorder has been tried for quicker response

PHARMACOKINETICS

- Completely absorbed from the gastrointestinal tract
- Large percentage metabolized by first-pass effect
- Peak plasma levels occur more rapidly with tertiary tricyclics, like amitriptyline (1–3 h) than with secondary tricyclics like desipramine and nortriptyline (4–8 h)
- Highly lipophilic; concentrated primarily in myocardial and cerebral tissue
- Highly bound to plasma protein
- Metabolized primarily by the liver
- Most tricyclics have linear pharmacokinetics, i.e., a change in dose leads to a proportional change in plasma concentration
- Elimination half-life: see pp. 55–56; steady state reached in about 5 days
- Pharmacokinetics may vary between males and females; data suggest that plasma levels of tricyclic antidepressants may dip in female patients prior to menstruation

ONSET AND DURATION OF ACTION

- Tricyclics and related drugs are long-acting; they may be given in a single daily dose, usually at bedtime (except protriptyline, which is usually given in the morning)
- Therapeutic effect is seen after 7–28 days
- Sedative effects are seen within a few hours of oral administration, with lessened sleep disturbance after a few days
- Occasionally patients may lose response to antidepressant after several months ("poop-out syndrome") [Check compliance with therapy; optimize dose (plasma level may be useful); may need to change drug]

ADVERSE EFFECTS

- The pharmacological and side effect profile of cyclic antidepressants is dependent on their affinity for and activity on neurotransmitters/receptors (see table p. 40)
- See chart p. 42 for incidence of adverse effects at therapeutic doses of specific agents; incidence of adverse effects may be greater in early days of treatment; patients adapt to many side effects over time

1. CNS Effects

- A result of antagonism at histamine H_1-receptors and α_1-adrenoreceptors
- Occur frequently

a) Cognitive Effects

- Drowsiness (most common adverse effect) [Management: prescribe bulk of dose at bedtime]
- Weakness, lethargy, fatigue
- Conversely, excitement, agitation, restlessness, and insomnia have occurred
- Decrease REM sleep (except for trimipramine); vivid dreaming or nightmares can occur, especially if all the medication is given at bedtime
- Confusion, disturbed concentration, disorientation
- Precipitation of hypomania or mania (risk 11–50% in patients with a history of BAD – less frequent in patients receiving lithium), psychosis, panic reactions, anxiety, or euphoria may occur

b) Neurological Effects

- Fine tremor
- Akathisia (rare – check serum iron for deficiency); can occur following abrupt drug withdrawal; reported with amoxapine, imipramine and desipramine
- Tardive dyskinesia (reported primarily with amoxapine, but also seen on rare occasions with other antidepressants)
- Seizures (more common in children and patients with eating disorder) can occur following abrupt drug increase or after drug withdrawal; risk increases with high plasma levels
- Tinnitus – more likely with serotonergic agents
- Paresthesias reported with tricyclics (approximate risk 4%)
- Myoclonus – more likely with serotonergic agents; includes muscle jerks of lower extremities, jaw, and arms, and nocturnal myoclonus – may be severe in up to 9% of patients [If severe, clonazepam, valproate or carbamazepine may be of benefit]
- Dysphasia, stuttering
- Disturbance in gait, parkinsonism, dystonia

2. Anticholinergic Effects

- A result of antagonism at muscarinic receptors (ACh)
- Occur frequently, esp. in elderly patients
- Dry mucous membranes; may predispose patient to monilial infections [Management: sugar-free gum and candy, oral lubricants (e.g., MoiStir, OraCare D), pilocarpine tablets (10–15 mg/day) or mouthwash (4 drops 4% solution to 12 drops water swished in mouth and spat out), bethanechol]
- Blurred vision [Management: pilocarpine 0.5% eye drops]
- Dry eyes; may be of particular difficulty in the elderly or those wearing contact lenses [Management: artificial tears, but employ caution with patients wearing contact lenses; these patients should have their dry eyes managed with their usual wetting solutions or comfort drops]
- Constipation (frequent in children on therapy for enuresis) [Management: increase bulk and fluid intake, fecal softener, bulk laxative]
- Urinary retention, delayed micturition [Management: bethanechol 10–30 mg tid]
- Excessive sweating [Management: daily showering, talcum powder; in severe cases: Drysol solution, terazosin 1–10 mg daily, oxybutynin up to 5 mg bid, clonidine 0.1 mg bid; drug may need to be changed]
- Confusion, disorientation, delirium, delusions, hallucinations (more common in the elderly, especially with higher doses)
- Dental caries due to decreased salivation, changes in buffer capacity of saliva, and bacterial environment [Management: maintain oral hygiene]

3. Cardiovascular Effects

- A result of antagonism at α_1-adrenoreceptors, muscarinic, 5-HT_2 and H_1-receptors and inhibition of sodium fast channels
- More common in elderly

Non-Selective Cyclic Antidepressants (cont.)

- Risk increases with high plasma levels
- Tachycardia; may be more pronounced in younger patients
- Orthostatic hypotension [Management: sodium chloride tablets, caffeine, fludrocortisone (0.1–0.5 mg/day), midodrine (2.5–10 mg tid), use of support stockings]
- Prolonged conduction time; contraindicated in heart block or post-myocardial infarction
- Arrhythmias, syncope, thrombosis, thrombophlebitis, stroke, and congestive heart failure have been reported on occasion
- May cause hypertension in patients with bulimia

4. GI Effects

- A result of inhibition of 5-HT uptake and ACh antagonism
- Anorexia, nausea, vomiting, diarrhea
- Weight gain (up to 30% patients with chronic use; average gain of up to 7 kg – weight gain is linear over time and is often accompanied by a craving for sweets) [Management: nutritional counseling, exercise, dose reduction, changing antidepressant]
- Constipation (see anticholinergic effects)
- Peculiar taste, "black tongue," glossitis

5. Sexual Side Effects

- A result of altered dopamine (D_2) activity, 5-HT_2 blockade, inhibition of 5-HT reuptake, α_1-blockade, and ACh blockade
- Decreased libido, impotence [Management: amantadine (100–400 mg prn), bethanechol (10 mg tid or 10–25 mg prn), neostigmine (7.5–15 mg prn), cyproheptadine (4–16 mg prn), yohimbine (5.4–16.2 mg prn]
- Testicular swelling, painful ejaculation, retrograde ejaculation, increased libido and priapism; spontaneous orgasm with yawning (clomipramine)
- Breast engorgement and breast tissue enlargement in males and females
- Anorgasmia [Management: amantadine (100–400 mg prn), cyproheptadine (4–16 mg prn), yohimbine (5.4–10.8 mg od or prn), ginseng, ginkgo biloba (180–900 mg)]

6. Endocrine Effects

- Both increases and decreases in blood sugar levels reported
- Carbohydrate craving reported in up to 87% of patients on maintenance therapy – may result in weight gain
- Menstrual irregularities, amenorrhea and galactorrhea (amoxapine)
- Can induce syndrome of SIADH with hyponatremia; risk increased with age

7. Allergic Reactions

- Rare
- Jaundice, hepatitis, rash, urticaria, pruritis, edema, blood dyscrasias
- Photosensitivity, skin pigmentation (imipramine, desipramine)
- Case reports of thrombocytopenia

8. Other Adverse Effects

- Rare reports of alopecia with tricyclics

WITHDRAWAL

- Reported incidence: 20–80% – likely due to cholinergic and adrenergic rebound
- Abrupt withdrawal from high doses may cause a "flu-like" syndrome consisting of fever, fatigue, sweating, coryza, malaise, myalgia, headache; psychological symptoms: anxiety, agitation, hypomania or mania, insomnia, vivid dreams, as well as dizziness, nausea, vomiting; akathisia and dyskinesia also reported
- Most likely to occur 24–48 h after withdrawal, or after a large dosage decrease
- Rebound depression can occur (even in individuals not previously depressed – such as patients with obsessional disorders)
- Paradoxical mood changes reported on abrupt withdrawal, including hypomania or mania

☞ **THESE MEDICATIONS SHOULD THEREFORE BE WITHDRAWN GRADUALLY AFTER PROLONGED USE**

Management

- Reinstitute drug (at slightly lower dose) and gradually taper dose over several days (e.g., by 25 mg every 3–5 days)

- Alternatively, can treat specific symptoms:
  - Cholinergic rebound (e.g., nausea, vomiting, sweating) – ginger, benztropine 0.5–4 mg prn, atropine 1–4 mg tid to qid
  - Anxiety, agitation, insomnia – benzodiazepine (e.g., lorazepam 0.5–2 mg prn)
  - Dizziness – meclizine 12.5–25 mg q6h prn, dimenhydrinate 25–50 mg q6h prn
  - Neurological symptoms: Akathisia – propranolol 10–20 mg tid–qid; Dyskinesia – clonazepam 0.5–2 mg prn; Dystonia – benztropine 0.5–4 mg prn

PRECAUTIONS

- Use cautiously in patients in whom excess anticholinergic activity could be harmful (e.g., prostatic hypertrophy, urinary retention, narrow-angle glaucoma)
- Use with caution in patients with respiratory difficulties, since antidepressants can dry up bronchial secretions and make breathing more difficult
- May lower the seizure threshold; therefore, administer cautiously to patients with a history of convulsive disorders, organic brain disease, or a predisposition to convulsions (e.g., alcohol withdrawal)
- May impair the mental and physical ability to perform hazardous tasks (e.g., driving a car or operating machinery); will potentiate the effects of alcohol
- May induce manic reactions in up to 50% of patients with bipolar affective disorder; because of risk of increased cycling, bipolar affective disorder is a relative contraindication
- Combination of cyclic antidepressants with SSRIs can lead to increased plasma level of the cyclic antidepressant. Combination therapy has been used in the treatment of resistant patients; use of serotonergic cyclic antidepressants with SSRIs can cause a serotonergic reaction
- Use caution when switching from a cyclic antidepressant to fluoxetine and vice versa (see Interactions, pp. 37–39 and Switching Antidepressants, p. 57)
- Concurrent ingestion of a cyclic antidepressant with high fiber foods or laxatives (e.g., bran, psyllium) can decrease absorption of the antidepressant

TOXICITY

- The therapeutic margin is low (lethal dose is about 3 times the maximum therapeutic dose); prescribe limited quantities
- Symptoms of toxicity are extensions of the common adverse effects: anticholinergic, CNS stimulation followed by CNS depression, myoclonus, hallucinations, respiratory depression and seizures
- Cardiac irregularities occur and are most hazardous; duration of QRS complex on the electrocardiogram (ECG) reflects the severity of the overdose; if it equals or exceeds 0.12 s, it should be considered a danger sign (normal range 0.08–0.11 s)

Management

- Activated charcoal (1–2 g/kg initially followed by 2 or 3 more doses several hours apart) decreases tricyclic antidepressant absorption and lowers its blood level
- Cathartics (sorbitol or magnesium citrate) will aid in drug evacuation. Give together with charcoal. Monitor bowel sounds to avoid impaction
- DO NOT GIVE IPECAC due to possibility of rapid neurological deterioration and high incidence of seizures
- Supportive treatment, with patient closely monitored in hospital
- Physostigmine salicylate
- Diazepam IV is the drug of choice for convulsions
- Forced diuresis and dialysis are of little benefit

PEDIATRIC CONSIDERATIONS

- Antidepressants are used in enuresis, insomnia and parasomnias, attention deficit hyperactivity disorder (ADHD), major depressive disorder, obsessional disorder, panic disorder, school phobia, separation anxiety disorder, bulimia, and Tourette's syndrome (clomipramine); value of tricyclics in treating depression in children is questioned
- Start drug at a low dose (10–25 mg) and increase gradually by 10–25 mg every 4–5 days to a maximum dose of 3–5 mg/kg (tricyclics)
- Half life of imipramine is shorter than in adults (hepatic metabolism is greater than in adults)
- Prior to treatment, a baseline ECG is recommended. When an effective daily dose is reached, a steady state serum level and ECG should be done. Do a follow-up ECG at any dose change and a plasma level every few months

Non-Selective Cyclic Antidepressants (cont.)

- The U.S. FDA defines the following ECG and examination values as unsafe in children treated with tricyclics: (a) PR interval > 200 ms, (b) QRS interval > 30% above a baseline (or > 120 ms), (c) BP > 140 mmHg systolic or 90 mmHg diastolic, (d) Heart rate > 130 beats/min at rest
- Efficacy and toxicity appear to be dose-related
- Abrupt dose increase can precipitate seizures
- Children being treated for enuresis may experience drowsiness, anxiety, emotional instability, nervousness, and sleep disorder
- Sudden death (rarely) reported with desipramine, even with therapeutic plasma levels; plasma levels may be higher by 42% in children than adults, at the same dose
- Hypertension (rarely) reported with imipramine
- Cardiac complications reported in children who smoke marihuana while on antidepressants

GERIATRIC CONSIDERATIONS

- Initiate dose lower and slower than in younger patients; elderly patients may take longer to respond and may require trials of up to 12 weeks before response is noted
- Monitor for excessive CNS and anticholinergic effects; use an antidepressant least likely to cause these effects (e.g., nortriptyline, desipramine)
- Caution when combining with other drugs with CNS and anticholinergic properties; additive effects can result in confusion, disorientation, and delirium; elderly are sensitive to anticholinergic effects
- Caution regarding cardiovascular side effects: orthostatic hypotension (can lead to falls), tachycardia, and conduction slowing
- Cognitive impairment can occur, including decreased word-recall and facial recognition

USE IN PREGNANCY

- Antidepressants have not been demonstrated to have teratogenic effects
- If possible, avoid during first trimester
- Dosage required to achieve therapeutic plasma level may increase during the third trimester of pregnancy
- Urinary retention in neonate has been associated with antidepressant use in third trimester

Breast milk

- Antidepressants are excreted into breast milk and it is estimated that the baby will receive up to 4% of the mother's dose; half-life of antidepressant increased in neonate 3–4-fold
- Doxepin metabolite concentration reported to reach similar plasma level in infant as in mother
- The American Academy of Pediatrics classifies antidepressants as drugs "whose effects on nursing infants are unknown but may be of concern"

NURSING IMPLICATIONS

- Psychotherapy and education are also important in the treatment of depression
- Monitor therapy by watching for adverse side effects, mood and activity level changes; keep physician informed
- Be aware that the medication reduces the degree of depression and may increase psychomotor activity; this may create concern about suicidal behavior
- Expect a lag time of 7–28 days before antidepressant effects will be noticed
- Check for constipation; increase fluids and increase bulk in diet to lessen constipation
- Check for urinary retention; if required the physician may order bethanechol orally or by sc injection
- Reassure patient that drowsiness and dizziness usually subside after first few weeks; if dizzy, patient should get up from lying or sitting position slowly, and dangle legs over edge of bed before getting up
- Excessive use of caffeinated foods, drugs, or beverages may increase anxiety and agitation and confuse the diagnosis
- Expect a dry mouth; suggest frequent mouth rinsing with water, and sour or sugarless hard candy or gum
- Artificial tears may be useful for patients who complain of dry eyes (or wetting solutions for those wearing contact lenses)

PATIENT INSTRUCTIONS

For detailed patient instructions on cyclic antidepressants, see the Patient Information Sheet on p. 246.

- Avoid driving a car or operating hazardous machinery until response to drug has been determined
- Alcohol or other CNS depressants will cause an increase in sleepiness, dizziness, and lightheadedness
- Avoid exposure to extreme heat and humidity as these drugs may affect the body's ability to regulate temperature
- Check with your doctor before taking other medication, including over-the-counter drugs, such as cold remedies
- These drugs may interact with medication used by a dentist, so let him know the name of the drug you are taking
- Avoid ingesting high fiber foods or laxatives (e.g., bran) concurrently with medication, as this may reduce the antidepressant level

DRUG INTERACTIONS

- Clinically significant interactions are listed below

Class of Drug	Example	Interaction Effects
ACE-inhibitor	Enalapril	Increased plasma level of clomipramine due to decreased metabolism
Alcohol		Short-term or acute use reduces first-pass metabolism of antidepressant and increases its plasma level; chronic use induces metabolizing enzymes and decreases its plasma level
Anesthetic	Enflurane	Report of seizures with amitriptyline
Anorexiant	Dexfenfluramine, fenfluramine	Increased plasma level of nortriptyline, imipramine, amitriptyline and desipramine
Antiarrhythmic	Quinidine, procainamide Propafenone, quinidine	Prolonged cardiac conduction Increased plasma level of desipramine (by 500%) and imipramine (by 30%)
Anticholinergic	Antiparkinsonian agents, antihistamines, neuroleptics	Increased anticholinergic effect; may increase risk of hyperthermia, confusion, urinary retention, etc.
Anticonvulsant	Carbamazepine, barbiturates, phenytoin Valproate, divalproex, valproic acid Phenobarbital	Decreased plasma level of tricyclics due to enzyme induction Increased plasma level of tricyclic antidepressant Increased plasma level of phenobarbital with clomipramine
Anticoagulant	Warfarin	Increased prothrombin time with tricyclics
Antidepressant		
Irreversible MAOI	Phenelzine, tranylcypromine	If used together, do not add cyclic antidepressants to MAOI: start cyclic antidepressant first or simultaneously with MAOI; for patients already on MAOI, discontinue MAOI 10–14 days before starting combination therapy Combined cyclic and MAOI therapy has additive antidepressant effects in treatment-resistant patients
RIMA	Moclobemide	Additive antidepressant effect in treatment-resistant patients
NDRI	Bupropion	Additive antidepressant effect in treatment-resistant patients Elevated imipramine level (by 57%), desipramine level (by 82%) and nortriptyline level (by 200%) with combination
SSRI	Fluoxetine, fluvoxamine, paroxetine, sertraline	Elevated tricyclic plasma level (due to release from protein binding and inhibition of oxidative metabolism); monitor plasma level and for signs of toxicity Additive antidepressant effect in treatment-resistant patients
Antifungal	Ketoconazole, fluconazole	Increased plasma level of antidepressant due to inhibited metabolism (89% with amitriptyline; 70% with nortriptyline); 20% increase with imipramine and no increase with desipramine

Non-Selective Cyclic Antidepressants (cont.)

Class of Drug	Example	Interaction Effects
Antihistamine	Terfenadine, astemizole	Inhibited metabolism of antihistamine by nortriptyline (via CYP3A4) leading to accumulation of parent compound and resultant adverse cardiac effects; potentiation of QT prolongation (loratidine, cetirizine and fexofenadine levels elevated, but considered safe)
Antihypertensive	Bethanidine, clonidine, debrisoquin, methyldopa, guanethidine, reserpine	Decreased antihypertensive effect due to inhibition of α-adrenergic receptors
	Acetazolamide, thiazide diuretics	Hypotension augmented
	Labetalol	Increased plasma level of imipramine (by 54%) and desipramine
Antipsychotic	Chlorpromazine, haloperidol, perphenazine	Increased plasma level of either agent
Ca-channel blocker	Nifedipine	May antagonize the efficacy of antidepressant drugs
	Diltiazem, verapamil	Increased imipramine plasma level by 30% and 15%, respectively; increased level of trimipramine
Cannabis/marihuana		Case reports of tachycardia, lightheadedness, confusion, mood lability and delirium with nortriptyline and desipramine; may evoke cardiac complications in youth
CNS depressant	Hypnotics, antihistamines, benzodiazepines	Increased sedation, CNS depression
Cholestyramine		Decreased absorption of antidepressant, if given together
Cimetidine		Increased plasma level of antidepressant; for desipramine, inhibition of hydroxylation occurs only in rapid metabolizers
Grapefruit juice		Decreased conversion of clomipramine to metabolite due to inhibition of CYP3A4
Insulin		Decreased insulin sensitivity reported with amitriptyline
Lithium		Additive antidepressant effect
Methylphenidate		Increased plasma level of imipramine and clomipramine due to decreased metabolism; additive antidepressant effect
L-Tryptophan		Additive antidepressant effect
MAO-B inhibitor	L-deprenyl (selegiline)	Reports of serotonergic reactions
Narcotic	Methadone	Increased plasma level of desipramine (by about 108%)
	Morphine	Enhanced analgesic effect
Omeprazole		Increased plasma level of antidepressant due to inhibited metabolism
Oral contraceptive	Estrogen/progesterone	Increased plasma level of antidepressant due to decreased metabolism
Oxybutynin		Increased metabolism of clomipramine (may be due to induction of CYP3A4)

Class of Drug	Example	Interaction Effects
Phenylbutazone		Decreased gastric emptying with desipramine leading to impaired absorption of phenylbutazone
Propoxyphene		Increased plasma level of doxepin due to decreased metabolism
Protease inhibitor	Ritonavir	Increased plasma levels of tricyclic antidepressant due to decreased metabolism (AUC of desipramine increased by 145%; peak plasma level increased 22%)
Rifampin		Decreased plasma level of antidepressant due to increased metabolism
Smoking – cigarettes		Increased clearance of antidepressant due to induction of CYP1A2
Stimulant	Methylphenidate	Plasma level of antidepressant may be increased Used together to augment antidepressant effect Cardiovascular effects increased with combination, in children – monitor Case reports of neurotoxic effects with imipramine, but considered rare – monitor
Sulfonylurea	Tolbutamide	Increased hypoglycemia
Sympathomimetic	Epinephrine, norepinephrine (levarterenol), phenylephrine Isoproterenol	Enhanced pressor response from 2- to 8-fold; benefit may outweigh risks in anaphylaxis May increase likelihood of arrhythmias
Tamoxifen		Decreased plasma level of doxepin by 25% due to induced metabolism via CYP3A4
Thyroid drug	Triiodothyronine (T_3-liothyronine), L-thyroxine (T_4)	Additive antidepressant effect in treatment-resistant patients
Triptan	Sumatriptan, zolmitriptan	Possible serotonergic reaction when combined with antidepressants with serotonergic activity (e.g., clomipramine)

Effects of Antidepressants on Neurotransmitters/Receptors*

	Amitriptyline	Clomipramine	Desipramine	Doxepin	Imipramine	Nortriptyline	Protriptyline	Trimipramine	Amoxapine	Maprotiline
NE reuptake	+++	+++	+++++	+++	+++	++++	+++++	++	++++	++++
5-HT reuptake	+++	++++	++	++	+++	++	++	+	++	+
DA reuptake	+	+	+	+	+	+	+	+	+	+
Blockade 5-HT$_1$	++	+	+	++	+	++	+	+	++	+–
Blockade 5-HT$_2$	+++	+++	++	+++	+++	+++	+++	+++	+++++	++
Blockade ACh	+++	+++	++	+++	+++	++	+++	+++	++	++
Blockade H$_1$	++++	+++	++	+++++	+++	+++	+++	+++++	+++	++++
Blockade α_1	+++	+++	++	+++	+++	+++	++	+++	+++	+++
Blockade α_2	++	+	+	+	+	+	+	+	+	+
Blockade D$_2$	+	++	+	+	+	+	+	++	++	++
Selective	NE>5-HT	NE<5-HT	NE>5-HT	NE>5-HT	NE>5-HT	NE>5-HT	NE>5-HT	NE>5-HT	NE>5-HT	NE>5-HT

	Trazodone	Nefazodone	Bupropion	Venlafaxine	Citalopram	Fluoxetine	Fluvoxamine	Paroxetine	Sertraline	Mirtazapine
NE reuptake	+	++	+	++	+	++	++	+++	++	+
5-HT reuptake	++	++	+–	+++	++++	+++	++++	+++++	++++	+
DA reuptake	+–	+	++	+	+–	+	+	+	++	–
Blockade 5-HT$_1$	+++	+++	+–	+–	+–	+–	+–	+–	+–	–
Blockade 5-HT$_2$	++++	+++	+–	+–	+	++	+	+–	+	++++
Blockade ACh	–	+–	+–	–	–	+	+–	++	++	++
Blockade H$_1$	++	+–	+	–	++	+	–	+–	+–	+++++
Blockade α_1	+++	+++	+	–	+	+	+	+	++	++
Blockade α_2	++	++	+–	+–	+–	+–	+	+	+	+++
Blockade D$_2$	+	++	–	–	+–	+	++	+–	+–	+
Selective	NE<5-HT	NE<5-HT	NE>5-HT	NE<5-HT	NE<5-HT	NE<5-HT	NE<5-HT	NE<5-HT	NE<5-HT	NE = 5HT

* The ratio of K_i values (intrinsic dissociation constant) between various neurotransmitters/receptors determines the pharmacological profile for any one drug

Key: K_i (nM) > 100,000 = –; 10,000–100,000 = +–; 1000–10,000 = +; 100–1000 = ++; 10–100 = +++; 1–10 = ++++; 0.1–1 = +++++

1/K_i (M) < 0.001 = –; 0.001–0.01 = +–; 0.01–0.1 = +; 0.1–1 = ++; 1–10 = +++; 10–100 = ++++; 100–1000 = +++++

Adapted from Seeman, P., Receptor Tables Vol. 2: Drug Dissociation Constants for Neuroreceptors and Transporters. 1993. SZ Research, Toronto; Richelson, E., Synaptic effects of antidepressants. *Journal of Clinical Psychopharmacology* 16:3 (Suppl. 2) 1–9, 1996

Pharmacological Effects of Antidepressants on Neurotransmitters/Receptors

NE Reuptake Block

- Antidepressant effect
- Side effects: tremors, tachycardia, sweating, insomnia, erectile and ejaculation problems
- Potentiation of pressor effects of NE (e.g., sympathomimetic amines)
- Interaction with guanethidine (blockade of antihypertensive effect)

5-HT Reuptake Block

- Antidepressant, anti-obsessional effect
- Can increase or decrease anxiety, depending on dose
- Side effects: dyspepsia, nausea, headache, nervousness, akathisia, sexual side effects, anorexia
- Potentiation of drugs with serotonergic properties (e.g., L-tryptophan); caution regarding "serotonin syndrome"

DA Reuptake Block

- Antidepressant, antiparkinsonian effect
- Side effects: psychomotor activation, aggravation of psychosis

H_1 Blockade

- Most potent action of cyclic antidepressants
- Side effects: sedation, postural hypotension, weight gain
- Potentiation of effects of other CNS drugs

ACh Blockade

- Second most potent action of cyclic antidepressants
- Side effects: dry mouth, blurred vision, constipation, urinary retention, sinus tachycardia, QRS changes, memory disturbances, sedation
- Potentiation of effects of drugs with anticholinergic properties

α_1 Blockade

- Side effects: postural hypotension, dizziness, reflex tachycardia, sedation
- Potentiation of antihypertensives acting via α_1 blockade (e.g., prazosin)

α_2 Blockade

- CNS arousal; possible decrease in depressive symptoms
- Side effect: sexual dysfunction, priapism
- Antagonism of antihypertensives acting as α_2 stimulants (e.g., clonidine, methyldopa)

5-HT_1 Blockade

- Antidepressant, anxiolytic and antiaggressive action

5-HT_2 Blockade

- Anxiolytic (5-HT_{2C}), antidepressant (5-HT_{2A}), antipsychotic, antimigraine effect, improved sleep
- Side effects: hypotension, ejaculatory problems, sedation, weight gain (5-HT_{2C})

D_2 Blockade

- Antipsychotic effect
- Side effects: extrapyramidal (e.g., tremor, rigidity), endocrine changes, sexual dysfunction (males)

Frequency of Adverse Reactions to Cyclic Antidepressants at Therapeutic Doses

Reaction	Amitriptyline	Clomipramine	Desipramine	Doxepin	Imipramine	Nortriptyline	Protriptyline	Trimipramine	Amoxapine	Maprotiline
CNS Effects										
Drowsiness, sedation	> 30%	> 2%	> 2%	> 30%	> 10%	> 2%	< 2%	> 30%	> 10%	> 10%
Insomnia	> 2%	> 10%	> 2%	> 2%	> 10%	< 2%	> 10%	> 2%[b]	> 10%	< 2%
Excitement, hypomania*	< 2%	< 2%	> 2%	< 2%	> 10%	> 2%	> 10%	< 2%	> 2%	> 2%
Disorientation/confusion	> 10%	> 2%	–	< 2%	> 2%	> 10%	–	> 10%	> 2%	> 2%
Headache	> 2%	> 2%	< 2%	< 2%	> 10%	< 2%	–	> 2%	> 2%	< 2%
Asthenia, fatigue	> 10%	> 2%	> 2%	> 2%	> 10%	> 10%	> 10%	> 2%	> 2%	> 2%
Anticholinergic Effects										
Dry mouth	> 30%	> 30%	> 10%	> 30%	> 30%	> 10%	> 10%	> 10%	> 30%	> 30%
Blurred vision	> 10%	> 10%	> 2%	> 10%	> 10%	> 2%	> 10%	> 2%	> 2%	> 10%
Constipation	> 10%	> 10%	> 2%	> 10%	> 10%	> 10%	> 10%	> 10%	> 30%	> 10%
Sweating	> 10%	> 10%	> 2%	> 2%	> 10%	< 2%	> 10%	> 2%	> 2%	> 2%
Delayed micturition**	> 2%	> 2%	–	< 2%	> 10%	< 2%	< 2%	< 2%	> 10%	> 2%
Extrapyramidal Effects										
Unspecified	> 2%[a]	< 2%[a]	< 2%	> 2%[a]	< 2%	–	–	< 2%	> 2%[a]	> 2%
Tremor	> 10%	> 10%	> 2%	> 2%	> 10%	> 10%	> 2%	> 10%	> 2%	> 10%
Cardiovascular Effects										
Orthostatic hypotension/ dizziness	> 10%	> 10%	> 2%	> 10%	> 30%	> 2%	> 10%	> 10%	> 10%	> 2%
Tachycardia, palpitations	> 10%	> 10%	> 10%	> 2%	> 10%	> 2%	> 2%	> 2%	> 10%	> 2%
ECG changes***	> 10%[e]	> 10%[e]	> 2%[e]	> 2%[e]	> 10%[e]	> 2%[e]	> 10%[e]	> 10%[e]	< 2%[e]	< 2%[e]
Cardiac arrhythmia	> 2%	> 2%	> 2%	> 2%	> 2%	> 2%	> 2%	> 2%	< 2%	< 2%
GI distress	> 2%	> 10%	> 2%	< 2%	> 10%	< 2%	–	< 2%	> 2%	> 2%
Dermatitis, rash	> 2%	> 2%	> 2%	< 2%	> 2%	< 2%	< 2%	< 2%	> 10%	> 10%
Weight gain (over 6 kg)	> 30%	> 10%	> 2%	> 10%	> 10%	> 2%	< 2%	> 10%	< 2%	> 10%
Sexual disturbances	> 2%	> 30%	> 2%	> 2%	> 30%	< 2%	< 2%	< 2%	> 2%	< 2%
Seizures[c]	< 2%	< 2%[d]	< 2%	< 2%	< 2%	< 2%	< 2%	< 2%	< 2%[d]	> 2%[d]

– None reported in literature perused, * More likely in bipolar patients, ** Primarily in the elderly, *** ECG abnormalities usually without cardiac injury
(a) Tardive dyskinesia reported (rarely), (b) No effect on REM sleep, (c) In non-epileptic patients, (d) Higher incidence if dose above 250 mg daily clomipramine, 225 mg daily maprotiline or 300 mg daily amoxapine, (e) Conduction delays: increased PR, QRS or QT_c interval

Frequency of Adverse Reactions to Cyclic Antidepressants at Therapeutic Doses (cont.)

Reaction	SARI				SSRIs					
	Trazodone	Nefazodone	Bupropion	Venlafaxine	Citalopram	Fluoxetine	Fluvoxamine	Paroxetine	Sertraline	Mirtazapine(l)
CNS Effects										
Drowsiness, sedation	> 30%	> 10%	> 2%	> 10%	> 10%	> 10%	> 10%	> 10%	> 10%	> 30%(n)
Insomnia	> 2%	> 2%	> 10%	> 10%(i)	> 10%	> 10%(i)	> 10%	> 10%	> 10%	> 2%
Excitement, hypomania*	–(e)	> 2%	> 10%(e)	> 10%(e)	> 2%	> 2%	> 10%	> 2%	> 10%	> 2%
Disorientation/confusion	< 2%	> 10%	> 2%	> 2%	< 2%	> 10%	> 2%	< 2%	< 2%	> 2%
Headache	> 2%	> 10%	> 10%	> 10%	> 10%	> 10%	> 10%	> 10%	> 10%	> 2%
Asthenia, fatigue	> 10%	> 10%	> 2%	> 10%	> 10%	> 10%	>10%	> 10%	> 2%	> 10%
Anticholinergic Effects										
Dry mouth	> 10%	> 10%	> 10%	> 10%	> 10%	> 10%	> 10%	> 10%	> 10%	> 30%
Blurred vision	> 2%(d)	> 10%	> 10%	> 2%	> 2%	> 2%	> 2%	> 2%	> 2%	> 10%
Constipation	> 2%	> 10%	> 10%	> 10%	> 2%	> 2%	> 10%	> 10%	> 2%	> 10%
Sweating	–	> 2%	> 10%	> 10%	> 10%	> 2%	> 10%	> 10%	> 2%	> 2%
Delayed micturition**	< 2%	< 2%	> 2%	< 2%	> 2%	> 2%	> 2%	> 2%	< 2%	> 2%
Extrapyramidal Effects										
Unspecified	> 2%(b)	< 2%	> 2%	> 2%	< 2%	> 2%(b)	> 2%	> 2%	> 2%	< 2%
Tremor	> 2%	< 2%	> 10%	> 2%	> 2%	> 10%	> 10%	> 10%	> 10%	> 2%
Cardiovascular Effects										
Orthostatic hypotension/ dizziness	> 10%(f)	> 10%	> 2%(m)	> 10%(m)	> 2%	> 10%	> 2%	> 10%	> 10%	> 2%
Tachycardia, palpitations	> 2%	< 2%(j)	> 2%	> 2%	> 2%(j)	< 2%(j)	< 2%(j)	> 2%(j)	> 2%(j)	> 2%
ECG changes***	> 2%	< 2%	< 2%	< 2%	< 2%	< 2%	< 2%	< 2%	< 2%	< 2%
Cardiac arrhythmia	> 2%(g)	< 2%	< 2%	< 2%	< 2%	< 2%(o)	< 2%	< 2%	< 2%	< 2%
GI distress	> 10%	> 10%	> 10%	> 30%	> 10%	> 10%	> 30%	> 10%	> 30%	> 2%
Dermatitis, rash	< 2%	< 2%	> 2%	> 2%	< 2%	> 2%	> 2%	< 2%	> 2%	< 2%
Weight gain (over 6 kg)(r)	> 2%	> 2%	< 2%(k)	< 2%(k)	> 2%	> 2%(k)	> 2%(k)	> 10%(k)	> 2%(k)	> 30%
Sexual disturbances	< 2%(h)	> 2%	< 2%(p)(h)	> 30%(h)	> 30%	> 30%(h)	> 30%	> 30%(h)	> 30%(h)	> 10%
Seizures(a)	< 2%	< 2%	< 2%(c)	< 2%	< 2%	< 2%	< 2%	< 2%	< 2%	< 2%

* More likely in bipolar patients, ** Primarily in the elderly, *** ECG abnormalities usually without cardiac injury. (a) In non-epileptic patients; risk increased with elevated plasma levels, (b) Tardive dyskinesia reported (rarely), (c) Higher incidence if doses used above 450 mg/day of bupropion or in patients with bulimia, (d) Found to lower intraocular pressure, (e) Less likely to precipitate mania, (f) Less frequent if drugs given after meals, (g) Patients with pre-existing cardiac disease have a 10% incidence of premature ventricular contractions, (h) Priapism reported, (i) Especially if given in the evening, (j) Decreased heart rate reported, (k) Weight loss reported initially, (l) Not marketed in Canada, (m) Hypertension reported; may be more common in patients with pre-existing hypertension, (n) sedation decreased at higher doses (above 15 mg), (o) Slowing of sinus node and atrial dysrhythmia, (p) Improved sexual functioning, (r) with chronic treatment

Monoamine Oxidase Inhibitors

GENERAL COMMENTS

- Monoamine oxidase inhibitors can be classified as follows:

Chemical Class	Agent	Page
Reversible Inhibitor of MAO-A (RIMA)	Moclobemide	See p. 44
Irreversible MAOIs	Isocarboxazid Phenelzine Tranylcypromine	See p. 48 See p. 48 See p. 48

Reversible Inhibitor of MAO-A (RIMA)

PRODUCT AVAILABILITY

Chemical Class	Generic Name	Trade Name[(A)]	Dosage Forms and Strengths
Reversible Inhibitor of MAO-A (RIMA)	Moclobemide[(C)]	Manerix	Tablets: 150 mg, 300 mg

[(A)] Generic preparations may be available, [(C)] Not marketed in USA

INDICATIONS*

▲ • Major depression
▲ • Chronic dysthymia
- Preliminary data suggest improved concentration and attention in children with ADHD
- Preliminary data suggest efficacy in seasonal affective disorder, social phobia and chronic fatigue syndrome; and a positive effect on learning and memory in cognitive disorders
- Possible role in obsessive compulsive disorder
- Suggested to modulate impulsivity/aggression and affective instability in borderline personality disorder
- Data contradictory as to efficacy in social phobia
- Early data suggest moclobemide may aid in smoking cessation

PHARMACOLOGY

- Benzamide derivative chemically distinct from irreversible MAOIs
- Inhibits the action of MAO-A enzyme that metabolizes the neurotransmitters serotonin, norepinephrine, and dopamine; in chronic doses over 400 mg daily, will produce 20–30% inhibition of MAO-B in platelets
- Inhibition is reversible (within 24 h)
- Combined therapy with cyclic antidepressants or lithium may increase antidepressant effect

DOSING

- Starting dose, 300–450 mg daily given in divided dose; usual dose range, 300–600 mg daily; some patients respond to 150 mg daily, but most require doses above 450 mg/day

* ▲ Approved indications

- Dosing is not affected by age or renal function; should be decreased in patients with liver disorder
- Should be taken after meals to minimize tyramine-related responses (e.g., headache)
- Preliminary data suggest once daily dosing as effective as divided dosing

PHARMACOKINETICS

- See p. 56
- Relatively lipophilic, but at low pH is highly water-soluble
- Rapidly absorbed from gut, high first-pass effect; peak effect seen between 0.7 and 3 h
- Has low plasma-protein binding (50%)
- Plasma level increases in proportion to dose; blockade of MAO-A correlates with plasma concentration
- Metabolized by oxidation primarily via CYP2C19; elimination half-life 1–3 h; clearance decreased as dosage increased because of auto-inhibition or metabolite-induced inhibition
- Age has no effect on pharmacokinetics

ONSET AND DURATION OF ACTION

- Suggested that onset of antidepressant action may be quicker than with other antidepressants

ADVERSE EFFECTS

- See table p. 54

1. CNS Effects
   - Most common: insomnia, headache and sedation
   - Increased stimulation (restlessness, anxiety, agitation, and aggressivity) can occur – dose related
   - Hypomania reported especially in patients with bipolar disorder
2. Anticholinergic Effects
   - Dry mouth
   - Blurred vision
3. Cardiovascular Effects
   - Hypotension
4. GI Effects
   - Nausea
   - Both weight loss and weight gain
5. Endocrine Effects
   - Reports of galactorrhea in females

WITHDRAWAL

- None known

PRECAUTIONS

- Hypertensive patients should avoid ingesting large quantities of tyramine-rich foods
- Hypertensive reactions may occur in patients with thyrotoxicosis or pheochromocytoma
- Patients prescribed doses above 600 mg/day should minimize the use of tyramine-rich foods
- Use caution when combining with serotonergic drugs as "serotonin syndrome" has been reported (see p. 7) with CNS irritability, increased muscle tone, myoclonus, diaphoresis, and elevated temperature (see Interactions, pp. 46–47)
- Reduce dose by 1/2 to 2/3 in patients with severe liver impairment

TOXICITY

- Symptoms same as side effects, but intensified: drowsiness, disorientation, stupor, hypotension, tachycardia, hyperreflexia, grimacing, sweating, agitation and hallucinations; serotonin syndrome reported
- Fatalities have occurred when combined with citalopram or clomipramine in overdose

Management
- Gastric lavage, emesis, activated charcoal may be of benefit
- Monitor vital functions, supportive treatment

PEDIATRIC CONSIDERATIONS

- Preliminary data suggest improved concentration and attention in children with ADHD

Reversible Inhibitor of MAO-A (RIMA) (cont.)

GERIATRIC CONSIDERATIONS

- Dosing not affected by age or renal function
- Improvement in cognitive functioning in elderly depressed patients has been noted

USE IN PREGNANCY

- Data on safety in pregnancy is lacking
- Animal studies have not shown any particular adverse effects on reproduction

Breast milk

- Moclobemide is secreted into breast milk at about 1% of maternal dose

NURSING IMPLICATIONS

- If patient has difficulty sleeping, ensure last dose of moclobemide is no later than 1700 h
- It is not necessary to maintain a special diet when on moclobemide; however, excessive amounts of foods with high tyramine content can lead to headache

PATIENT INSTRUCTIONS

For detailed patient instructions on moclobemide, see the Patient Information Sheet on p. 248.

- Take moclobemide after food to minimize side effects. Do not eat a big meal after taking your medication
- It is not necessary to maintain a special diet with this drug, but excessive amounts of foods containing tyramine (e.g., aged cheese, sausage, sauerkraut, etc.) can cause a headache
- Take no other drug (including over-the-counter medication) without consulting your doctor or pharmacist; avoid all products containing dextromethorphan
- This drug may interact with medication used by a dentist, so let him know the name of the drug you are taking

FOOD INTERACTIONS

- No particular precautions are required; however, excessive consumption of tyramine-containing food should be avoided to minimize hypertension risk

DRUG INTERACTIONS

- Clinically significant interactions are listed below

Class of Drug	Example	Interaction Effects
Anticholinergic	Antiparkinsonian drugs	Increased atropine-like effects
Antidepressant		
Cyclic (non-selective)	Desipramine, nortriptyline	Additive antidepressant effect in treatment-resistant patients Potentiation of weight gain, hypotension, and anticholinergic effects
	Clomipramine	Enhanced serotonergic effects – **AVOID**
SNRI, SARI	Venlafaxine, nefazodone	Enhanced effects of serotonin and/or norepinephrine; no data on safety with combination
SSRI	Fluoxetine, citalopram	Use cautiously and monitor for serotonergic adverse effects, especially with citalopram Higher incidence of insomnia may occur; increased headache reported with fluvoxamine Fluoxetine and fluvoxamine can inhibit the metabolism of moclobemide
Anxiolytic	Buspirone	Serotonergic reaction possible
Cimetidine		Decreased metabolism of moclobemide; plasma level can double
Lithium		Additive antidepressant effect in treatment-resistant patients

Class of Drug	Example	Interaction Effects
L-Tryptophan		"Serotonin syndrome" possible (see p. 7)
MAO-B inhibitor	L-Deprenyl (selegiline)	Caution – dietary restrictions recommended as both A + B MAO enzymes inhibited with combination
Narcotic	Meperidine, pentazocine, dextropropoxyphene, dextromethorphan	Serotonergic reaction, increased restlessness, potentiation of analgesic effect – **AVOID**
NSAID	Ibuprofen	Enhanced effect of ibuprofen
Sympathomimetic amine		
Indirect-acting	Ephedrine, amphetamine, methylphenidate, L-dopa, etc.	Increased blood pressure and enhanced effects if used over prolonged periods or at high doses
Direct-acting	Salbutamol, epinephrine, etc.	As above
Triptan	Sumatriptan, zolmitriptan	Possibly increased serotonergic effects
	Rizatriptan	Decreased metabolism of rizatriptan; AUC and peak plasma level increased by 119% and 41%, respectively, and AUC of metabolite increased by 400%

Irreversible Monoamine Oxidase Inhibitors

PRODUCT AVAILABILITY

Chemical Class	Generic Name	Trade Name[(A)]	Dosage Forms and Strengths
Hydrazine derivative	Isocarboxazid[(B)] Phenelzine	Marplan Nardil	Tablets: 10 mg Tablets: 15 mg
Non-hydrazine derivative	Tranylcypromine	Parnate	Tablets: 10 mg

[(A)] Generic preparations may be available, [(B)] Not marketed in Canada

INDICATIONS*

- ▲ "Atypical" depression (patients showing hypochondriasis, somatic anxiety, irritability)
- ▲ Major depression unresponsive to other antidepressants
- ▲ Phobic anxiety states or social phobia
- Atypical (anergic) bipolar depression
- Panic disorder prophylaxis
- Obsessive-compulsive disorder
- Depression in patients with borderline personality disorder
- Chronic dysthymia
- Efficacy in posttraumatic stress disorder reported
- May improve negative symptoms in chronic schizophrenia
- Possible antiherpetic effect

PHARMACOLOGY

- Inhibit the action of MAO-A and B enzymes that metabolize the neurotransmitters responsible for stimulating physical and mental activity (serotonin, norepinephrine, dopamine); cause down-regulation of β-adrenoceptors
- Inhibition is irreversible and lasts about 10 days
- Combined therapy with cyclic antidepressants or lithium may increase antidepressant effect
- Best response to MAOIs occurs at dosages that reduce MAO enzyme activity by at least 80%; may require up to 2 weeks to reach maximum MAO inhibition

DOSING

- See p. 56
- Due to short half-life, bid dosing required; give doses in the morning and mid-day to avoid overstimulation and insomnia (occasionally cause sedation)

PHARMACOKINETICS

- See p. 56
- Rapidly absorbed from the GI tract, metabolized by the liver and excreted almost entirely in the urine
- Peak plasma level of tranylcypromine occurs within 1–2 h and correlates with elevations in supine blood pressure, orthostatic drop of systolic blood pressure, and rise in pulse rate. Blood pressure elevation correlates with dose
- With long-term use, irreversible MAOIs can impair own metabolism resulting in nonlinear pharmacokinetics and potential for drug accumulation

* ▲ Approved indications

ONSET AND DURATION OF ACTION

- May require up to two weeks to reach maximum MAO inhibition
- Energizing effect often seen within a few days
- Tolerance to antipanic effects reported

ADVERSE EFFECTS

- See p. 54

1. CNS Effects

a) Cognitive Effects

- Drowsiness
- Stimulant effect (insomnia, restlessness, anxiety) can occur [trazodone 50 mg beneficial as a hypnotic]
- REM sleep decreased with phenelzine
- Headache
- Hypomania and mania: in patients with bipolar disorder, risk up to 35%; concomitant use of a mood stabilizer recommended; in unipolar disorder, risk about 4%

b) Neurological Effects

- Paresthesias or "electric shock-like" sensations; carpal tunnel syndrome (numbness) reported; may be due to vitamin B6 deficiency [Management: pyridoxine 50–150 mg/day]
- Myoclonic jerks, especially during sleep (10–15%), tremor, muscle tension, cramps, akathisia (dose-related) [cyproheptadine may be helpful for cramps or jerks; clonazepam or valproate are useful for nocturnal myoclonus]

2. Anticholinergic Effects

- Constipation common [Management: increase bulk and fluid intake, fecal softener, bulk laxative]
- Dry mouth
- Urinary retention

3. Cardiovascular Effects

- Dizziness, weakness, orthostatic hypotension [Management: fludrocortisone 0.1–0.5 mg/day]
- Occasionally, hypertensive patients may experience a rise in blood pressure
- Edema in lower extremities [restrict sodium; support hose; amiloride 5–10 mg bid, hydrochlorothiazide up to 50 mg/day]

4. GI Effects

- The most common are anorexia, nausea and vomiting
- Increased appetite and weight gain

5. Sexual Side Effects

- Impotence, anorgasmia, decreased libido, ejaculation difficulties [Management: amantadine, bethanechol, neostigmine, cyproheptadine, yohimbine – see SSRIs, p. 6, for doses]
- May diminish sperm count
- Rarely priapism

6. Endocrine Effects

- Hyponatremia and SIADH reported

7. Other Adverse Effects

- Rare reports of liver toxicity
- Rare reports of hair loss with tranylcypromine
- Case reports of thrombocytopenia

HYPERTENSIVE CRISIS

- Can occur with irreversible MAOIs due to ingestion of incompatible foods (containing elevated levels of tyramine) or drugs (see lists pp. 51–53)
- Not related to dose of drug

Signs and Symptoms

- Occipital headache, neck stiffness or soreness, nausea, vomiting, sweating (sometimes with fever and sometimes with cold, clammy skin), dilated pupils and photophobia, sudden nose bleed, tachycardia, bradycardia, and constricting chest pain

Management

- Withhold medication and notify physician immediately
- Monitor vital signs, ECG
- Nifedipine 10 mg bitten and swallowed, may decrease blood pressure (occasionally drastically – monitor)
- Phentolamine is an alternative parenteral treatment

Irreversible Monoamine Oxidase Inhibitors (cont.)

- Patient should stand and walk, rather than lie down, during a hypertensive reaction; BP will drop somewhat

WITHDRAWAL

- Occur occasionally 1–4 days after abrupt withdrawal
- Reports of muscle weakness, agitation, vivid nightmares, headache, palpitations, nausea, sweating, irritability, and myoclonic jerking; acute organic psychosis with hallucinations reported
- REM rebound occurs
- Maintain dietary and drug restrictions for at least 10 days after stopping MAOI

PRECAUTIONS

- Should not be administered to patients with cerebrovascular disease, cardiovascular disease, or a history of hypertension
- Should not be used alone in patients with marked psychomotor agitation
- When changing from one MAOI to another, or to a tricyclic antidepressant, allow a minimum of 10 medication-free days
- Need 10–14 days to be excreted from the system before an incompatible drug or food is given, or before surgery or ECT
- Hypertensive crisis can occur if given concurrently with certain drugs or foods (see lists below)
- Use caution when combining with serotonergic drugs as "serotonin syndrome" has been reported (see p. 7)

TOXICITY

- Symptoms same as side effects but intensified
- Severe cases progress to extreme dizziness and shock
- Overdose, whether accidental or intentional, can be fatal: patient may be symptom-free up to 6 h, then progress to restlessness-coma-death – therefore, close medical supervision is indicated for 48 h following an overdose

PEDIATRIC CONSIDERATIONS

- MAOIs are prescribed in panic disorder/agoraphobia, separation anxiety, major depressive disorder, selective mutism, and attention-deficit hyperactivity disorder
- Dose should be carefully titrated and maintained between 0.3 and 1 mg/kg
- Ability to comply with restrictions as to diet and drugs should be assessed before prescribing

GERIATRIC CONSIDERATIONS

- Suggested that MAOIs may have particular efficacy in the elderly, as monoamine oxidase activity in the brain increases with age
- Orthostatic hypotension may be problematic, use divided doses [Management: support stockings, sodium chloride tablets, fludrocortisone]

USE IN PREGNANCY

- Avoid; increased incidence of malformations demonstrated with use in first trimester

Breast milk

- The American Academy of Pediatrics considers tranylcypromine compatible with breast feeding
- No data on phenelzine

NURSING IMPLICATIONS

- The incidence of orthostatic hypotension is high, esp. in the elderly and at the start of treatment: tell patient to get out of bed slowly
- Educate patient regarding foods and drugs to avoid; a diet sheet should be provided for each patient
- Warn patient not to self-medicate, but to consult physician or pharmacist to prevent drug-drug interactions
- Educate patient to report headache; measure pulse and blood pressure, and report increases to physician immediately
- If patient has difficulty sleeping, ensure last dose of MAOI is no later than 1500 h

PATIENT INSTRUCTIONS

For detailed patient instructions on MAOIs, see the Patient Information Sheet on p. 250.

- Be aware of foods to avoid with this medication
- Take no other drug (including over-the-counter medication) without consulting your doctor or pharmacist
- This drug may interact with medication used by a dentist, so let him know the name of the drug you are taking
- This drug may impair the mental and physical abilities required for driving a car or operating machinery
- Alcohol or other CNS depressants will cause an increase in sleepiness, dizziness, and lightheadedness

FOOD INTERACTIONS

There are many serious food and drug interactions that may precipitate a hypertensive crisis; maintain dietary and drug restrictions for at least 10 days after stopping MAOI

Foods to avoid:
- All matured or aged cheeses (e.g., cheddar, brick, mozzarella, parmesan, blue, gruyere, stilton, brie, Swiss, Roquefort, camembert)
- Broad bean pods (e.g., Fava) – contain dopamine
- Overripe bananas (banana peel)
- Meat extract (e.g., Bovril, Oxo), concentrated yeast extracts (e.g., Marmite)
- Dried salted fish
- Sauerkraut
- Sausage (if aged, especially salami, mortadella, pepperoni, pastrami)
- Soya sauce or soybean condiments, tofu
- Tap (draft) beer, alcohol-free beer

It is SAFE to use in moderate amounts (only if fresh):
- Cottage cheese, cream cheese, farmer's cheese, processed cheese, Cheez Whiz, ricotta, Havarti, Boursin
- Liver (as long as it is fresh), fresh or processed meats (e.g., hot dogs)
- Spirits (in moderation)
- Soy milk
- Salad dressings
- Worcestershire sauce
- Yeast-leavened bread

Reactions have also been reported with:
- Pickled herring, smoked fish
- Sour cream, yogurt
- Meat tenderizers
- Caviar, snails, tinned fish, shrimp paste
- Homemade red wine, Chianti, canned/bottled beer, sherry, champagne
- Tea, coffee, cola
- Tinned and packet soup (especially miso)
- Sausage: bologna, summer sausage, or other unrefrigerated fermented meats; game meat that has been hung
- Chocolate
- Overripe fruit, avocados, raspberries
- Oriental foods
- Spinach
- Nuts

☞ **MAKE SURE ALL FOOD IS FRESH, STORED PROPERLY, AND EATEN SOON AFTER BEING PURCHASED – products stored even under refrigeration will show an increase in tyramine content after several days**
- Never touch food that is fermented or possibly "off"
- Avoid restaurant sauces, gravy, and soup

Over-the-counter drugs: DO NOT USE without prior consultation with doctor or pharmacist:
- Cold remedies, decongestants (including nasal sprays and drops), some antihistamines and cough medicines
- Narcotic painkillers (e.g., products containing codeine)
- All stimulants including pep-pills (Wake-ups, Nodoz)
- All appetite suppressants

Irreversible Monoamine Oxidase Inhibitors (cont.)

- Anti-asthma drugs (Primatine P)
- Sleep aids and sedatives (Sominex, Nytol)
- Yeast, dietary supplements (e.g., Ultrafast, Optifast)

DRUG INTERACTIONS

- Clinically significant interactions are listed below

Class of Drug	Example	Interaction Effects
Anesthetic, general		May enhance CNS depression
Anorexiant	Fenfluramine, dexfenfluramine	"Serotonin syndrome" (see p. 7); **AVOID**
Anticholinergic	Antiparkinsonian agents, antipsychotics	Increased atropine-like effects
Anticonvulsant	Carbamazepine	Possible decrease in metabolism and increased plasma level of carbamazepine with phenelzine
Antidepressant		
Cyclic (non-selective)	Amitriptyline, desipramine	If used together, do not add cyclic antidepressants to MAOI. Start cyclic antidepressant first or simultaneously with MAOI. For patients already on MAOI, discontinue the MAOI for 10–14 days before starting combination therapy Combined cyclic and MAOI therapy has increased antidepressant effects and will potentiate weight gain, hypotension and anticholinergic effects
	Clomipramine	"Serotonin syndrome" reported; **AVOID** (see p. 7)
SARI	Trazodone	Low doses of trazodone (25–50 mg) used to treat antidepressant-induced insomnia Combined therapy has additive antidepressant effects; monitor for serotonergic effects
SNRI	Venlafaxine	Metabolism of serotonin and norepinephrine inhibited; **AVOID**
SSRI	Fluoxetine , paroxetine, sertraline	"Serotonin syndrome" and death reported with serotonergic antidepressants; **AVOID**
NDRI	Bupropion	Metabolism of dopamine inhibited; **AVOID**
NaSSA	Mirtazapine	Possible serotonergic reaction; **AVOID**
Antihypertensive	Ace-inhibitors, α-blockers, β-blockers Guanethidine	Enhanced hypotension Antihypertensive effects of guanethidine decreased
Antipsychotic	Phenothiazines, clozapine	Additive hypotension
Atropine		Prolonged action of atropine
Anxiolytic	Buspirone	Several cases of increased blood pressure reported
Bromocriptine		Increased serotonergic effects
CNS depressant	Barbiturates, sedatives, alcohol	May enhance CNS depression
Ginseng		May cause headache, tremulousness or hypomania; case report of irritability and visual hallucinations with combination
Insulin		Enhanced hypoglycemic response through stimulation of insulin secretion and inhibition of gluconeogenesis

Class of Drug	Example	Interaction Effects
L-Dopa		Increased blood pressure; increased serotonergic effects Use carbidopa/L-dopa combination to inhibit peripheral decarboxylation
L-Tryptophan		Reports of "serotonin syndrome," with hyperreflexia, tremor, myoclonic jerks, and ocular oscillations (see p. 7); **AVOID**
Lithium		Increased serotonergic effects Additive antidepressant effect in treatment-resistant patients
MAO-B inhibitor	L-deprenyl (selegiline)	Increased serotonergic effects
Muscle relaxant	Succinylcholine	Phenelzine may prolong muscle relaxation by inhibiting metabolism
Narcotics and related drugs	Meperidine, dextromethorphan, diphenoxylate, tramadol Propoxyphene	Excitation, sweating, and hypotension reported; may lead to development of encephalopathy, convulsions, coma, respiratory depression, and "serotonin syndrome." If a narcotic is required, meperidine should not be used; other narcotics should be instituted cautiously Potentiation of catecholamine-release reported, resulting in anxiety, confusion, ataxia, hypotension
Reserpine		Central excitatory syndrome and hypertension reported due to central and peripheral release of catecholamines
Sibutramine		Increased noradrenergic and serotonergic effects possible. DO NOT COMBINE
Stimulant	MDMA ("Ecstasy")	Case reports of "serotonin syndrome" (see p. 7)
Sulfonylureas		Enhanced hypoglycemic response
Sympathomimetic amine	*Indirect acting:* amphetamine, methylphenidate, ephedrine, pseudoephedrine, phenylpropanolamine, dopamine, tyramine *Direct acting:* epinephrine, isoproterenol, norepinephrine (levarterenol), methoxamine, salbutamol *Phenylephrine*	Release of large amounts of norepinephrine with hypertensive reaction; **AVOID** No interaction Increased pressor response
Tetrabenazine		Central excitatory syndrome and hypertension reported due to central and peripheral release of catecholamines
Triptan	Sumatriptan, zolmitriptan, rizatriptan	"Serotonin syndrome" (see p. 7); **AVOID;** recommend that 2 weeks elapse after discontinuing an irreversible MAOI and using sumatriptan

Frequency (%) of Adverse Reactions to MAOI Antidepressants at Therapeutic Doses

Reaction	Isocarboxazid	Phenelzine	Tranylcypromine	Moclobemide
CNS Effects				
Drowsiness, sedation	> 2%	> 10%	> 10%	> 2%
Insomnia	> 2%[a]	> 10%[a]	> 10%[a]	> 10%[a]
Excitement, hypomania**	> 2%	> 10%	> 10%	> 10%
Disorientation/confusion	> 2%	> 2%	> 2%	> 2%
Headache	> 10%	> 2%	–	> 10%
Asthenia	> 2%	< 2%	< 2%	< 2%
Anticholinergic Effects				
Dry mouth	> 10%	> 30%	> 10%	> 10%
Blurred vision	> 2%	> 10%	> 2%	> 10%
Constipation	> 2%	> 10%	> 2%	> 2%
Sweating	< 2%	> 2%	–	> 2%
Delayed micturition*	> 2%	> 2%	> 2%	< 2%
Extrapyramidal Effects				
Unspecified	> 2%	> 10%	< 2%	< 2%
Tremor	> 10%	> 10%	> 2%	> 2%
Cardiovascular Effects				
Orthostatic hypotension/dizziness	> 10%	> 10%	> 10%	> 10%
Tachycardia	–	> 10%[d]	> 10%[d]	> 2%
ECG changes***	> 2%	< 2%[e]	< 2%[e]	> 2%
Cardiac arrhythmia	> 2%	< 2%	< 2%	> 2%
GI distress (nausea)	> 10%	> 10%	> 2%	> 10%
Dermatitis, rash	> 2%	< 2%	> 2%	> 2%
Weight gain (over 6 kg)	> 2%	> 10%	> 2%	< 2%
Sexual disturbances	> 2%	> 30%[f]	> 2%[f]	> 2%
Seizures[c]	–	< 2%	–[b]	< 2%

* Primarily in the elderly, ** More likely in bipolar patients, *** ECG abnormalities usually without cardiac injury
(a) Especially if given in the evening, (b) May have anticonvulsant activity, (c) In non-epileptic patients, (d) Decreased heart rate reported, (e) Shortened QTc interval, (f) Priapism reported

Antidepressant Doses

Drug	Therapeutic Dose Range (mg)	Comparable Dose (mg)	Suggested Plasma Level (nmol/L**)	Protein Binding	Bioavail-ability	Elimination Half-life (h)	CYP-450 Metabolizing Enzymes[g]	CYP-450 Inhibition [h]
SSRIs								
Citalopram (Celexa)	10–60	10		80%	80%	23–45	3A4, 2C19, 2D6	1A2[w], 2D6[w], 2C19[w]
Fluoxetine (Prozac)	10–80[c]	10		94%	72–85%	24–144 (parent) 200–330 (metabolite)	2D6[i], 3A4, **2C9**[j]	1A2[m], 2D6[p], 3A4([pi]), 2C19[m]
Fluvoxamine (Luvox)	50–300[c]	50		77–80%	60%	9–28	2D6, 3A4	1A2[p], 2D6[w], 3A4[p], 2C9, 2C19[m]
Paroxetine (Paxil)	10–60[c]	10		95%	?	3–65	**2D6**[j]	1A2[w], 2D6[p], 3A4[w], 2C9[w], 2C19[w]
Sertraline (Zoloft)	50–200[c]	25		98%	70%	22–36 (parent) 62–104 (metabolite)	2D6, **3A4**[j], 2C9, 2C19, 2B6	1A2[w], 2D6[w], 3A4[w], 2C9[w], 2C19[m]
NDRI								
Bupropion (Wellbutrin)[b] Bupropion SR (Wellbutrin SR, Zyban)	225–450[d] 150–300 mg[d]	200[d]	75–350*	80–85%	?	10–14 (parent) 20–27 (metabolites)	1A2, 2D6[i], 3A4, 2C9, **2B6**[j], 2E1, 2A6	2D6
SNRI								
Venlafaxine (Effexor) Venlafaxine XR (Effexor XR)	75–375	50		27%	?	3–7 (parent) 9–13 (metabolite) 9–12 (absorption half-life)	**2D6**[j], 3A4[i], 2E1 2C9, 2C19	1A2[w], 2D6[w], 3A4[w], 2C[w]
SARI								
Nefazodone (Serzone)	100–600	100		> 99%	15–23%	2–5[e] (parent) 3–18 (metabolites)	2D6[i], **3A4**[j]	1A2[w], 2D6[w], 3A4[p]
Trazodone (Desyrel)	150–600	100		93%	?	4–9	1A2, 2D6[i], **3A4**[j]	2D6[w]
NaSSA								
Mirtazapine (Remeron)	15–60	15		85%	50%	20–40	1A2, **2D6**[i,j], **3A4**[j], 2C	2D6[w], 3A4[w]
NONSELECTIVE CYCLIC AGENTS								
Tricyclic								
Amitriptyline (Elavil)	75–300	50	250–825*[f]	92–96%	43–48%	10–46	1A2, 2D6, 3A4, 2C	2D6[m]
Clomipramine (Anafranil)	75–300	50	300–1000	98%	48%	17–37	1A2, 2D6, 3A4, 2C	2D6[m]

Antidepressant Doses (cont.)

Drug	Therapeutic Dose Range (mg)	Comparable Dose (mg)	Suggested Plasma Level (nmol/L**)	Protein Binding	Bioavail-ability	Elimination Half-life (h)	CYP-450 Metabolizing Enzymes[g]	CYP-450 Inhibition [h]
Desipramine (Norpramin)	75–300	50	400–1000[f]	73–92%	50–68%	12–76	1A2, **2D6**[j]	2D6[m]
Doxepin (Sinequan, Triadapin)	75–300	50	500–950*	89%	25%	8–36	1A2	–
Imipramine (Tofranil)	75–300	50	500–800*[f]	89%	29–77%	4–34	**1A2**[j], 2D6, 3A4, 2C	2D6[m]
Nortriptyline (Aventyl, Pamelor)	40–200	25	150–500[f]	89–92%	64%	13–88	**2D6**[j]	2D6, 3A4, 2C
Protriptyline (Triptil, Vivactil)	20–60	15	350–700			54–124	–	–
Trimipramine (Surmontil)	75–300	50	500–800	95%	40%	7–30	1A2, 2D6	–
Dibenzoxazepine								
Amoxapine (Asendin)	100–600	100				8	–	–
Tetracyclic								
Maprotiline (Ludiomil)	100–225	50	200–950*	88%	66–100%	27–58	1A2, 2D6	–
RIMA								
Moclobemide (Manerix)[a]	300–600	150		50%	50–80%	1–3	2D6, **2C19**[j]	1A2, 2D6[w], 2C19
MAOI (irreversible)								
Isocarboxazid (Marplan)[b]	30–50	10		?	?		–	–
Phenelzine (Nardil)	45–90	15		?	?	1.5–4	2E1	–
Tranylcypromine (Parnate)	20–60	10		?	?	2.4	–	2D6, 2C19[p], 2A6

Monograph doses are just a guideline, and each patient's medication must be individualized.

* Includes sum of drug and its metabolites. ** Approximate conversion: nmol/L = 3.5 × ng/mL.

(a) Not marketed in USA, (b) Not marketed in Canada, (c) SSRIs have a flat dose response curve. For depression most patients respond to the initial (low) dose. Higher doses are used in the treatment of OCD, (d) Give in divided doses (maximum of 150 mg per dose), (e) Dose-dependent, (f) Established ranges for efficacy in major depressive disorder, (g) Cytochrome P450 isoenzymes involved in drug metabolism, (h) CYP-450 isoenzymes inhibited by the drug, (i) Specific to metabolite, (j) Main isoenzyme involved in metabolism, where known, (p) Potent inhibition of isoenzyme, (m) Moderate inhibition of isoenzyme, (w) Weak inhibition of isoenzyme.

Switching Antidepressants

Switching from		Switching to	Wash-out Period[a]
Non-selective cyclic	→	Non-selective Cyclic	No washout – use dose equivalents for switching (pp. 55–56)
	→	SSRI	5 half-lives of cyclic antidepressant (caution: see Interactions, p. 9)[b]
	→	NDRI	5 half-lives of cyclic antidepressant
	→	SNRI or SARI, NaSSA	No washout – taper[b]
	→	Irrev. MAOI	5 half-lives of cyclic antidepressant
	→	RIMA	5 half-lives of cyclic antidepressant
SSRI or SARI	→	Non-selective Cyclic	5 half-lives of SSRI or SARI (caution: with fluoxetine due to long half-life of active metabolite)[b]
	→	NDRI	No washout – taper (caution: with fluoxetine)[b]
	→	SNRI	No washout – taper (caution: with fluoxetine)[b], monitor for serotonergic effects
	→	Irrev. MAOI	5 half-lives of SSRI or SARI (caution: with fluoxetine) – DO NOT COMBINE
	→	RIMA	5 half-lives of SSRI or SARI (caution: with fluoxetine)
	→	SSRI or SARI, NaSSA	No washout – taper first drug over 2–5 days then start second drug (use lower doses of second drug if switching from fluoxetine; longer taper may be necessary if higher doses of fluoxetine used); monitor for serotonergic effects
Irrev. MAOI	→	Non-selective Cyclic	10 days – CAUTION
	→	SSRI or SARI	10 days – DO NOT COMBINE
	→	NDRI	10 days – DO NOT COMBINE
	→	SNRI	Minimum of 14 days – DO NOT COMBINE. Caution: case reports of serotonin syndrome after 14 days washout
	→	NaSSA[c]	10 days – DO NOT COMBINE
	→	RIMA	Start the next day if changing from low to moderate dose; taper from a high dose. Maintain dietary restrictions for 10 days
	→	Irrev. MAOI	10 days – DO NOT COMBINE
RIMA	→	Non-selective Cyclic	2 days – CAUTION
	→	SSRI, SARI or NaSSA	2 days – CAUTION
	→	NDRI	2 days – CAUTION
	→	SNRI	2 days – CAUTION
	→	Irrev. MAOI	Can start the following day at a low dose
NDRI	→	Non-selective Cyclic	2 days
	→	SSRI or SARI	No washout – taper (caution with fluoxetine)[b]
	→	SNRI , NaSSA	No washout – taper[b]; monitor for noradrenergic effects
	→	RIMA	5 half-lives of NDRI (3–5 days) – DO NOT COMBINE
	→	Irrev. MAOI	5 half-lives of NDRI (3–5 days) – DO NOT COMBINE
SNRI	→	Non-selective Cyclic	No washout – taper[b]
	→	SSRI or SARI	No washout – taper[b]; monitor for serotonergic effects
	→	NDRI, NaSSA	No washout – taper[b]; monitor for noradrenergic effects
	→	Irrev. MAOI	5 half-lives of SNRI (3 days) – DO NOT COMBINE
	→	RIMA	5 half-lives of SNRI (3 days) – CAUTION

(a) Recommendations pertain to out-patients. More rapid switching may be used in in-patients (except from an irreversible MAOI or RIMA) with proper monitoring of plasma levels and synergistic effects; (b) Taper first drug over 3 to 7 days prior to initiating second antidepressant; consider starting second drug at a reduced dose; (c) Data on NaSSa (mirtazapine) are limited. To concur with current practice, 5 half-lives should serve as an adequate washout when switching to or from mirtazapine (except from Irrev. MAOI).

Antidepressant Augmentation Strategies

ANTIDEPRESSANT NON-RESPONSE

- Ascertain diagnosis is correct
- Ascertain patient is compliant with therapy
- Ensure dosage prescribed is therapeutic; measure plasma level
- Ensure there has been an adequate trial period, i.e., up to 6 weeks at a reasonable dose

Factors Complicating Response

- Concurrent medical or psychiatric illness, e.g., hypothyroidism, obsessive compulsive disorder
- Concurrent prescription drugs may interfere with efficacy, e.g., calcium channel blockers
- Metabolic enhancers (e.g., carbamazepine) or inhibitors (e.g., erythromycin) will affect plasma level of antidepressant
- Drug abuse may make management difficult, e.g., cocaine
- Psychosocial factors may affect response
- Personality disorders lead to poor outcome; however, depression may evoke personality problems which may disappear when the depression is alleviated

Switching Antidepressants

- Up to 65% of treatment-resistant patients are reported to respond when a different class of antidepressant is tried; studies suggest response best when switch to an irreversible MAOI
- Use caution when switching to or from irreversible MAOIs (see Switching Antidepressants p. 57)
- Switching from one SSRI to another can offer enhanced response in up to 71% of previously non-responsive patients
- Switching between tricyclic agents is of questionable benefit

AUGMENTATION STRATEGIES

Antidepressant Combinations

- Combining antidepressants which affect different neurotransmitter systems may produce a better antidepressant response than either drug alone

MAOI + Cyclic

- Six open series cases report response rates of 54–100%
- Combination therapy should be started together, or MAOI can be added to the cyclic drug. Use caution with serotonergic agents (see Interactions; pp. 52–53)
- Require 6 weeks at adequate doses

☞ **DO NOT COMBINE AN IRREVERSIBLE MAOI WITH (1) SSRI, (2) SNRI, (3) NDRI, (4) SARI, or (5) RIMA**

SSRI + Cyclic

- Up to 50% of patients may respond to combination – data contradictory
- Use lower doses of TCA and monitor TCA levels to prevent toxicity (see Interactions, pp. 9–13)
- Combination of an SSRI and a noradrenergic cyclic drug (e.g., desipramine) reported to cause greater downregulation of β-adrenergic receptors and a more rapid response

RIMA + Cyclic

- Monitor for serotonergic adverse effects

RIMA + SSRI

- Up to 67% of refractory patients may respond to combination
- Monitor for serotonergic adverse effects

NDRI + SSRI
NDRI + SNRI

- Up to 35% of partial responders to either drug may have a marked response to the combination; however, adverse effects (e.g., tremor, panic attacks) may limit dosage (see Interactions, pp. 17–18)
- Bupropion may mitigate SNRI- or SSRI-induced sexual dysfunction

NaSSA + SSRI

- Response reported in 64% of refractory patients after mirtazapine 15–30 mg was added to SSRI treatment
- Reported to alleviate insomnia; may have an activating effect; weight gain and sedation also reported

Thyroid Hormone (T_3)(T_4)	• Up to 60% of non-responsive patients may respond within 1–2 weeks; dosage: 25–50 µg/day of liothyronine or 0.15–0.5 mg/day levothyroxine – if ineffective, discontinue after 3 weeks; T_3 considered to be more effective than T_4 (T_3 augmentation may be more effective in woman than in men) (see p. 211) • Mixed results reported
Lithium	• Up to 60% of patients may respond to combined treatment (lower response rates with SSRIs); response may occur within 48 h, but usually within 3 weeks • Unclear if there is a correlation between lithium level and clinical improvement when used as augmentation therapy; however, plasma level above 0.4 mmol/L is suggested for efficacy; usual dose: 600–900 mg/day • Response more likely in probable bipolar patients (with a first-degree relative with bipolar disorder or with a history of hypomania)
Anticonvulsants, e.g., Carbamazepine	• Monitor TCA levels due to increased metabolism with carbamazepine • With SSRI, monitor carbamazepine level (see Interactions) • There is no significant correlation between anticonvulsant plasma level and clinical improvement
Buspirone	• Beneficial response reported in depression and in OCD; effect observed within 2–4 weeks • Up to 65% of depressed patients reported to respond to combination with antidepressant – data contradictory • May help alleviate SSRI-induced sexual dysfunction • Monitor for adverse effects due to serotonergic excess • Usual dose: 15–60 mg/day
Psychostimulants	• Methylphenidate (10–40 mg) or d-amphetamine (5–40 mg) used as augmentation therapy with cyclic agents, SSRIs, SNRI or irreversible MAOIs • Rapid symptom resolution reported in up to 78% of patients in open trials; response was sustained (no tolerance observed) • May also be of value in depressed patients with ADHD • Caution: observe for activation and blood pressure changes • Irritability, anxiety and paranoia reported – use caution in patients who are anxious or agitated
Electroconvulsive Treatment	• May be used with antidepressant for acute treatment • Maintenance therapy with antidepressant or with lithium may be required
Tryptophan	• Data suggests efficacy when combined with cyclics, SSRIs or MAOIs; monitor for increased serotonergic effects
Pindolol	• Blocks serotonin autoreceptors and increases serotonin concentration at postsynaptic sites (see p. 210) • Four out of 5 controlled studies show a more rapid antidepressant response when pindolol used in combination with SSRIs and nefazodone; two out of the 5 studies suggest that pindolol augments the antidepressant effect • Usual dose: 2.5 mg tid • Monitor blood pressure and heart rate; caution in patients with asthma or cardiac conduction problems • Cases of hypomania and psychosis reported in bipolar patients
Second Generation Antipsychotics	• Early data suggest that low doses of risperidone (0.5–2 mg/day) or olanzapine (5–20 mg/day) can augment SSRIs in patients with MDD or OCD; reported to decrease anxiety, irritability and insomnia

Electroconvulsive Therapy (ECT)

DEFINITION

- The induction of grand mal convulsions, by means of an externally applied electric stimulus, for the treatment of certain mental disorders
- **Not** the administration of subconvulsive electric stimuli, referred to as cranial electrostimulation or electrosleep therapy; **not** the administration of aversive electric stimuli as a behavior modification protocol; and not transcranial magnetic stimulation (TMS; preliminary comparison of TMS with ECT indicates that TMS may be effective for major depression, but not with psychotic symptoms)
- Sometimes called electro-shock therapy and, in the animal research literature, referred to as electroconvulsive shock (ECS)

INDICATIONS

- Major depression; especially when associated with high suicide risk, inanition/dehydration, depressive stupor, catatonia, delusions, non-response to one or more adequate trials of antidepressants or intolerance of therapeutic dosages
- Prophylaxis or attenuation of recurrent major depression; i.e., "maintenance" ECT after response to an acute/index course of ECT, if previous antidepressants have not prevented recurrence
- Prevention of relapse of major depression, i.e., "continuation" ECT for up to 6 months after response to an acute/index course of ECT, if previous antidepressants have not prevented rapid relapse; may provide better outcome than antidepressants alone following an acute/index course
- Secondary depression concurrent with other mental or medical illnesses
- Depressed phase of bipolar affective disorder
- Manic phase of bipolar affective disorder; adjunct to mood stabilizers and antipsychotics for severe mania (manic "delirium") and rapid-cycling illness
- Dysphoric mania ("mixed bipolar")
- Post-partum psychoses; secondary line of treatment after non-response to antidepressants and/or antipsychotics
- Schizophrenia; especially with concurrent catatonic and/or affective symptoms; adjunct to adequate dosage of antipsychotics for non-responsive "positive" symptoms; after failed clozapine trial
- Schizoaffective disorder, delusional disorder, first-episode psychosis; non-response to one or more adequate drug trials
- Reports of effectiveness for Parkinson's disease ("on-off" phenomenon), neuroleptic malignant syndrome, status epilepticus, tardive dyskinesia and affective/psychotic disorders associated with mental retardation
- Efficacy in refractory obsessive compulsive disorder reported (probably indicated only when concurrent depression warrants ECT)
- Reports of efficacy in phencyclidine-induced psychosis

GENERAL COMMENTS

- Consider ECT early in the treatment algorithm, in the presence of very severe illness (do not regard as treatment of last resort)

THERAPEUTIC EFFECTS

- Vegetative symptoms of depression, such as insomnia and fatigue, and catatonic symptoms may respond initially; later improvement of affective symptoms, such as depressed mood and anhedonia; followed by improvement of cognitive symptoms, such as impaired self-esteem, helplessness, hopelessness, suicidal and delusional ideation
- Manic symptoms which respond include agitation, euphoria, motor overactivity, and thought disorder
- Some "positive" symptoms of schizophrenia and other psychoses may respond
- Most effective treatment for severe depression in that a substantial proportion of non-responders to antidepressants do recover with ECT; "melancholic" and "psychotic" presentations respond best

MECHANISM OF ACTION

- Exact mechanism unknown

- Affects almost all neurotransmitters implicated in the pathogenesis of the mental disorders (norepinephrine, serotonin, acetylcholine, dopamine, GABA)
- Neurophysiological effects include increased permeability of the blood-brain barrier, suppression of regional cerebral blood flow and neurometabolic activity; "anticonvulsant" effects may be related to outcome (inhibitory neurotransmitters are increased by ECT)
- Affects neuroendocrine substances (CRF, ACTH, TRH, prolactin, vasopressin, metenkephalins, beta endorphins)

DOSAGE

- "Dosage" may be some combination of the electrical energy/charge of the stimulus, electrode placement, seizure duration and the total number of convulsions induced; the precise duration of seizure required is unknown (perhaps must be at least 15 s) because there is no clear correlation between seizure duration and outcome; augmenting agents (e.g., caffeine) are rarely necessary
- Bilateral stimulus electrode placement (regardless of the stimulus energy/charge) has been found more effective than unilateral placement; "high-energy" bilateral may be effective for non-response to "threshold" bilateral treatment
- Unilateral electrode placement is effective for many patients but, when used, the stimulus energy/charge should be substantially greater than that which is just necessary to induce a convulsion (threshold stimulus); if no response after 4 to 6 treatments, recommend switch to bilateral (preliminary evidence suggests that unilateral treatment with a multiple of 5 to 6 times the threshold stimulus may be as effective as bilateral and cause fewer cognitive side effects)
- Gender, age and electrode placement affect seizure threshold: males have higher thresholds than females, thresholds increase with age and are greater with bilateral than unilateral ECT
- Total number of treatments required for a full therapeutic effect may range from approximately 6 to 20; if there is absolutely no therapeutic effect after 12 to 15 treatments, it is unlikely that further treatments will be effective

ONSET AND DURATION OF ACTION

- Therapeutic effect may be evident within three treatments but onset may require as many as 12 treatments in some cases
- Relapse rate following discontinuation is high (30–70%) within 1 year, partly dependent on degree of medication resistance pre-ECT; prophylactic antidepressants should be administered in almost all cases; "continuation" ECT for up to 6 months if antidepressant prophylaxis of rapid relapse ineffective; lithium plus antidepressant may decrease relapse of major depression following ECT

PROCEDURE

- Administer three times per week on alternate days; decrease frequency to twice weekly, if necessary, to reduce cognitive side effects
- ECT must always be administered under general anesthesia with partial neuromuscular blockade
- Induce light "sleep" anesthesia with sodium thiopental; little clinical advantage seen with newer agents such as propofol (more expensive and almost always results in much briefer convulsions; may also raise the seizure threshold; reserve for patients with post-treatment delirium or severe nausea unresponsive to antinauseants)
- Induce neuromuscular blockade with succinylcholine or a short-acting non-depolarizing agent. Post-ECT myalgia may be due to insufficient relaxation or fasciculations (attenuate the latter with adjunctive non-depolarizing muscle relaxant (e.g., rocuronium) which necessitates a higher dosage of succinylcholine)
- Pretreat with atropine or glycopyrrolate if excess oral secretions and/or significant bradycardia anticipated (i.e., patient on a β-blocker); post-treat with atropine if bradycardia develops
- Pretreat any concurrent physical illness which may complicate anesthesia (i.e., antihypertensives, gastric acid/motility suppressants, hypoglycemics); special circumstances require anesthesia and/or internal medicine consultation
- If possible, withhold all psychopharmaceuticals with anticonvulsant properties (i.e., benzodiazepines, carbamazepine, valproate) for at least the night before and morning of each treatment
- Continue all other psychopharmaceuticals, except MAOIs (see Contraindications), when clinically necessary
- Outpatient treatment can be administered if warranted by the clinical circumstances if there is no medical anesthesia contraindication and if the patient can comply with the pre- and post-treatment procedural requirements

ADVERSE EFFECTS

- Memory loss occurs to some degree during all courses of ECT
  - significant, patchy amnesia for the period during which ECT is administered; may persist indefinitely
  - retrograde amnesia for some events up to a number of months pre-ECT; may be permanent; uncommonly, longer periods of retrograde amnesia
  - patchy anterograde amnesia for 3–6 months post-ECT; no evidence of permanent anterograde amnesia

Electroconvulsive Therapy (ECT) (cont.)

  - patients may rarely complain of permanent anterograde memory impairment; unknown if this is a residual effect of the ECT or an effect of residual symptoms of the illness for which ECT was prescribed
- Mortality rate; between two and four deaths per 100,000 treatments; higher risk in those with concurrent cardiovascular disease
- Post-treatment delirium uncommon; usually of short duration
  - reported in elderly patients; when more than one electric stimulus is used to induce a convulsion; after prolonged seizures
  - due to concurrent drug toxicity (e.g., lithium carbonate; clozapine – see Interactions)
  - if occurs consider propofol anesthesia for subsequent treatments
- Tachycardia and hypertension may be pronounced; duration several minutes post-treatment
- Bradycardia (to the point of asystole) and hypotension may be pronounced if stimulus is subconvulsive
  - increased risk if patient on a β-blocker
  - attenuated by the subsequent convulsion, atropine and medication with anticholinergic effect
- Prolonged seizures and status epilepticus rare; monitor treatment with EEG until convulsion ends; seizures should be terminated after 3 min duration (with anesthetic dosage of the induction agent, repeated if necessary, or a benzodiazepine)
- Spontaneous seizures
  - incidence of post-ECT epilepsy is approximately that found in the general population
- Headache and muscle pain common but not usually severe
  - pretreat with rocuronium bromide (approximately 3 mg) for severe muscle pain
- Temporo-mandibular joint pain; may be reduced with bifrontal electrode placement (compared to standard bitemporal placement)

PRECAUTIONS

- Obtain pretreatment anesthesia and/or internal medicine consultation for all patients with significant pre-existing cardiovascular disease, potential gastro-esophageal reflux, compromised airway, and other circumstances which may complicate the procedure (i.e., personal or family history of significant adverse effects, or delay in recovery from general anesthesia); treat as indicated
- Monitor by EKG, pulse oximetry and blood pressure, before and after ECT
- Patients with insulin-dependent diabetes mellitus may have a reduced need for insulin after ECT, as ECT reduces blood glucose levels for several hours (may be related to pretreatment fasting)
- 10–30% of bipolar depressed patients can switch to hypomania or mania following ECT

CONTRAINDICATIONS

Note: all contraindications should be regarded in the context of, and relative to, the risks of withholding ECT

- Rheumatoid arthritis complicated by erosion of the odontoid process
- Recent myocardial infarction
- Increased intracranial pressure
- Recent intracerebral hemorrhage/unstable aneurysm
- Extremely loose teeth which may be aspirated if dislodged
- Threatened retinal detachment
- Other disorders associated with increased anesthetic risk (American Society of Anesthesiologists level 3 or 4)
- Concurrent administration of an irreversible MAOI, which may interact with anesthetic agents (although most reports have implicated meperidine as the interacting drug). Severe impairment in cardiac output and hypotension during ECT may require resuscitation with a pressor agent; the choice may be limited in the presence of an irreversible MAOI. The literature therefore recommends that MAOIs be discontinued 14 days prior to elective anesthesia; if there are compelling reasons to continue the MAOI, or start ECT prior to this waiting period, obtain anesthesia consultation. The potential for a hypertensive response is much less in the presence of a selective, reversible MAOI (RIMA) such that their concurrent administration is acceptable
- Concurrent drug toxicity
- Clozapine (see Interactions)

PEDIATRIC CONSIDERATIONS

- May be necessary for childhood or early adolescent onset of severe affective disorder with suicide risk, if antidepressants are ineffective
- Should never be prescribed without consultation by a specialist in child and adolescent psychiatry

GERIATRIC CONSIDERATIONS

- No specific risks, benefits, or contraindications attributable to age
- Concurrent early dementia is not a contraindication
- Suggestions that response to ECT is more favorable than in younger patients

USE IN PREGNANCY

- Safe in all trimesters; obtain obstetrical consultation
- Fetal monitoring recommended
- Precaution: increased risk of gastro-esophageal reflux

NURSING IMPLICATIONS

- Patients must be kept NPO (especially for solid food) for approximately 8 h before treatment; continuous observation may be required
- Dentures must be removed before treatment
- Observe and monitor vital signs until patient is recovered, oriented and alert before discharge from recovery room
- When possible avoid prn benzodiazepines the night prior to and the morning of treatment

PATIENT INSTRUCTIONS

- "Nothing by mouth" (NPO) after midnight, except for specified medication (e.g., antihypertensives) with sip of water
- Do not operate a motor vehicle or machinery the day of each treatment; outpatients must be escorted home after treatment
- Limit the use of prn sedatives and hypnotics the night before and the morning of treatment

PRETREATMENT WORK-UP AND DOCUMENTATION

- Assess patient's capacity to consent to treatment; answer patient's questions about ECT; obtain signed and witnessed consent form (valid consent requires full disclosure to the patient of the nature of the procedure, all material risks and expected benefit of ECT and those of alternative available treatments, and the prognosis if no treatment is given); if patient incapable, get written consent from eligible substitute
- Physical examination
- Hb, WBC and differential for all patients over age 60 and when clinically indicated
- Electrolytes and creatinine for all patients on any diuretic, on lithium, or with insulin-dependent diabetes, and as clinically indicated, including patients with a history of water intoxication
- EKG for all patients over age 45, those being treated for hypertension, or with a history of cardiac disease and as clinically indicated
- Chest x-rays for patients with myasthenia gravis and spinal x-rays for those patients with a history of compression fracture or other injury, significant pain, and as clinically indicated; cervical spine x-rays for all patients with rheumatoid arthritis
- Sickle cell screening of all black patients; infectious hepatitis screening as clinically indicated
- Blood glucose on day of each treatment for all patients with diabetes mellitus/patients on hypoglycemic agents
- Prothrombin time and partial thromboplastin time for all patients on anticoagulants

DRUG INTERACTIONS

- Clinically significant interactions are listed below

Class of Drug	Example	Interaction Effects
Anticonvulsant	Carbamazepine, valproate	Increased seizure threshold with potential adverse effects of subconvulsive stimuli; it is possible to over-ride the anticonvulsant effect with a modest increase in energy of electric stimulus

Class of Drug	Example	Interaction Effects
Antidepressant		
Irreversible MAOI	Phenelzine	Possible need of a pressor agent for resuscitation requires that this combination be avoided
SARI, NDRI, SSRI	Trazodone, bupropion, fluoxetine	Prolonged seizures reported; clinical significance unknown. Concurrent administration not contraindicated
	Trazodone	Rare case reports of cardiovascular complications in patients with and without cardiac disease – more likely to occur at high dosages (i.e., >300 mg/day)
Antihypertensive	β-blockers, e.g., propranolol	May potentiate bradycardia and hypotension with subconvulsive stimuli Confusion reported with combined use
Benzodiazepine	Lorazepam, diazepam	Increased seizure threshold with potential adverse effects of subconvulsive stimuli or abbreviated seizure
Caffeine		Increased seizure duration Reports of hypertension, tachycardia, and cardiac dysrhythmia
Clozapine		Spontaneous (tardive) seizures reported following ECT Delirium reported with concurrent, or shortly following clozapine treatment; however, there are many case reports of uncomplicated concurrent use
Lithium		Lithium toxicity may occur, perhaps due to an increased permeability of the blood-brain barrier; decrease or discontinue lithium and monitor patient. Concurrent administration not contraindicated if lithium level within the therapeutic range
L-Tryptophan		Increased seizure duration
Propofol		Decreased seizure duration (may be very substantial); may increase seizure threshold
Theophylline		Increased seizure duration, status epilepticus. Concurrent administration not contraindicated if serum level within the therapeutic range

ANTIPSYCHOTICS (NEUROLEPTICS)

GENERAL COMMENTS

- Antipsychotics can be classified as follows:

Chemical Class	Agent	Page
"Second Generation" Antipsychotics[A]		
Benzisoxazole	Risperidone	See p. 73
Dibenzodiazepine	Clozapine	See p. 73
Dibenzothiazepine	Quetiapine	See p. 73
Thienobenzodiazepine	Olanzapine	See p. 73
Benzothiazolylpiperazine	Ziprasidone[E]	See p. 73
"Conventional" Antipsychotics[B]		
Butyrophenone	Haloperidol Droperidol[C] [E]	See p. 79
Dibenzoxazepine	Loxapine[D]	See p. 79
Dihydroindolone	Molindone[D][E]	See p. 79
Diphenylbutylpiperidine	Pimozide	See p. 79
Phenothiazines		
– aliphatic	Example: chlorpromazine	See p. 79
– piperazine	Example: trifluoperazine	See p. 79
– piperidine	Example: thioridazine	See p. 80
Thioxanthenes	Example: thiothixene	See p. 80

[A] Formerly called "atypical," which describes antipsychotics that have a decreased incidence of EPS at therapeutic doses (do not cause catalepsy in animals); the boundaries, however, between "typical" and "atypical" neuroleptics are not definitive. "Atypical" neuroleptics (1) may have low affinity for D_2 receptors and are readily displaced by endogenous dopamine in striatum (e.g., clozapine, molindone, quetiapine); (2) may have high D_2 blockade and high muscarinic blockade-anticholinergic activity (e.g., thioridazine); (3) may block both D_2 and 5-HT_2 receptors (e.g., risperidone, clozapine, olanzapine, quetiapine); (4) may have high D_4 blockade (e.g., clozapine, olanzapine, loxapine); (5) may reduce negative symptoms by blocking α_1 and α_2 adrenergic receptors (e.g., clozapine, risperidone, methotrimeprazine, quetiapine); (6) may lack a sustained increased prolactin response (e.g., clozapine, quetiapine, olanzapine); (7) show mesolimbic selectivity (e.g., olanzapine, clozapine, quetiapine); (8) may block D_2 loosely (e.g., clozapine, quetiapine).
[B] Formerly called "typical."
[C] Injectable drug used primarily in the emergency setting (see below)
[D] "Typical" antipsychotics with "atypical" features.
[E] Not available in Canada.

- Significant pharmacological characteristics of antipsychotics:
  - antipsychotic activity
  - absence of deep coma or anesthesia with administration of large (not toxic) doses
  - absence of physical or psychic dependence
- The term "tranquilizer" was introduced to describe the psychic effects of reserpine (which is rarely used for this indication now); the term is outmoded
- Appear to control symptoms of schizophrenia such as thought disorder, hallucinations, delusions, alterations in affect, autism, ideas of influence, and ideas of reference

Antipsychotics (Neuroleptics) (cont.)

- In mania, reduce euphoria, excitement, irritability, expansiveness, energy, thought disorder, and pressure of ideas; some suggestion that "conventional" agents may predispose to secondary depression or enhance cycling in BAD
- Negative symptoms (e.g., anhedonia, amotivation, poverty of speech, cognitive impairment) may respond better to "second generation" antipsychotics (this may be related to an improved side effect profile or secondary to decreased positive symptoms)
- Some clinicians suggest that onset of action with some "second generation" agents may be slower than with "conventional" drugs due to the need for slow titration of dose – prn doses are not considered useful, by some
- Non-compliance with antipsychotic therapy estimated to be 15–35% in inpatients and up to 65% in outpatients with oral medication; with depot agents 10–15% non-compliance within 2 years and 40% within 7 years – results in high incidence of relapse
- Droperidol is available only as an injectable and is marketed as an adjunct to anesthesia; it is used for sedation/behavior control of acutely psychotic patients

PHARMACOLOGY

- Exact mechanism of action unknown – primary action has been attributed to D_2 blockade, although "second generation" compounds have suggested a role for other dopamine receptors (e.g., D_3 and D_4) and other neurotransmitters (e.g., serotonin, glutamate)
- Receptor specificity varies with different antipsychotics: e.g., clozapine, olanzapine, quetiapine, risperidone and ziprasidone have greater 5-HT_2 blockade than D_2 blockade (see p. 86)
- Clozapine, quetiapine and olanzapine selectively block mesolimbic (A_{10}) dopamine neurons; other antipsychotics block both A_{10} and A_9 (nigrostriatal neurons)
- Ziprasidone is a moderate inhibitor of 5HT and NE reuptake

DOSING

- Current opinion suggests use of lower doses (i.e., haloperidol 2–10 mg daily, or equivalent); clinical efficacy correlated with D_2 binding above 60% (see pp. 90–93); outcome studies show patient response at low doses similar to high doses, with decreased adverse effects
- Acute patients may require slightly higher doses than chronic patients; manic patients may need even higher doses; maintenance doses for bipolar patients tend to be about half those used in schizophrenia
- Lower doses are recommended in the elderly, in children, and in patients with compromised liver or renal function
- Lower doses are used in first-episode patients
- Dosage requirements of olanzapine may be higher in young males who smoke and lower in older, non-smoking females

BLOOD LEVELS

- The usefulness of serum levels is still unclear; it is suggested that a curvilinear relationship is true with some antipsychotics, and they may be effective within a narrow plasma level range (therapeutic window, e.g., haloperidol)
- Threshold plasma level suggested for response to clozapine (350 ng/ml, or 1050 nmol/L suggested by some; 250 ng/ml or 750 nmol/L by others)
- Threshold plasma level may be important for response to olanzapine in acutely ill schizophrenic patients (9 ng/ml or 27 nmol/L)

PHARMACOKINETICS

- Varies with individual agents

Oral

- Peak plasma levels of oral doses reached 1–4 h after administration
- Highly bound to plasma proteins
- Most phenothiazines and thioxanthenes have active metabolites
- Metabolized extensively in the liver; specific agents inhibit cytochrome P-450 metabolizing enzymes (see pp. 90–93)
- Once-daily dosing is appropriate because of long elimination half-life; recommended that doses of clozapine above 300 mg be divided due to seizure risk; it is recommended that quetiapine be given twice daily (due to short half-life; D_2 receptor occupancy maintained up to 12 h)
- Differences in plasma concentration between males and females demonstrated with clozapine (40–50% increase in females) and with olanzapine (30% increase in females)

- On discontinuation, clozapine and quetiapine are rapidly eliminated from the plasma and brain – may result in rapid re-emergence of symptoms

Dissolving Tablets

- Supralingual preparation of olanzapine (Zydis) dissolves in saliva within 15 seconds and is absorbed in approximately 2 minutes (can be swallowed with or without liquid) – bioequivalent to oral tablet

IM

- Generally peak plasma level reached sooner than with oral preparation
- Bioavailability usually greater than with oral drug; dosage should be adjusted accordingly (loxapine excepted)
- With loxapine, single IM doses produce lower concentrations of active metabolite, for first 12–16 h, than does oral therapy – this may result in a different balance between D_2 and $5HT_2$ blockade

Depot IM

- See chart on pp. 94–95
- Bioavailability is greater than with oral agents (by a factor of at least 2)
- Presence of "free" fluphenazine in multi-dose vials of fluphenazine decanoate is responsible for high peak plasma level seen within 24 hours of injection – monitor for EPS

Zuclopenthixol Acuphase

- Short-acting depot injection (see p. 93)
- Peak plasma level: 24–36 h; elimination half-life = 36 h (mean)

ADVERSE EFFECTS

- See "second generation" antipsychotics (pp. 74–77), "conventional" antipsychotics (pp. 81–84) and charts (pp. 88–89)

LABORATORY TESTS

- Routine laboratory tests are not indicated except:
  - with fever, rigidity and diaphoresis – monitor white blood cell count and CPK (rule out neuroleptic malignant syndrome)
  - with pruritis or signs of jaundice – do liver function tests; some clinicians suggest annual liver tests
  - with seizures, polydipsia – do electrolytes
  - with galactorrhea, amenorrhea – do prolactin level
  - serum potassium and magnesium prior to prescribing thioridazine, mesoridazine and ziprasidone, and periodically during course of therapy
  - weights, fasting blood glucose and lipids with clozapine and olanzapine at baseline and periodically during course of treatment

☞ **Clozapine monitoring: WBC* and granulocyte counts must be done weekly (after 6 months can be done bi-weekly in Canada if patient had no abnormalities). "Green": WBC ≥ 3.5 × 10^9/L or ANC** ≥ 2.0 × 10^9/L; "Yellow": WBC 2–3.5 × 10^9/L or ANC 1.5–2 × 10^9/L – do blood work twice weekly till normal; "Red": WBC < 2 × 10^9/L or ANC < 1.5 × 10^9/L – STOP clozapine and monitor bloodwork and clinical symptoms for 4 weeks. DO NOT rechallenge**

Monitoring

- See Laboratory Tests
- Blood pressure and pulse during dosage titration with clozapine, risperidone, quetiapine, chlorpromazine, thioridazine
- ECG: prior to prescribing thioridazine, mesoridazine and ziprasidone, and periodically during course of therapy; DO NOT PRESCRIBE these drugs if patient's QT_c > 450 ms
- EEG: if seizures or myoclonus occurs. May also be used to determine need for prophylactic valproate with clozapine
- Slit lamp ophthalmic examinations recommended with quetiapine, at baseline and at 6-month intervals, as per product monograph – risk is low
- Thyroid function tests (T_4, TSH) with quetiapine, especially in patients at risk for hypothyroidism
- Body mass index and weight during course of treatment
- Blood glucose, triglyceride and cholesterol levels upon initiation of "second generation" antipsychotic (especially in obese, non-white males), and periodically thereafter

PEDIATRIC CONSIDERATIONS

- The use of conventional antipsychotics should be confined to disturbed children or those who have not responded to other types of medication; "second generation" agents may be preferred due to lesser risk of extrapyramidal and dysphoric effects
- Antipsychotics found useful for the following indications: pervasive developmental disorder (autism), schizophrenia, conduct disorders, and tic disorders

* WBC = white blood count
** ANC = absolute neutrophil count

Antipsychotics (Neuroleptics) (cont.)

- Used in managing aggression, temper tantrums, psychomotor excitement, stereotypies, and hyperactivity unresponsive to other therapy
- Early studies suggest efficacy of risperidone and olanzapine in the management of pervasive developmental disorders
- Clozapine found effective in childhood schizophrenia; increased risk of side effects including drowsiness, tachycardia, hypersalivation, diarrhea, blood dyscrasias and seizures
- Open label study suggests efficacy of olanzapine for mixed or manic phase of BAD in children
- Start doses low and increase slowly; limit dose and duration of therapy; assess dosage requirements and continued need for drug and monitor for early signs of tardive dyskinesia; higher incidence of tardive dyskinesia with conventional antipsychotics (in up to 51% of patients) – see page 98 for risk factors
- Behavioral toxicity can occur when high doses used; this includes: worsening of symptoms, impairment of learning, apathy, irritability, tics, or hallucinations
- Children and adolescents may be more sensitive to side effects
- Children may be more prone to weight gain with "second generation" antipsychotics – may be of concern in individuals with juvenile onset diabetes mellitus, Prader-Willi syndrome, Turner's syndrome or Trisomy-21
- Adolescents prescribed clozapine have up to 60% risk of EEG abnormalities (dose-related)
- Children and adolescents may be more sensitive to prolactin-elevating effects of "second generation" and conventional antipsychotics

GERIATRIC CONSIDERATIONS

- Start dose low and increase slowly; elimination half-life tends to be increased in the elderly
- Monitor for excessive CNS and anticholinergic effects; utilize drugs least likely to cause these effects, e.g., low dose haloperidol, loxapine, risperidone, and olanzapine
- Elderly are more sensitive to extrapyramidal reactions. Balance need for antiparkinsonian drug with type of antipsychotic used
- Caution when combining with other drugs with CNS and anticholinergic properties; additive effects can result in confusion, disorientation, delirium
- As most "second generation" antipsychotics and some conventional agents (e.g., phenothiazines) can cause orthostatic hypotension, use caution during dosage titration and when other hypotensive agents are prescribed
- Elderly have a very high incidence of tardive dyskinesia with conventional antipsychotics – risk about 30% per year in persons over age 45
- Higher risk of agranulocytosis with clozapine reported in the elderly

USE IN PREGNANCY

- Antipsychotics have not been clearly demonstrated to have teratogenic effects
- If possible, avoid during first trimester; suggested that high-potency agents offer less risk
- Use of moderate to high doses in last trimester may produce extrapyramidal reactions in newborn and impair temperature regulation after birth
- Caution with clozapine – concentration of clozapine in plasma of fetus exceeds that in the mother; floppy infant syndrome and neonatal seizures reported

Breast milk

- Antipsychotics have been detected in breast milk in concentrations of 0.2–11%; clinical significance in the newborn is unclear
- The American Academy of Pediatrics classifies antipsychotics as drugs "whose effect in the nursing infant is unknown but may be of concern"
- Suggested that patients taking clozapine not breast feed as concentration of drug in breast milk exceeds that in mother's plasma

MEDICOLEGAL ISSUES

- Antipsychotic therapy has been a source of litigation
- Be frank with patients; antipsychotics are not innocuous; however, continuing psychosis is very destructive
- Provide educational material, drug education groups, answer questions of family and patients

- Keep educating and re-educating patients about their illness and their medication as levels of retention of material are low; a policy of ongoing education is better than written consent, though in some jurisdictions written consent is necessary
- No antipsychotic is perfectly safe; for tardive dyskinesia some may be safer than others (e.g., clozapine, quetiapine, risperidone and olanzapine seem less harmful and are felt to have antidyskinetic effects; document a baseline assessment for movement disorders, and monitor regularly (e.g., every 6–12 months)

NURSING IMPLICATIONS

- Careful observation, data collection, and documentation of patient behavior patterns prior to drug administration, as well as during therapy, are essential nursing measures
- Care is essential in minimizing side effects; patients should be educated and reassured about side effects to promote positive attitudes towards taking medication; allow patient to ventilate fears about medication. Unrecognized and untreated side effects (e.g., akathisia, sexual dysfunction) may play a major role in noncompliance with treatment
- Prn antiparkinsonian agents may be required liberally during first few weeks of treatment with conventional antipsychotics; patient should take antiparkinsonian agents (e.g., Cogentin, Kemadrin) only for the extrapyramidal (EPS) side effects of antipsychotics; excess use of these agents may precipitate an anticholinergic (toxic) psychosis. Prophylactic antiparkinsonian agents may be required on a temporary basis, by young males, or by individuals with a history of EPS on low doses of antipsychotics, when given "conventional" antipsychotics
- Blurred vision is usually transient; near vision only is affected; if severe, pilocarpine eye drops or neostigmine tablets may be prescribed
- A gain in weight may occur in some patients receiving antipsychotics (especially "second generation" agents); proper diet, exercise and avoidance of calorie-laden beverages is important; monitor weight and body mass index during course of treatment
- Monitor patient's intake and output; urinary retention can occur, especially in the elderly; bethanechol (Urecholine) can reverse this
- Anticholinergics reduce peristalsis and decrease intestinal secretions leading to constipation; increasing fluids and bulk (e.g., bran, salads), as well as fruit in the diet is beneficial; if necessary, bulk laxatives (e.g., Metamucil, Prodiem) or a stool softener (e.g., Surfak) can be used; lactulose is effective in chronic constipation
- Do not mistake akathisia for anxiety or psychotic agitation
- Hold dose and notify physician if patient develops acute dystonia, severe persistent extrapyramidal reactions (longer than a few hours), or has symptoms of jaundice or blood dyscrasias (fever, sore throat, infection, cellulitis, weakness)
- Check patients on depot injections for indurations
- Recommend patient visit general practitioner yearly for a physical examination, including ophthalmological and neurological examination
- If half tablets of olanzapine are required, store broken tablet in tight, light-resistant container (tablet discolors), and use within 7 days. Avoid exposure to powder as dermatitis, eye irritation and allergic reactions reported
- "Older" multi-punctured vials of fluphenazine decanoate may contain hydrolyzed ("free") fluphenazine, which can result in higher peak plasma levels within 24 hours of injection – monitor for EPS
- Screen for symptoms suggesting obstructive sleep apnea in overweight patients

PATIENT INSTRUCTIONS

For detailed patient instructions on antipsychotics and clozapine, see the Patient Information Sheets on pp. 254 and 256.

- Avoid photosensitivity reactions by using sunscreen agents and protective clothing until response to sun has been determined; wear UV-protective sunglasses in bright sunlight
- Avoid exposure to extreme heat and humidity as antipsychotics affect the body's ability to regulate temperature
- Show caution about driving a car or operating machinery until response to drug is determined; drowsiness and dizziness usually subside after the first few weeks; caution should be used when combining antipsychotics with alcohol or other depressants
- Dry mouth can be alleviated by drinking water, sucking sour candy, or chewing sugarless gum; patient should rinse mouth periodically and brush teeth regularly; caution patient about the use of calorie-laden or caffeine-containing beverages (e.g., colas); excess use of caffeine may cause anxiety and agitation and counteract the beneficial effects of antipsychotics
- Do not break or crush tablets unless you have been advised to do so by your doctor. If you are advised to break an olanzapine tablet in half, do so carefully and avoid touching the powder – wash your hands after this procedure. Store the unused half tablet in a light-resistant, closed container and use the half tablet within 7 days

Antipsychotics (Neuroleptics) (cont.)

- Take medication with meals or with water, milk or orange juice. Avoid apple or grapefruit juice as they may interfere with drug effects.
- Report immediately to the physician the appearance of muscle stiffness/spasms, lethargy, weakness, fever, sore throat, flu-like symptoms, or any other signs of infection
- Get up slowly from lying or sitting position to avoid dizziness or lightheadedness

DRUG INTERACTIONS

- Clinically significant interactions are listed below

Class of Drug	Example	Interaction Effects
Adsorbent	Antacids, activated charcoal, cholestyramine, attapulgite (kaolin-pectin)	Oral absorption decreased significantly when used simultaneously; give at least 1 h before or 2 h after the antipsychotic
Anesthetic	Enflurane	Additive hypotension with chlorpromazine
Antiarrhythmic	Quinidine	Increased plasma level of clozapine, risperidone and haloperidol due to inhibited metabolism via CYP2D6
	Quinidine, procainamide, amiodarone, disopyramide, bretylium	Additive cardiac depression and impaired conduction with thioridazine, mesoridazine, chlorpromazine, pimozide – DO NOT COMBINE
Antibiotic	Ciprofloxacin	Increased clozapine (by up to 80%) and olanzapine level due to inhibited metabolism via CYP1A2
	Clarithromycin	Decreased clearance of pimozide by 80%; DO NOT COMBINE due to effects on cardiac conduction – deaths reported
	Erythromycin	Increased plasma level and decreased clearance of clozapine (by 33–54%) and of quetiapine due to inhibition of metabolism via CYP3A4
Anticholinergic	Antiparkinsonian drugs, antidepressants, antihistamines	Potentiate atropine-like effects causing dry mouth, blurred vision, constipation, etc.; may produce inhibition of sweating, and may lead to paralytic ileus; high doses can bring on a toxic psychosis Variable effects seen on metabolism, plasma level, and efficacy of antipsychotic
Anticoagulant	Warfarin	Decreased PT ratio or INR response with haloperidol and quetiapine
Anticonvulsant	Carbamazepine	Increased level of carbamazepine and metabolite with loxapine and haloperidol Increased clearance and decreased antipsychotic plasma level (up to 100% with haloperidol, 63% with clozapine; 44% with olanzapine; also with risperidone, ziprasidone, zuclopenthixol and flupenthixol) Avoid clozapine due to risk of agranulocytosis with either agent
	Phenytoin, phenobarbital	Decreased antipsychotic plasma level due to induction of metabolism; reported with haloperidol, phenothiazines, and quetiapine (5-fold) With phenobarbital, plasma level of clozapine decreased by 35% and ratio of metabolite to parent drug increased
	Valproate (divalproex, valproic acid)	Increased neurotoxicity, sedation, and other side effects due to decreased clearance of valproic acid (by 14%) Increased plasma level of haloperidol by an average of 32% Both increased and decreased clozapine levels reported; changes in clozapine/norclozapine ratio. Case report of hepatic encephalopathy Combination of valproate and olanzapine associated with a high rate of weight gain

Class of Drug	Example	Interaction Effects
Antidepressant		
Cyclic, SARI	Amitriptyline, trimipramine, trazodone	Additive sedation, hypotension, and anticholinergic effects Increased plasma level of either agent
SARI	Nefazodone	Increased plasma level of quetiapine and clozapine due to inhibited metabolism via CYP3A4
SSRI	Fluoxetine, paroxetine, fluvoxamine, sertraline	Increased plasma level of antipsychotic (up to 100% increase with haloperidol, 2–7-fold increase with fluoxetine and clozapine and 2–10-fold increase with fluvoxamine and clozapine (increased AUC by 119% and decreased clearance by 50% of olanzapine, with fluvoxamine); 3-fold increase in plasma level of thioridazine and mesoridazine with fluvoxamine). DO NOT COMBINE thioridazine or mesoridazine with fluoxetine, fluvoxamine or paroxetine Increased EPS and akathisia Combination of SSRI and novel antipsychotic found beneficial in refractory MDD or OCD (see p. 59). Reported to decrease negative symptoms of schizophrenia
Irrev. MAOI, RIMA	Tranylcypromine, moclobemide	Additive hypotension
Antifungal	Ketoconazole	Increased clozapine, olanzapine, quetiapine, ziprasidone and pimozide levels due to inhibition of metabolism via CYP3A4; monitor for effects on cardiac conduction with clozapine, ziprasidone and pimozide
Antihistamine	Terfenadine, astemizole	Potentiation of QT prolongation leading to torsades de pointes. Caution with mesoridazine, thioridazine, pimozide
Antihypertensive	Methyldopa, enalapril, clonidine	Additive hypotensive effect
	Guanethidine	Reversal of antihypertensive effect with chlorpromazine, haloperidol and thiothixene (not reported with molindone) due to blockade of guanethidine uptake into postsynaptic neurons
Antipsychotic combination	Clozapine, risperidone	Competitive inhibition of clozapine with risperidone for CYP2D6 metabolism resulting in elevated total clozapine level
	Thioridazine, quetiapine	Increased clearance of quetiapine by 65%
	Thioridazine, fluphenazine, haloperidol	Increase in plasma of free (unbound) fluphenazine or haloperidol (by 30% and 50%, respectively) when combined with thioridazine
	Olanzapine, clozapine, pimozide	Potential for cardiac side effects with combination of novel drug with pimozide, due to competition for metabolism via CYP1A2 and risk of elevated plasma level
Antitubercular drug	Isoniazid	Increased plasma level of haloperidol due to inhibited metabolism
	Rifampin	Decreased clozapine level (by 600%) and decreased haloperidol plasma level due to induction of metabolism
Anxiolytic		
Benzodiazepines	Alprazolam	Increased plasma level of haloperidol (by 19%)
	Diazepam	Increased sedation and orthostatic hypotension with olanzapine
	Clonazepam, lorazepam	Increased incidence of dizziness (collapse) and sedation when combined with clozapine; ECG changes, delirium and respiratory arrest reported – more likely to occur early in treatment when clozapine added to benzodiazepine regimen Synergistic effect with antipsychotics; used to calm agitated patients

Antipsychotics (Neuroleptics) (cont.)

Class of Drug	Example	Interaction Effects
Buspirone		May increase extrapyramidal reactions Increased haloperidol and metabolite plasma level (by 26% and 83%, respectively)
β-Blocker	Propranolol	Increased plasma level of both chlorpromazine and propranolol reported Thioridazine level increased 3–5-fold – DO NOT COMBINE
	Pindolol	Increased plasma level of both thioridazine and pindolol reported – DO NOT COMBINE
Ca-channel blocker	Diltiazem, verapamil	Increased plasma level of quetiapine due to inhibited metabolism via CYP3A4 Additive Ca-channel blocking effects with thioridazine and pimozide – caution, as may lead to conduction abnormalities
Caffeine	Coffee, tea, cola	Increased plasma levels of clozapine due to competition for metabolism via CYP1A2
Cimetidine		Inhibited metabolism of clozapine, olanzapine , risperidone, quetiapine and thiothixene, with resultant increase in plasma level and adverse effects
CNS depressant	Antidepressants, hypnotics, antihistamines Alcohol	Increased CNS effects Alcohol may worsen EPS, increase in olanzapine absorption Additive CNS effects and orthostatic hypotension with olanzapine and quetiapine
Disulfiram		Decreased plasma level of perphenazine and an increase in its metabolite Decreased metabolism and increased plasma level of clozapine
Donepezil		Exacerbation of EPS with combination possible
Grapefruit juice		Increased plasma level of pimozide, clozapine and quetiapine due to inhibition of metabolism via CYP3A4; AVOID
Lithium		Increased neurotoxicity at therapeutic doses; may increase EPS; increased plasma level of molindone and haloperidol; possibly increased risk of agranulocytosis and seizures with clozapine
Metoclopramide		Increased risk of EPS
Oral contraceptive		Estrogen potentiates hyperprolactinemic effect of antipsychotics
Protease inhibitor	Ritonavir	Decreased metabolism and increased plasma level of clozapine and pimozide due to inhibited metabolism via CYP3A4; AVOID due to effects on cardiac conduction Moderate increase in AUC of chlorpromazine, haloperidol, perphenazine, risperidone and thioridazine
Smoking – cigarettes		Decreased plasma level of antipsychotic (clozapine, chlorpromazine, haloperidol, fluphenazine, olanzapine, thiothixene) by 20–100% due to induction of metabolism
Stimulant	Amphetamine Methylphenidate	Antipsychotics can counteract many signs of stimulant toxicity Case reports of worsening of tardive movement disorder and prolongation or exacerbation of withdrawal dyskinesia following antipsychotic discontinuation
Sympathomimetic	Epinephrine, norepinephrine	May result in paradoxical fall in blood pressure (due to α-adrenergic block produced by antipsychotics); benefits may outweigh risk in anaphylaxis; phenylephrine is a safe substitute for hypotension

"Second Generation" Antipsychotics (Neuroleptics)

PRODUCT AVAILABILITY

Chemical Class	Generic Name	Trade Name[(A)]	Dosage Forms and Strengths
Benzisoxazole	Risperidone	Risperdal	Tablets: 0.25 mg[(B)], 0.5 mg[(B)], 1 mg, 2 mg, 3 mg, 4 mg Oral solution: 1 mg/ml
Dibenzodiazepine	Clozapine	Clozaril	Tablets: 25 mg, 100 mg
Thienobenzodiazepine	Olanzapine	Zyprexa Zyprexa Zydis	Tablets: 2.5 mg, 5 mg, 7.5 mg, 10 mg, 15 mg[(B)], 20 mg[(B)] Oral dissolving tablets: 5 mg, 10 mg, 15 mg[(B)], 20 mg[(B)]
Dibenzothiazepine	Quetiapine	Seroquel	Tablets: 25 mg, 100 mg, 150 mg[(B)], 200 mg
Benzothiazolylpiperazine	Ziprasidone[(B)]	Geodon	Capsules: 20 mg, 40 mg, 60 mg, 80 mg

[(A)] Generic preparations may be available, [(B)] Not marketed in Canada, [(C)] Not marketed in USA

INDICATIONS*

▲ • Treat symptoms of acute and chronic psychoses (i.e., schizophrenia, manic phase of bipolar disorder, delusional disorder)
▲ • Prophylaxis of schizophrenia
▲ • Treatment-resistant schizophrenia (clozapine)
▲ • Maintenance of treatment response in schizophrenia (olanzapine)
▲ • Prophylaxis of bipolar affective disorder
▲ • Agitated aggressive behavior of dementia; reported to decrease psychotic and behavioral symptoms in patients with dementia or Alzheimer's disease (olanzapine, risperidone, quetiapine)
▲ • Acute mania (olanzapine – USA)

- Clozapine, olanzapine and risperidone may have antimanic, antidepressant and mood-stabilizing properties; early data suggest clozapine may be effective in refractory bipolar affective disorder and rapid-cycling bipolar disorder
- Delusional major depression
- Psychosis associated with Parkinson's disease
- Augmentation in refractory obsessive-compulsive disorder and related disorders (risperidone, olanzapine, clozapine) – occasional reports of worsening of OCD symptoms
- Efficacy reported in the management of pervasive developmental disorders (risperidone, clozapine, quetiapine)
- Preliminary evidence suggests efficacy in tic disorders, Tourette's syndrome and trichotillomania (risperidone, olanzapine, quetiapine)
- Psychosis associated with psychostimulant use (risperidone)
- Self-mutilation and aggression in psychotic patients (with and without borderline personality disorder)
- Early data suggest benefit as augmentation strategy in refractory depression
- Clozapine reported to decrease motor symptoms in a number of movement disorders (e.g., tremor, dyskinesia and bradykinesia of Parkinson's disease, essential tremor, akinetic disorders, Huntington's chorea, blepharospasm, Meige syndrome, etc.)
- Clozapine suggested to decrease addictive behaviors (e.g., smoking, alcoholism, drug-abuse)
- Studies suggest clozapine and olanzapine decrease suicidality in patients with schizophrenia
- Early data suggest a role in the treatment of delirium (quetiapine, risperidone, olanzapine)
- Early data suggest benefit in anorexia nervosa (olanzapine)

* ▲ Approved indications

"Second Generation" Antipsychotics (Neuroleptics) (cont.)

ADMINISTRATION

Oral Medication

- Medication may be given with meals or followed by a glass of water, milk or orange juice; avoid apple or grapefruit juice as they may interfere with drug effect
- Food increases the bioavailability of ziprasidone; fatty foods increase the absorption of ziprasidone
- Do not give oral medication within 2 h of an antacid or antidiarrheal drug, as absorption of the antipsychotic will be decreased

ADVERSE EFFECTS

- See chart on p. 89 for incidence of adverse effects
- Many adverse effects are transient; persistent symptoms often have remedies, but are best dealt with by change of dose or drug

1. CNS Effects

- A result of antagonism at H_1, ACh and α_1-receptors
- Headache (risperidone, olanzapine – 10 to 15%; quetiapine – 19% incidence)

a) Cognitive Effects

- Sedation and fatigue common, especially during the first 2 weeks of therapy (primarily with clozapine, quetiapine and olanzapine) [Management: prescribe bulk of dose at bedtime; some clinicians recommend stimulants if symptoms persist (controversial)]
- Insomnia (risperidone, olanzapine); vivid dreams, nightmares (risperidone, clozapine)
- Confusion, disturbed concentration, disorientation (more common with high doses, or in elderly); toxic delirium reported with clozapine
- Dysphoria
- May improve cognition: e.g., attention/information processing, reaction time and verbal fluency (clozapine); attention, executive functioning, and working memory (risperidone); verbal learning and memory, verbal fluency and executive functioning (olanzapine)
- May cause exacerbation of obsessive-compulsive symptoms (higher doses)
- Risperidone more likely to produce insomnia, anxiety, and agitation; hypomania and mania have been reported with risperidone and olanzapine in patients with bipolar-type schizoaffective disorder – may be resistant to mood stabilizers
- Increased agitation, aggression reported with olanzapine
- Case reports of new onset panic attacks with olanzapine and risperidone

b) Neurological Effects

- A result of antagonism at dopamine D_2 receptors (extrapyramidal reactions correlated with D_2 binding above 80%)
- Lowered seizure threshold; caution in patients with a history of seizures. May occur if dose increased rapidly or may be secondary to hyponatremia in SIADH. Risk of seizures with clozapine 1% (doses below 300 mg), 2.7% (300–600 mg) and 4.4% (above 600 mg); may be preceded by myoclonus; 4% risk of seizures and up to 60% risk of EEG abnormalities in adolescents with clozapine [Management: valproate or topiramate in therapeutic doses – recommended as prophylaxis in patients on doses of clozapine over 550 mg daily]; nonspecific EEG abnormalities reported with olanzapine, including cases of seizures; seizures rare with quetiapine (0.8%) and risperidone (0.3%)
- Myoclonic jerks, tics or cataplexy reported with clozapine; may be precursor of generalized seizure [decrease dose or add anticonvulsant]
- Extrapyramidal reactions less common with "second generation" antipsychotics and are dose-dependent with olanzapine, risperidone and ziprasidone (see p. 89) (low iron may predispose to akathisia). Clozapine and quetiapine have the lowest risk of EPS and may ameliorate existing symptoms
- Loss of gag reflex (especially in males)
- Dysphagia (difficulty swallowing); of greater concern in males; sialorrhea (especially with clozapine) – see GI Effects
- Urinary incontinence (overflow incontinence); enuresis reported with clozapine (up to 42%); case reports with olanzapine and risperidone [Desmopressin or DDAVP 10 µg nasal spray or tablets 0.2 mg, oxybutynin 5–15 mg, ephedrine 25–150 mg/day, pseudoephedrine 60 mg or tolterodine 1–4 mg/day may be useful]
- Pain reported with olanzapine (8% incidence)
- Paresthesias or "burning sensations" reported with risperidone
- Tardive dyskinesia (TD) (see p. 98). Risk lower with "second generation" antipsychotics, and these drugs may reduce TD symptoms.

Clozapine has the lowest TD risk, based on current data and has demonstrated a significant reduction in existing TD, often within 1–4 weeks (sometimes up to 12 weeks)

2. Anticholinergic Effects

- A result of antagonism at muscarinic receptors (ACh)
- Common; effects are additive if given concurrently with other anticholinergic agents
- Dry mucous membranes [Management: sugar-free gum and candy, oral lubricants (e.g., MoiStir, OraCare D), pilocarpine mouth wash – see p. 33]; may predispose patient to monilial infection
- Blurred vision, dry eyes [Management: artificial tears, wetting solutions; pilocarpine 0.5% eye drops]
- Constipation [Management: increase bulk and fluid intake, fecal softener (e.g., Surfak), bulk laxative (e.g., Prodiem, Metamucil)]
- Urinary retention [Management: bethanechol]
- Use of high doses or in combination with other anticholinergic drugs may result in anticholinergic toxicity with both central and peripheral effects including disorientation, confusion, memory loss, fever, tachycardia, etc.

3. Cardiovascular Effects

- A result of antagonism at α_1-adrenergic and muscarinic receptors
- Hypotension. **DO NOT USE EPINEPHRINE**, as it may further lower the blood pressure; phenylephrine may be used. Risperidone, quetiapine or clozapine dosing increases should be gradual to minimize hypotension as well as sinus and reflex tachycardia [Increase fluid and salt intake, use support hose, midodrine, fludrocortisone, dihydroergotamine]
- Transient increases in blood pressure, tachycardia reported with clozapine (usually during treatment initiation) – more common in the elderly; rare cardiac deaths
- ECG changes (T-wave inversion, ST segment depression, QT_c lengthening – may increase risk of arrhythmias) reported with ziprasidone and clozapine at higher doses and rarely with risperidone and quetiapine
- Rare reports of arrhythmias, myocardial infarction with olanzapine
- Sudden death of patients on antipsychotics is rare and probably due to arrhythmias, especially torsades de pointes
- Cases of collapse (with respiratory or cardiac arrest) reported at initiation of clozapine (benzodiazepines were used concomitantly in several cases)
- Cardiomyopathy, pericarditis and myocarditis with clozapine (0.06% incidence) – deaths have been reported. DO NOT USE in patients with severe cardiac disease
- Case reports of edema with olanzapine

4. GI Effects

- Weight gain (a result of multiple systems including 5-HT_{1B}, 5-HT_{2C}, α_1, and H_1 blockade, prolactinemia, gonadal and adrenal steroid imbalance – clozapine and olanzapine increase circulating leptin; may be related to insulin resistance (increased blood glucose); may also be due to carbohydrate craving and excessive intake of high-calorie beverages to alleviate drug-induced thirst and dry mouth);
  - Common with most "second generation" antipsychotics; not seen with ziprasidone, moderate risk with quetiapine and frequent with clozapine and olanzapine. Weight gain has been correlated with treatment response – data inconclusive
  - Approx. 50% patients gain an average of 20% of their weight (primarily fat). Patients with low BMI tend to gain more weight than patients with higher BMI at baseline. Maximal increase occurs in first 6 weeks of treatment (except with clozapine). Occurs more frequently in females and adults with mental retardation; may be dose-related; caution in women with polycystic ovaries. Weight gain suggested to plateau with risperidone and quetiapine
  - Weight gain may predispose to coronary artery disease, hyperglycemia (see p. 76) and obstructive sleep apnea [Management: diet, exercise, amantadine (100–300 mg/day), bromocriptine, topiramate, nizatidine (300 mg bid)]
- Anorexia, dyspepsia, dysphagia, occasionally diarrhea
- Reflux esophagitis (approx. 11% incidence reported with clozapine)
- Peculiar taste, glossitis
- Loss of gag reflex (more likely to be significant in males)
- Sialorrhea, difficulty swallowing, gagging (with clozapine up to 80%; case reports with olanzapine and risperidone) – may be due to stimulation of M_4 muscarinic or α_2 receptors in salivary glands [preliminary evidence suggests amitriptyline 25–100 mg, benztropine 2–4 mg, pirenzepine 25–50 mg, clonidine 0.1–0.4 mg daily, terazosin (2 mg daily) or atropine "eye" drops (1 drop sublingually 1–2 times a day) may be effective in treatment]; parotitis reported with clozapine

"Second Generation" Antipsychotics (Neuroleptics) (cont.)

- Severe constipation with clozapine has resulted in cases of gastrointestinal complications including fecal impaction, mucosal necrosis (rarely leading to death)

5. Sexual Side Effects

- A result of altered dopamine (D_2) activity, ACh blockade, α_1 blockade, H_1 blockade + 5-HT_2 blockade
- Decreased libido [Management: neostigmine or cyproheptadine 30 minutes before intercourse]
- Erectile difficulties, impotence [Management: bethanechol, yohimbine]
- Inhibition of ejaculation, abnormal ejaculation, retrograde ejaculation (risperidone) [ephedrine 25–150 mg], anorgasmia [Management: bethanechol (10 mg tid or 10–25 mg prn), neostigmine (7.5–15 mg prn), cyproheptadine (8 mg od or 4–12 mg prn), amantadine (100–200 mg daily)]
- Case reports of priapism

6. Endocrine Effects

- Prolactin level may be elevated (related to >50% D_2 occupancy) – increases occur several hours after dosing and normalize by 12–24 hours with clozapine, olanzapine and quetiapine; occurs for longer periods with risperidone (incidence 8–15%); adolescents and children may be at higher risk; prolactin levels may be associated with sexual side effects and infertility
- In women: breast engorgement and lactation (may be more common in women who have previously been pregnant), amenorrhea (with risk of infertility), menstrual irregularities, changes in libido, hirsutism (due to increased testosterone) and possibly osteoporosis (due to decreased estrogen) [Management: change antipsychotic; bromocriptine (low doses) or amantadine if prolactin level elevated]
- In men: gynecomastia, rarely galactorrhea, decreased libido and erectile or ejaculatory dysfunction [Management: bromocriptine if prolactin level elevated]
- Increased appetite, weight gain (see GI Effects, above). Hyperinsulinemia and enhanced insulin secretion may be associated with weight gain
- Hyperglycemia, glycosuria, and high or prolonged glucose tolerance tests (up to 33% incidence with clozapine, 6% with risperidone, and up to 27% incidence with olanzapine with chronic use); cases of exacerbation of "type 2" diabetes as well as de novo onset, and diabetic ketoacidosis in nondiabetic patients, reported with clozapine, risperidone, and olanzapine (induce dose-dependent insulin resistance). Impairment of glycemic control and new onset diabetes reported with quetiapine. Risk factors include obese, middle-aged non-white male
- Hyperlipidemia reported with clozapine, olanzapine and quetiapine: cholesterol and triglyceride concentrations have been correlated with blood glucose and insulin levels; a positive correlation reported between insulin and leptin (see weight gain p. 75); ziprasidone reported to lower levels of cholesterol and triglycerides independent of changes in body mass index
- SIADH – hyponatremia with polydipsia and polyuria; increased risk in the elderly, smokers and alcoholics; risk may be decreased with clozapine. Monitor sodium levels to decrease risk of seizures in chronically treated patients (especially with clozapine) [Management: fluid restriction, demeclocycline up to 1200 mg/ day, captopril 12.5 mg/day, propranolol 30–120 mg/day; replace electrolytes]
- Dose-dependent decrease in total T_4 and free T_4 concentrations reported with quetiapine

7. Ocular Effects

- Lens changes can occur after chronic use of quetiapine (reported incidence of 0.005%) – slit lamp examinations recommended, in monograph, at start of therapy and at 6-month intervals
- Case report of palinopsia with risperidone
- Case report of esotropia (form of strabismus) with olanzapine

8. Hypersensitivity Reactions

- Usually appear within the first few months of therapy (but may occur after the drug is discontinued)
- Photosensitivity and photoallergy reactions including sunburn-like erythematous eruptions which may be accompanied by blistering
- Skin reactions, rashes, rarely abnormal skin pigmentation (risperidone)
- Cholestatic jaundice (reversible if drug stopped)

- occurs in less than 0.1% of patients on antipsychotics within first 4 weeks of treatment, with most antipsychotics
- signs include yellow skin, dark urine, pruritis
- Transient asymptomatic transaminase elevations (ALT/SGPT 2–3 times the upper limit of normal) reported with olanzapine (in up to 6% of patients), clozapine (up to 37%), quetiapine (up to 9%)
- Reports of pancreatitis with risperidone, olanzapine and clozapine (possibly secondary to hypertriglyceridemia)
- Rare reports of interstitial nephritis and acute renal failure with clozapine
- Agranulocytosis
  - occurs in less than 0.1% of patients within first 12 weeks of treatment
  - occurs in about 1–2% of patients on clozapine (0.38% risk with monitoring), may be due to metabolite formed via CYP3A4 pathway; monitor WBC and differential; risk factors include older age, female gender and certain ethnic groups (i.e., Ashkenazi Jews)
  - mortality high if drug not stopped and treatment initiated
  - signs include sore throat, fever, weakness, mouth sores
  - recurrence of previous clozapine-induced neutropenia reported after olanzapine started
- Eosinophilia reported with clozapine frequently between weeks 3 and 5 of treatment; higher incidence in females. Neutropenia can occur concurrently. Transient eosinophilia also reported with olanzapine (5.7%)
- Transient leukocytosis – 41% risk with clozapine
- Case reports of thrombocytopenia with olanzapine, risperidone and clozapine; cases of thrombocytosis with clozapine
- Case reports of pulmonary embolism and venous embolism with clozapine
- Rarely, asthma, laryngeal, angioneurotic or peripheral edema, and anaphylactic reactions occur
- Neuroleptic malignant syndrome (NMS) – rare disorder characterized by muscular rigidity, tachycardia, hyperthermia, altered consciousness, autonomic dysfunction, and increase in CPK
  - can occur with any class of antipsychotic agent, at any dose, and at any time (increased risk in hot weather); other risk factors include organic brain syndromes, mood disorders, dehydration, exhaustion, agitation
  - NMS with clozapine may present with fewer extrapyramidal symptoms, a lower rise in CPK and increased autonomic effects
  - potentially fatal unless recognized early and medication is stopped; supportive therapy must be instituted as soon as possible, especially fluid and electrolytes (mortality rate 4%)
  - dantrolene, amantadine and bromocriptine may be helpful

9. Temperature Regulation

- Altered ability of body to regulate response to changes in temperature and humidity; may become hyperthermic or hypothermic; more likely in temperature extremes due to inhibition of the hypothalamic control area
- Transient temperature elevation can occur with clozapine in up to 50% of patients, usually within the first three weeks of treatment; may be accompanied by an elevation in WBC

10. Other Adverse Effects

- Mild elevations in uric acid (olanzapine)
- Rhinitis (risperidone 15%; olanzapine 12%; also with clozapine) – incidence higher with risperidone in children
- Case reports of exacerbation of bulimia nervosa with risperidone and clozapine
- Case report of hyperventilation with quetiapine

WITHDRAWAL

- Most likely to occur 24–48 h after withdrawal, or after a large dosage decrease
- Abrupt cessation of high doses may rarely cause gastritis, nausea, vomiting, dizziness, tremors, feelings of warmth or cold, sweating, tachycardia, headache, and insomnia in some patients; symptoms begin 2–3 days after abrupt discontinuation of treatment and may last up to 14 days; agitation, aggression, delirium, worsening of psychosis, diaphoresis and abnormal movements associated with rapid clozapine withdrawal (suggested taper of 25–100 mg/week)

"Second Generation" Antipsychotics (Neuroleptics) (cont.)

- Rebound neurological symptoms may occur including akathisia, dystonia and parkinsonism (within the first few days), withdrawal dyskinesia reported within 1–4 weeks
- Tardive neurological symptoms may emerge
- Supersensitivity psychosis (acute relapse) has been described after acute withdrawal, in some patients – common with clozapine

☞ **THEREFORE THESE MEDICATIONS SHOULD BE WITHDRAWN GRADUALLY AFTER PROLONGED USE**

PRECAUTIONS

- Use with caution in the elderly, in the presence of cardiovascular disease, chronic respiratory disorder, hypoglycemia, convulsive disorders
- Caution in prescribing to patients with known or suspected hepatic disorder; monitor clinically and measure transaminase level (ALT/SGPT), periodically
- Should be used very cautiously in patients with narrow angle glaucoma or prostatic hypertrophy
- Monitor if QT interval exceeds 420 ms and reduce dose if exceeds 500 ms. DO NOT USE ziprasidone in patients with a history of QTc prolongation, recent myocardial infarction or uncompensated heart failure. Patients with hypokalemia or hypomagnesia may also be at risk
- Do not use clozapine in patients with severe cardiac disease. In patients with a family history of heart failure, perform a thorough cardiac evaluation prior to starting therapy
- Cigarette smoking is reported to induce the metabolism and decrease the plasma level of most antipsychotics
- Rapid elimination of clozapine from plasma and brain following abrupt discontinuation may result in early and severe relapse
- Allergic cross-reactivity (rash) between chlorpromazine and clozapine reported

TOXICITY

- Symptoms of toxicity are extensions of common adverse effects: anticholinergic, extrapyramidal, CNS stimulation followed by CNS depression
- Postural hypotension may be complicated by shock, coma, cardiovascular insufficiency, myocardial infarction, and arrhythmias
- Convulsions appear late, except with clozapine; symptoms may persist as drug elimination may be prolonged following intoxication
- Supportive treatment should be given

LABORATORY TESTS/ MONITORING

- See p. 67
- Specific guidelines apply to clozapine (p. 67)

"Conventional" Antipsychotics (Neuroleptics)

PRODUCT AVAILABILITY

Chemical Class	Generic Name	Trade Name(A)	Dosage Forms and Strengths
Butyrophenone	Haloperidol	Haldol	Tablets: 0.5 mg, 1 mg, 2 mg, 5 mg, 10 mg, 20 mg Oral solution: 2 mg/ml Injection: 5 mg/ml
		Haldol Decanoate	Injection (depot): 50 mg/ml, 100 mg/ml
Dibenzoxazepine	Loxapine	Loxapine(C), Loxitane(B)	Tablets(C): 5 mg, 10 mg, 25 mg, 50 mg Capsules(B): 5 mg, 10 mg, 25 mg, 50 mg Oral solution: 25 mg/ml Injection: 50 mg/ml
Dihydroindolone	Molindone(B)	Moban	Capsules: 5 mg, 10 mg, 25 mg, 50 mg, 10 mg Oral solution: 20 mg/ml
Diphenylbutylpiperidine	Pimozide	Orap	Tablets: 2 mg, 4 mg
Aliphatic phenothiazine	Chlorpromazine	Largactil(C), Thorazine(B)	Tablets: 10 mg, 25 mg, 50 mg, 100 mg, 200 mg Capsules(B): 30 mg, 75 mg, 150 mg Oral solution: 30mg/ml(B), 100 mg/ml(B), 5 mg/ml(C), 20 mg/ml(C), 40 mg/ml(C) Oral syrup: 10 mg/ml(B) Injection: 25 mg/ml Suppositories: 25 mg, 100 mg
	Methotrimeprazine	Nozinan	Tablets: 2 mg, 5 mg, 25 mg, 50 mg Oral solution: 5 mg/ml, 40 mg/ml Injection: 25 mg/ml,
	Triflupromazine(B)	Vesprin	Injection: 10 mg/ml, 20 mg/ml
Piperazine phenothiazine	Fluphenazine	Moditen(C), Prolixin(B)	Tablets: 1 mg, 2.5 mg, 5 mg, 10 mg Oral solution: 2.5 mg/ml, 5 mg/ml(B) Injection: 2.5 mg/ml
		Moditen enanthate(C) Prolixin enanthate(B)	Injection (depot): 25 mg/ml
		Modecate(C), Prolixin decanoate(B)	Injection (depot): 25 mg/ml, 100 mg/ml
	Perphenazine	Trilafon	Tablets: 2 mg, 4 mg, 8mg, 16 mg Oral solution: 16 mg/5ml Injection: 5 mg/ml
	Thioproperazine	Majeptil	Tablets: 10 mg
	Trifluoperazine	Stelazine	Tablets: 1 mg, 2 mg, 5 mg, 10 mg Oral solution: 10 mg/ml Injection: 2 mg/ml

"Conventional" Antipsychotics (Neuroleptics) (cont.)

Piperidine phenothiazine	Mesoridazine	Serentil	Tablets: 10 mg, 25 mg, 50 mg, 100 mg[(B)] Oral solution[(B)]: 25 mg/ml Injection[(B)]: 25 mg/ml
	Pericyazine	Neuleptil	Capsules: 5 mg, 10 mg, 20 mg Oral solution: 10 mg/ml
	Pipotiazine[(C)]	Piportil L4	Injection (depot): 25 mg/ml, 50 mg/ml
	Thioridazine	Mellaril	Tablets: 10 mg, 15 mg[(B)], 25 mg, 50 mg, 100 mg, 150 mg[(B)], 200 mg[(B)] Oral solution: 30 mg/ml, 100 mg/ml[(B)] Oral suspension: 10 mg/ml[(C)], 25 mg/5ml[(B)], 100 mg/5 ml[(B)]
Thioxanthene	Flupenthixol	Fluanxol Fluanxol Depot[(C)]	Tablets: 0.5 mg, 3 mg Injection (depot): 20 mg/ml, 100 mg/ml
	Thiothixene	Navane	Capsules: 1 mg[(B)], 2 mg, 5 mg, 10 mg, 20 mg Oral solution: 5 mg/ml Powder for injection[(B)]: 5 mg/ml
	Zuclopenthixol[(C)]	Clopixol Clopixol Acuphase Clopixol Depot	Tablets: 10 mg, 25 mg, 40 mg Injection: 50 mg/ml Injection (depot): 200 mg/ml

(A) Generic preparations may be available, (B) Not marketed in Canada, (C) Not marketed in USA

INDICATIONS*

- ▲ Treatment of acute and chronic psychoses (i.e., schizophrenia, manic phase of bipolar disorder, delusional disorder, toxic psychosis)
- ▲ Prophylaxis of schizophrenia
- ▲ Prophylaxis of bipolar affective disorder
- ▲ Agitated aggressive behavior of dementia and mental retardation
- ▲ Severe behavioral problems in children (e.g., hyperexcitability, explosiveness, aggression)
- ▲ Control of impulsivity and aggression in psychosis (pericyazine, haloperidol)
- ▲ Tourette's syndrome (haloperidol, pimozide)
- ▲ Anti-emetic (chlorpromazine, trifluoperazine, perphenazine, methotrimeprazine)
- ▲ Porphyria (chlorpromazine)
- ▲ An adjunct to anesthesia, analgesia, refractory hiccups and in the treatment of tetanus (chlorpromazine, methotrimeprazine)
- ▲ Sedation (methotrimeprazine)
- Delirium (haloperidol)
- Agitation in major depression
- Augmentation for refractory obsessive-compulsive disorder and related disorders (e.g., pimozide); data suggest efficacy of haloperidol in trichotillomania
- Low doses of flupenthixol have been used in the treatment of depression (dose: 0.5–4.5 mg), borderline personality disorder and cocaine withdrawal
- Antipruritic, especially in neurodermatitis and eczema
- Potential antidepressant and anxiolytic action (loxapine – due to metabolites which are inhibitors of NE reuptake)
- Childhood autism (haloperidol)
- Huntington's disease

* ▲ Approved indications

ADMINISTRATION

Short-Acting Injections

- Watch for orthostatic hypotension, especially with parenteral administration of chlorpromazine or methotrimeprazine; keep patient supine or seated for 30 minutes afterwards; monitor BP before and after each injection
- Give IM into upper outer quadrant of buttocks or in the deltoid (deltoid offers faster absorption as it has better blood perfusion); alternate sites, charting (L) or (R); massage slowly after, to prevent sterile abscess formation; tell patient that injection may sting
- Prevent contact dermatitis by keeping drug solution off patient's skin and clothing and injector's hands
- Do not let drug stand in syringe for longer than 15 min as plastic may adsorb drug

Depot Injections

- Use a needle of at least 21 gauge; give deep IM into large muscle (using Z-track method); rotate sites and specify in charting
- SC administration can be used for fluphenazine
- Do not let drug stand in syringe for longer than 15 min as plastic may adsorb drug
- DO NOT massage injection site

Oral Medication

- Medication may be given with meals or followed by a glass of water, milk or orange juice. Avoid apple or grapefruit juice as they may interfere with drug effect
- Protect liquids from light
- Discard markedly discolored solutions; however, a slight yellowing does not affect potency
- Dilute liquids with milk, orange juice, or semisolid food just before administration as some drugs may be bitter in taste
- Some liquids such as chlorpromazine and methotrimeprazine have local anesthetic effects and should be well diluted to prevent choking
- Do not give oral medication within 2 h of an antacid or antidiarrheal drug, as absorption of the antipsychotic will be decreased
- If patient is suspected of not swallowing tablet medication, liquid medication can be given

ADVERSE EFFECTS

- See charts on pp. 88–89 for incidence of adverse effects; the incidence of adverse effects may differ between different dosage forms of the same drug (e.g., oral vs depot vs acuphase)
- Many adverse effects are transient; persistent symptoms often have remedies, but are best dealt with by change of dose or drug

1. CNS Effects

- A result of antagonism at H_1, ACh and α_1-receptors

a) Cognitive Effects

- Sedation common, especially during the first 2 weeks of therapy (primarily with aliphatics) [Management: prescribe bulk of dose at bedtime]
- Confusion, disturbed concentration, disorientation (more common with high doses, or in elderly)
- May improve attention/information processing; antipsychotics do not seem to affect memory or psychomotor performance unless anticholinergic effects prominent (e.g., chlorpromazine)
- Depression and enhanced cycling reported with prophylaxis of BAD with "conventional" agents (with or without lithium)

b) Neurological Effects

- A result of antagonism at dopamine D_2 receptors (extrapyramidal reactions correlated with D_2 binding above 75–80%)
- Lowered seizure threshold; caution in patients with a history of seizures. May occur if dose increased rapidly or may be secondary to hyponatremia in SIADH
- Extrapyramidal reactions (see p. 97) seen primarily with the high potency antipsychotics: dystonias, dyskinesias, "Pisa syndrome," akathisia, pseudoparkinsonism, perioral tremor, "rabbit syndrome," akinesia (low calcium levels may predispose to extrapyramidal reactions and low iron to akathisia). Suggested that patients who lack CYP2D6 isoenzyme may be at higher risk for chronic movement disorder
- Loss of gag reflex (especially in males)
- Dysphagia (difficulty swallowing); of greater concern in males; sialorrhea – see GI Effects
- Urinary incontinence (overflow incontinence) [Desmopressin or DDAVP 10 μg nasal spray or tablets 0.2 mg, oxybutynin 5–15 mg or ephedrine 25–150 mg/day, pseudoephedrine 60 mg or tolterodine 1–4 mg/day may be useful]
- Tardive dyskinesia (see p. 98). Risk in adults with schizophrenia: 38% after 5 years, 56% after 10 years; risk increased to 30% per year in persons over age 45. Spontaneous remissions: 14–24% after 5 years. Persistent or tardive dyskinesias appear late in therapy, rarely

"Conventional" Antipsychotics (Neuroleptics) (cont.)

sooner than 3–6 months, and often persist after termination of therapy; usually occur in the over-40 age group; females are affected twice as often as males; symptoms often appear only when the antipsychotic is discontinued or the dosage lowered; symptoms are not alleviated by antiparkinsonian medication and may be made worse by it; symptoms disappear during sleep and can be suppressed by voluntary effort and concentration; they are exacerbated by stress.

Greater vulnerability in patients with affective disorders and in non-insulin dependent diabetes mellitus (1-year hazard rate in patients with unipolar depression reported as 13.5% vs. 5% for adults with schizophrenia; lower hazard rate reported in patients on concomitant lithium therapy)

Other tardive syndromes include:

- Tardive dystonia (see p. 98)
- Tardive parkinsonism
- Tardive akathisia (some think this is indistinguishable from early akathisia) (see p. 98)
- Tardive ballismus
- Tardive Tourette's syndrome
- Tardive vomiting (especially in smokers)
- Tardive hypothalamic syndrome; associated with polydipsia

2. Anticholinergic Effects

- A result of antagonism at muscarinic receptors (ACh)
- Common; effects are additive if given concurrently with other anticholinergic agents
- Dry mucous membranes [Management: sugar-free gum and candy, oral lubricants (e.g., MoiStir, OraCare D), pilocarpine mouth wash – see p. 33]; may predispose patient to monilial infection
- Blurred vision, dry eyes [Management: artificial tears, wetting solutions; pilocarpine 0.5% eye drops]
- Constipation [Management: increase bulk and fluid intake, fecal softener (e.g., Surfak), bulk laxative (e.g., Prodiem, Metamucil), osmotic laxative (e.g., Lactulose)]
- Urinary retention [Management: bethanechol]
- Use of high doses or in combination with other anticholinergic drugs may result in anticholinergic toxicity with both central and peripheral effects including disorientation, confusion, memory loss, fever, tachycardia, etc.

3. Cardiovascular Effects

- A result of antagonism at α_1-adrenergic and muscarinic receptors
- Hypotension, most frequent with parenteral use. **DO NOT USE EPINEPHRINE**, as it may further lower the blood pressure; phenylephrine may be used
- Dizziness, fainting [change antipsychotic; if not possible: sodium chloride tablets, caffeine, use of elastic stockings]
- Tachycardia, nonspecific ECG changes (including ST segment depression, flattened T waves and increased U wave amplitude), QTc lengthening – in rare cases "torsades de pointes" arrhythmia has occurred (especially with mesoridazine, droperidol, thioridazine, and pimozide); electrolyte abnormalities including hypokalemia, hypomagnesia and hypocalcemia can contribute to the development of torsades de pointes
- Sudden death of patients on antipsychotics is probably due to arrhythmias (rare)

4. GI Effects

- Weight gain (a result of multiple systems including $5HT_{1B}$, $5HT_{2C}$, α_1, H_1 blockade, hyperprolactemia and gonadal and adrenal steroid imbalance; may be related to insulin resistance (increased blood glucose); may also be due to carbohydrate craving and excessive intake of high calorie beverages to alleviate drug-induced thirst and dry mouth): more likely to occur early in treatment; more common with low-potency agents (e.g., chlorpromazine – mean gain 3–5 kg), and may be dose-dependent; women reported to be at higher risk [Management: diet, exercise, amantadine, bromocriptine]; weight loss also reported
- Anorexia, dyspepsia, dysphagia, constipation, occasionally diarrhea
- Peculiar taste, glossitis
- Loss of gag reflex (more likely to be significant in males)

- Vomiting common after prolonged treatment, especially in smokers
- Sialorrhea, difficulty swallowing, gagging

5. Sexual Side Effects

- A result of altered dopamine (D_2) activity, ACh blockade, α_1 blockade
- Reported incidence in males is 16–60% and females 7–33%
- Decreased libido [Management: neostigmine (7.5–15 mg prn) or cyproheptadine (4–16 mg prn) 30 minutes before intercourse]
- Erectile difficulties, impotence [Management: bethanechol (10 mg tid or 10–50 mg prn), yohimbine (5.4–16.2 mg prn or 5.4 mg tid), sildenafil (25–100 mg prn), amantadine (100–400 mg prn)]
- Inhibition of ejaculation, retrograde ejaculation or absence of ejaculation (especially thioridazine), pain at orgasm (males and females) and anorgasmia [Management: bethanechol (10 mg tid or 10–50 mg prn), neostigmine (7.5–15 mg prn), cyproheptadine (4–16 mg prn), amantadine (100–400 mg prn)]
- Priapism (especially with thioridazine, chlorpromazine, mesoridazine)

6. Endocrine Effects

- Prolactin level may be elevated (related to 50–75% D_2 occupancy); incidence 10–95% depending on drug and dose – effect is sustained. High prolactin levels may be associated with sexual side effects, menstrual disturbances, infertility, reduced bone density as well as polydipsia (by increasing thirst and water consumption)
- In women: breast engorgement and lactation (may be more common with higher doses and in women who have previously been pregnant), amenorrhea, menstrual irregularities, changes in libido, hirsutism and possibly osteoporosis (due to decreased estrogen) [Management: re-evaluate dose, change antipsychotic; bromocriptine (low doses) or amantadine if prolactin level elevated]
- False positive pregnancy test
- In men: gynecomastia, rarely galactorrhea, decreased libido and erectile or ejaculatory dysfunction [Management: bromocriptine if prolactin level elevated]
- Increased appetite, weight gain (see GI Effects, p. 82)
- Hypoglycemia or hyperglycemia, glycosuria, and high or prolonged glucose tolerance tests (in 3% of patients on depot antipsychotics)
- SIADH (hypothalamic syndrome) – hyponatremia with polydipsia and polyuria; reported to occur in 6–20% of chronic patients; risk increased in the elderly, smokers and alcoholics; suggestion that risk may be increased with depot haloperidol; monitor sodium levels to decrease risk of seizures in chronically treated patients [Management: fluid restriction, demeclocycline up to 1200 mg/day, captopril 12.5 mg/day, propranolol 30–120 mg/day; replace electrolytes]
- Water intoxication can occur 1–10 years after onset of polydipsia; symptoms include cerebral edema with headache, blurred vision, nausea, vomiting, anorexia, diarrhea, muscle cramps, restlessness, psychosis, convulsions – can progress to renal and cardiac failure, coma and death

7. Ocular Effects

- Lenticular pigmentation
  - related to long-term use of antipsychotics (primarily chlorpromazine)
  - presents as glare, halos around lights or hazy vision
  - granular deposits in eye
  - vision usually is not impaired; may be reversible if drug stopped
  - often present in patients with antipsychotic-induced skin pigmentation or photosensitivity reactions
- Pigmentary retinopathy (retinitis pigmentosa)
  - primarily associated with chronic use of thioridazine or chlorpromazine [annual ophthalmological examination recommended]
  - reduced visual acuity (may occasionally reverse if drug stopped)
  - blindness can occur
- With chronic use, chlorpromazine can cause pigmentation of the endothelium and Descemet's membrane of the cornea; it can color the conjunctiva, sclera and eyelids a slate-blue color – may not be reversible when drug stopped
- Association reported between phenothiazine use and cataract formation

8. Hypersensitivity Reactions

- Usually appear within the first few months of therapy (but may occur after the drug is discontinued)
- Photosensitivity and photoallergy reactions including sunburn-like erythematous eruptions which may be accompanied by blistering

"Conventional" Antipsychotics (Neuroleptics) (cont.)

- Skin reactions, rashes, abnormal skin pigmentation
- Cholestatic jaundice (reversible if drug stopped)
  - occurs in less than 0.1% of patients within first 4 weeks of treatment, with most antipsychotics
  - occurs in less than 1% of patients on chlorpromazine
  - signs include yellow skin, dark urine, pruritis
- Low potency agents may be a risk factor for venous thrombosis in predisposed individuals – case reports of deep vein thrombosis in patients on chlorpromazine – usually occurs in first 3 months of therapy
- Transient asymptomatic transaminase elevations (ALT/SGPT 2–3 times the upper limit of normal) reported with haloperidol (up to 16% of patients)
- Agranulocytosis
  - occurs in less than 0.1% of patients within first 12 weeks of treatment with most antipsychotics
  - mortality high if drug not stopped and treatment initiated
  - signs include sore throat, fever, weakness, mouth sores
- Rare reports of thrombocytopenia
- Rarely, asthma, laryngeal, angioneurotic or peripheral edema, and anaphylactic reactions occur
- Neuroleptic malignant syndrome (NMS) – rare disorder characterized by muscular rigidity, tachycardia, hyperthermia, altered consciousness, autonomic dysfunction, and increase in CPK
  - can occur with any class of antipsychotic agent, at any dose, and at any time (more common in the summer); other risk factors include organic brain syndromes, mood disorders, dehydration, exhaustion, agitation, rapid or parenteral administration of antipsychotic
  - potentially fatal unless recognized early and medication is stopped; supportive therapy must be instituted as soon as possible, especially fluid and electrolytes (mortality rate 4%)
  - dantrolene, amantadine and bromocriptine may be helpful
- Hypersensitively reactions at injection site (especially haloperidol decanoate 100 mg/ml)
- Cases of systemic lupus erythematosus reported with chlorpromazine

9. Temperature Regulation

- Altered ability of body to regulate response to changes in temperature and humidity; may become hyperthermic or hypothermic in temperature extremes due to inhibition of the hypothalamic control area

WITHDRAWAL

- Most likely to occur 24–48 h after withdrawal, or after a large dosage decrease
- Abrupt cessation of high doses may rarely cause gastritis, nausea, vomiting, dizziness, tremors, feelings of warmth or cold, sweating, tachycardia, headache, and insomnia in some patients; symptoms begin 2–3 days after abrupt discontinuation of treatment and may last up to 14 days
- Rebound neurological symptoms may occur including akathisia, dystonia and parkinsonism (within the first few days), withdrawal dyskinesia reported within 1–4 weeks
- Tardive neurological symptoms may emerge
- Supersensitivity psychosis (acute relapse) has been described after acute withdrawal in some patients

☞ **THEREFORE THESE MEDICATIONS SHOULD BE WITHDRAWN GRADUALLY AFTER PROLONGED USE**

Management

- Maintain antiparkinsonian drug for a few days after stopping the antipsychotic to minimize EPS reactions

PRECAUTIONS

- Hypotension occurs most frequently with parenteral use, especially with high doses; the patient should be in supine position during short-acting IM administration and remain supine or seated for at least 30 minutes; measure the BP before each IM dose

- IM injections should be very slow; the deltoid offers faster absorption as it has better blood perfusion
- Use with caution in the elderly, in the presence of cardiovascular disease, chronic respiratory disorder, hypoglycemia, convulsive disorders
- Caution in prescribing to patients with known or suspected hepatic disorder; monitor clinically and measure transaminase level (ALT/SGPT), periodically
- Should be used very cautiously in patients with narrow angle glaucoma or prostatic hypertrophy
- Prior to prescribing thioridazine or mesoridazine, baseline ECG and serum potassium should be done, and monitored periodically during the course of therapy. DO NOT USE thioridazine in patients with QT_c interval over 450 ms
- Monitor if QT interval exceeds 420 ms and discontinue drug if exceeds 500 ms; do not exceed 800 mg thioridazine or 20 mg pimozide daily
- Cigarette smoking is reported to induce the metabolism and decrease the plasma level of most antipsychotics
- Allergic cross-reactivity (rash) between chlorpromazine and clozapine reported

TOXICITY

- Symptoms of toxicity are extensions of common adverse effects: anticholinergic, extrapyramidal, CNS stimulation followed by CNS depression
- Postural hypotension may be complicated by shock, coma, cardiovascular insufficiency, myocardial infarction, and arrhythmias
- Convulsions appear late
- Thioridazine overdosage should include continuous ECG monitoring; avoid drugs that produce additive QT prolongation (e.g. disopyramide, procainamide and quinidine)

Management

- Supportive treatment should be given

Effects of Antipsychotics on Neurotransmitters/Receptors*

	Chlorpromazine	Methotrimeprazine	Triflupromazine	Mesoridazine	Pericyazine	Pipotiazine	Thioridazine	Fluphenazine	Perphenazine	Thioproperazine	Trifluoperazine
Blockade D_1	+++	?	++	+++	?	?	+++	+++	+++	?	+++
Blockade D_2	+++	+++	++++	++++	++++	+++++	+++++	+++++	++++	+++++	+++++
Blockade D_3	++++	?	?	?	?	+++++	++++	+++++	?	++++	?
Blockade D_4	++++	?	?	?	?	?	++++	++++	?	+++	+++
Blockade H_1	+++	+++++	+++	++++	?	?	+++	+++	++++	?	++
Blockade M_1	+++	?	+++	+++	?	?	++++	+	+	?	+
Blockade α_1	++++	?	++++	++++	?	?	++++	+++	+++	?	+++
Blockade α_2	++	?	?	+	+	?	+	+	++	+	+
Blockade 5-HT_{1A}	+	+++	+	++	?	++	+	+	+	?	+
Blockade 5-HT_{2A}	++++	++++	++++	++++	?	+++	++++	++++	++++	++	++++
DA reuptake	+	?	?	?	?	?	+	+	+	?	?

	Haloperidol	Loxapine	Molindone	Pimozide	Flupenthixol	Thiothixene	Zuclopenthixol	Clozapine	Risperidone	Olanzapine	Quetiapine	Ziprasidone
Blockade D_1	+++	+++	+	++	++++	++	+++++	+++	+++	+++	+	+++
Blockade D_2	+++++	++++	++++	++++	++++	++++	+++++	++	+++++	+++	++	++++
Blockade D_3	++++	?	?	++++	++++	?	?	++	++	++++	++	++++
Blockade D_4	+++++	++++	+	+++	?	?	++++	++++	+++++	++++	–	+++
Blockade H_1	+	+++	+–	+	+++	+++	+++	++++	+++	++++	++++	+++
Blockade M_1	+	++	–	+	+++	+	++	+++	+–	++++	+++	–
Blockade α_1	+++	+++	+	+++	+++	++	++++	+++	++++	+++	++++	+++
Blockade α_2	+	+	++	++	++	++	++	+++	++++	++	+++	+–
Blockade 5-HT_{1A}	+	+	+	+–	+	+	+	++	++	+	++	++++
Blockade 5-HT_{2A}	+++	++++	+	+++	++++	+++	++++	++++	+++++	++++	++	+++++
DA reuptake	+	?	?	++	++	?	++	+–	+	?	?	?

* The ratio of K_i values between various neurotransmitters/receptors determines the pharmacological profile for any one drug.
Key: K_i (nM) > 100,000 = –; 10,000–100,000 = +–; 1000–10,000 = +; 100–1000 = ++; 10–100 = +++; 1–10 = ++++; 0.1–1 = +++++
$1/K_i$ < 0.001 = –; .001–.01 = +–; .01–.1 = +; .1–1 = ++; 1–10 = +++; 10–100 = ++++; 100–1000 = +++++
See p. 87 for Pharmacological Effects on Neurotransmitters.

Pharmacological Effects of Antipsychotics on Neurotransmitters/Receptors

Dopamine Blockade	• Additive or synergistic interactions occur between various dopamine receptor subtypes
D_1 Blockade	• May mediate antipsychotic effect
D_2 Blockade	• In mesolimbic area – antipsychotic effect: correlates with clinical efficacy in controlling positive symptoms of schizophrenia; an inverse relationship exists between D_2 blockade and therapeutic antipsychotic dosage (i.e., potent blockade = low mg dose) • In nigrostriatal tract – side effect: extrapyramidal (e.g., tremor, rigidity, etc.) • In tuberinfundibular area – side effect: prolactin elevation (e.g., galactorrhea, etc.)
D_3 Blockade	• May mediate antipsychotic effect on positive and negative symptoms of schizophrenia
D_4 Blockade	• May mediate antipsychotic effect on positive symptoms of schizophrenia
DA Reuptake Block	• Antidepressant, antiparkinsonian • Side effects: psychomotor activation, aggravation of psychosis
H_1 Blockade	• Anti-emetic effect • Side effects: sedation, drowsiness, postural hypotension, weight gain • Potentiation of effects of other CNS drugs
ACh Blockade	• Mitigation of extrapyramidal side effects • Side effects: dry mouth, blurred vision, constipation, urinary retention and incontinence, sinus tachycardia, QRS changes, memory disturbances, sedation • Potentiation of effects of drugs with anticholinergic properties
α_1 Blockade	• Side effects: postural hypotension, dizziness, reflex tachycardia, sedation, hypersalivation, urinary incontinence • Potentiation of antihypertensives acting via α_1 blockade (e.g., prazosin, labetalol)
α_2 Blockade	• May lead to increased release of acetylcholine and increased cholinergic activity • Side effect: sexual dysfunction • Antagonism of antihypertensives acting as α_2 stimulants (e.g., clonidine, methyldopa)
5-HT_1 Blockade	• Antidepressant, anxiolytic, and antiaggressive action
5-HT_2 Blockade	• May correlate with clinical efficacy in decreasing negative symptoms of schizophrenia (data speculative); may modulate (decrease) extrapyramidal effects caused by D_2 blockade • Anxiolytic (5-HT_{2C}), antidepressant (5-HT_{2A}) and antipsychotic effect • Side effects: hypotension, sedation, ejaculatory problems, weight gain

Frequency (%) of Adverse Reactions to Antipsychotics at Therapeutic Doses

	"CONVENTIONAL AGENTS"										
	Phenothiazines – Aliphatic			Phenothiazines – Piperidine				Phenothiazines – Piperazine			
Reaction	Chlorpromazine	Methotrimeprazine	Triflupromazine	Mesoridazine	Pericyazine	Pipotiazine	Thioridazine	Fluphenazine	Perphenazine	Thioproperazine	Trifluoperazine
Drowsiness, sedation	> 30	> 30	> 30	> 30	> 30	> 10	> 30	> 2	> 10	> 2	> 2
Insomnia, agitation	< 2	< 2	< 2	< 2	< 2	< 2	< 2	> 2	> 2	> 2	> 2
Extrapyramidal Effects											
Parkinsonism	> 10	> 10	> 10	> 10	> 2	> 30	> 2	> 30	> 30	> 30	> 30
Akathisia	> 2	> 2	> 2	> 30	> 2	> 10	> 2	> 30	> 30	> 30	> 30
Dystonic reactions	> 2	< 2	> 2	< 2	< 2	< 2	< 2	> 10	> 10	> 10	> 10
Cardiovascular Effects											
Orthostatic hypotension	> 30[c]	> 30[b,c]	> 30	> 30	> 10	> 2	> 30	> 2	> 2	> 2	> 10
Tachycardia	> 10	> 10	> 10	> 10	> 2	> 2	> 10	> 10	> 10	> 10	> 2
ECG abnormalities*	> 30[d]	> 10	> 10	> 10[d]	> 2	> 2	> 30[d]	> 2	> 2	> 2	> 2
QTc prolongation (> 450 ms)	> 2[d]	> 2	> 2	> 2[d]	> 2	> 2	> 10[d]	< 2[d]	–	–	< 2
Anticholinergic Effects	> 30	> 30	> 30	> 30	> 30	> 10	> 30	> 2	> 2	> 2	> 2
Endocrine Effects											
Sexual dysfunction[e]	> 2[f]	> 2[f]	> 2	> 10(f)	> 10[f]	> 10	> 30(f)	> 2[f]	> 2[f]	> 2	> 2[f]
Galactorrhea	> 30	> 30	> 30	> 30	> 10	> 30	> 30	> 10	> 10	> 10	> 10
Weight gain	> 30	> 10	> 30	> 30	> 10	> 10	> 30	> 30	> 10	> 10	> 10
Skin Reactions											
Photosensitivity	> 10	> 10	> 10	> 2	> 2	> 2	> 10[h]	< 2	< 2	< 2	> 2
Rashes	> 10	> 2	> 2	> 2	> 2	> 2	> 10	< 2	< 2	< 2	< 2
Pigmentation[a]	> 30[h]	< 2	< 2	–	–	–	> 2	–	–	–	–
Ocular Effects[a]											
Lenticular pigmentation	> 2	> 2	> 2	> 2	> 2	> 2	> 2	< 2	< 2	< 2	< 2
Pigmentary retinopathy	> 2[a]	> 2[a]	> 2	> 2	–	–	> 10[a]	–	< 2	< 2	< 2
Blood dyscrasias	< 2	< 2	< 2	< 2	< 2	< 2	< 2	< 2	< 2	< 2	< 2
Hepatic disorder	< 2	< 2	< 2	< 2	< 2	< 2	< 2	< 2	< 2	< 2	< 2
Seizures[g]	< 2[c]	< 2	< 2	< 2	< 2	< 2	< 2	< 2	< 2	< 2	< 2

Comparison of adverse effects are based on currently used/approved doses – usually dose related
– = None reported in literature perused, * = ECG abnormalities usually without cardiac injury including ST segment depression, flattened T waves and increased U wave amplitude
(a) Usually seen after prolonged use, (b) At start of therapy, (c) More frequent with rapid dose increase, (d) Higher doses pose greater risk, (e) Includes impotence, inhibition of ejaculation, anorgasmia, (f) Priapism reported, (g) In non-epileptic patients, (h) At higher doses

Frequency (%) of Adverse Reactions to Antipsychotics at Therapeutic Doses (cont.)

Reaction	"CONVENTIONAL" AGENTS							"SECOND GENERATION AGENTS"				
					Thioxanthenes							
	Haloperidol	Loxapine	Molindone	Pimozide	Flupenthixol	Thiothixene	Zuclopenthixol	Clozapine	Risperidone	Olanzapine	Quetiapine	Ziprasidone
Drowsiness, sedation	> 2	> 30	> 30	> 10	> 2	> 10	> 30	> 30	> 10[b]	> 30	> 10	> 10
Insomnia, agitation	> 10	< 2	> 2	> 2	< 2	> 10	> 10	> 2	> 10	> 10	> 10	> 2
Extrapyramidal Effects												
Parkinsonism	> 30[m]	> 30	> 30	> 10	> 30	> 30	> 30	> 2	> 10[i]	> 2	> 2	> 2
Akathisia	> 30	> 30	< 30	> 10	> 30	> 30	> 10	> 10	> 10[i]	> 10	> 2	> 2
Dystonic reactions	> 30[m]	> 10	> 30	> 2	> 10	> 2	> 10[m]	< 2	< 2[i]	< 2	< 2	> 2
Cardiovascular Effects												
Orthostatic hypotension	> 2	> 10	> 2	> 2	> 2	> 2	> 2	> 30	> 30[b]	> 2	> 10	> 2
Tachycardia	< 2	> 10	< 2	> 2	> 2	> 2	> 2	> 30	> 10	> 2	> 2	> 2
ECG abnormalities*	< 2	< 2	< 2	> 2[e]	> 2	< 2	< 2	> 30[p]	< 2	< 2	< 2	> 2[p]
QTc prolongation (>450 ms)	< 2[p]	–	–	> 2[e]	< 2	< 2	< 2	> 2[p]	< 2	< 2	< 2	< 2[p]
Anticholinergic Effects	> 2	> 10	> 10	> 2	> 10	> 2	> 10[f]	> 30[f]	> 2	> 10	> 2	> 2
Endocrine Effects												
Sexual dysfunction[j]	> 2[k]	> 2	< 2[k]	< 2	< 2[k]	< 2[k]	> 2[k]	< 2[k]	> 10[k]	> 2[k]	< 2[k]	< 2
Galactorrhea	< 2	< 2	< 2	< 2	–	< 2	–	< 2	> 2	< 2	–	–
Weight gain	> 2	< 2[d]	< 2[d]	> 2[d]	> 10	> 10	> 10	> 30	> 30	> 30	> 10	–
Skin Reactions												
Photosensitivity	< 2	< 2	–	–	< 2	< 2	< 2	< 2	> 2	–	–	–
Rashes	< 2	> 2	> 2	> 2	> 2	< 2	< 2	> 2	< 2	< 2	< 2	> 2
Pigmentation[a]	< 2	–	–	–	–	< 2	< 2	–	< 2	–	–	–
Ocular Effects[a]												
Lenticular pigmentation	< 2	< 2	–	< 2	< 2	< 2	< 2				< 2	–
Pigmentary retinopathy	–	< 2	–	–	< 2	< 2	–	–	–	–	–	–
Blood dyscrasias	< 2	< 2	< 2	< 2	< 2	< 2	< 2	< 2[n]	< 2	< 2	–	< 2
Hepatic disorder	< 2	< 2	> 2	< 2	< 2	< 2	< 2	> 2	< 2	> 2	< 2	–
Seizures[g]	< 2	< 2	> 2[h]	< 2	< 2	< 2	< 2	> 2[o]	< 2	< 2	< 2	–

Comparison of adverse effects are based on currently used/approved doses – usually dose related
– = None reported in literature perused, * = ECG abnormalities usually without cardiac injury including ST segment depression, flattened T waves and increased U wave amplitude
(a) Usually seen after prolonged use, (b) At start of therapy or with rapid dose increase, (c) More frequent with rapid dose increase, (d) Weight loss reported, (e) Pimozide above 20 mg daily poses greater risk, (f) Sialorrhea reported, (g) In non-epileptic patients, (h) Doses above 300 mg daily pose greater risk, (i) Increased risk with doses above 16 mg daily, (j) Includes impotence, inhibition of ejaculation, anorgasmia, (k) Priapism reported, (m) Lower incidence with depot preparation, (n) Risk < 2% with strict monitoring (legal requirement in North America), (o) Risk lower with doses below 300 mg, and increased at higher doses or single doses above 300 mg, (p) Higher doses pose greater risk

Antipsychotic Doses

Drug	Comparable Daily Dose (mg) (based on D_2 affinity and pharmacokinetics)	Apparent Clinical Equivalence in Schizophrenia (mg)*	Monograph Doses for Psychosis	Protein Binding	Bioavailability	Elimination Half-Life[h]	CYP-450 Metabolizing Enzymes[j]	CYP-450 Inhibitor[k]	%D_2 Receptor Occupancy[a] (dose & plasma level)[b]	%5-HT_{2A} Occupancy (dose)
SECOND GENERATION AGENTS **Benzisoxazole** Risperidone (Risperdal)	2.5**	2	1 mg bid to start and increase gradually Usual daily dose: 4–6 mg daily Doses above 10 mg/day do not usually produce further improvement	88–90%	60–80%	20–24	**2D6**[m], 3A4	2D6	60–75% (2–4 mg) 63–85% (2–6 mg; 36–252 nmol/L)	60–90% (1–4 mg)
Dibenzodiazepine Clozapine (Clozaril)[g]	50**	100	12.5–25 mg on day 1, 25–50 mg on day 2, then increase gradually by 25–50 mg increments up to 300–450 mg daily Doses not to exceed 900 mg daily Prescribing restrictions: – Canada: max of 7 day prescription for 6 months, then, if approved, can prescribe every 2 weeks – USA: max of 7 day prescription (Other countries may have less stringent regulations)	95%	40–60%	5–16	**1A2**[m] 2D6[o], 3A4[o], 2C9, 2C19[o]	–	38–68%[h] (300–900 mg; 600–2500 nmol/L)	85–94% (>125 mg)
Dibenzothiazepine Quetiapine (Seroquel)	50**	200	25 mg bid to start; increase by 25–50 mg bid per day, as tolerated, to a target dose of 300 mg per day (given bid) within 4–7 days Usual daily dose: 300–600 mg daily, in divided doses Doses above 800 mg/day not recommended	83%	10%	6–7	**3A4**[m]	–	20–44%[h] (300–700 mg)	21–80%[h] (150–600 mg)
Thienobenzodiazepine Olanzapine (Zyprexa)	10**	5	5–10 mg daily to start; target dose of 10 mg Further dose increases at intervals of not less than 1 week Doses above 20 mg/day not recommended	93%	57–80%	21–54	1A2, 2D6, 2C9, 2C19	–	55–80% (5–20 mg; 59–187 nmol/L) 83–88% (30–40 mg)	90–98% (5–20 mg)
Benzothiazolylpiperazine Ziprasidone (Geodon)[c]	?	40	80–160 mg daily	99%	30% (60% with food)	6.6 h	**3A4**[m]	2D6[w]	45–75% (40–80 mg)	80–90% (40–80 mg)

Drug	Comparable Daily Dose (mg) (based on D_2 affinity and pharmacokinetics)	Apparent Clinical Equivalence in Schizophrenia (mg)*	Monograph Doses for Psychosis	Protein Binding	Bioavailability	Elimination Half-Life[h]	CYP-450 Metabolizing Enzymes[j]	CYP-450 Inhibitor[k]	%D_2 Receptor Occupancy[a] (dose & plasma level)[b]	%5-HT_{2A} Occupancy (dose)
CONVENTIONAL AGENTS										
Butyrophenone										
Haloperidol (Haldol)	2	4	2–100 mg daily	92%	40–80%	12–36	1A2, 2D6, **3A4**[m]	2D6[p]	75–89% (4–6 mg; 6–13 nmol/L)	?
Haloperidol Decanoate (Haldol LA)	1.1 (30 mg q 4 weeks)	40 mg q 4 weeks	50 to 300 mg q 2–4 weeks	92%	–	p. 94	1A2, 2D6, **3A4**[m]	2D6[p]	60–85% (30–70 mg q 4 wks; 9 nmol/L)	
Dibenzoxazepine										
Loxapine (Loxapac, Loxitane)	15	40	60–100 mg daily, higher than 250 mg is not recommended	?	33%	8–30	1A2, 2D6, 3A4	–	60–80% (15–30 mg)	58–75% (10–30 mg) 75–90% (>30 mg)
Dihydroindolone										
Molindone (Moban)[c]	10	50	Usual daily dose: 50–200 mg	76%	?	6.5	2D6	–	?	?
Diphenylbutylpiperidine										
Pimozide (Orap)	2	2	2–20 mg daily; average dose: 6 mg/day Doses above 20 mg/day not recommended[d]	97%	15–50%	29–55 [f]	2D6, **3A4**[m]	2D6	77–79% (4–8 mg)	?
Phenothiazines – Aliphatic										
Chlorpromazine (Largactil, Thorazine)	100	100	Usual dose: Oral 75–1000 mg daily, IM: 30 to 150 mg daily	95–99%	25–65%	16–30	1A2, 2D6	2D6	78–80% (100–200 mg; 10 nmol/L)	?
Methotrimeprazine (Nozinan, Levopromazine)	70	Rarely used	For severe psychosis, doses up to 1 g or more daily, in divided doses	?	?	16–78	1A2, 2D6	2D6[p]	?	?
Triflupromazine (Vesprin)[c]	25	Rarely used	Usual dose: 60 mg IM up to a maximum of 150 mg/day	?	–	–	?	?	?	?

Antipsychotic Doses (cont.)

Drug	Comparable Daily Dose (mg) (based on D_2 affinity and pharmacokinetics)	Apparent Clinical Equivalence in Schizophrenia (mg)*	Monograph Doses for Psychosis	Protein Binding	Bioavail-ability	Elimi-nation Half-Life[h]	CYP-450 Metabol-izing Enzymes[j]	CYP-450 Inhibitor[k]	%D_2 Receptor Occupancy[a] (dose & plasma level)[b]	%5-HT_{2A} Occupancy (dose)
Phenothiazines – Piperazine										
Fluphenazine HCl (Moditen, Prolixin)	2	4	Up to 20 mg daily	90–99%	1–50%	13–58	1A2, 2D6	2D6[p]	?	?
Fluphenazine enanthate (Moditen inj., Prolixin enanthate)	0.93 (13 mg q 2 weeks)	16 mg q 4 weeks	12.5–100 mg q 1–3 weeks	90–99%	–	p. 94	1A2, 2D6	2D6[p]	?	?
Fluphenazine decanoate (Modecate, Prolixin decanoate)	0.46 (13 mg q 4 weeks)	15 mg q 4 weeks	2.5–50 mg q 2–4 weeks; doses up to 100 mg/injection may be necessary	90–99% R	–	p. 94	1A2, 2D6	2D6[p]	?	?
Perphenazine (Trilafon)	10	8	Usual dose: 12 to 64 mg daily	91–92%	25%	9–21	2D6	2D6[p]	79% (4–8 mg)	?
Thioproperazine (Majeptil)	5	10	5–40 mg daily; sometimes 90 mg or more daily may be needed	?	?	–	?	?	?	?
Trifluoperazine (Stelazine)	5	6	Up to 40 mg daily; doses up to 80 mg daily used rarely	95–99%	?	13	1A2		75–80% (5–10 mg)	R ?
Phenothiazines – Piperidine										
Mesoridazine (Serentil)[l]	50	Not recommended	Schizophrenia: 75–400 mg daily	70%	?	16–27	2D6	–	?	?
Pericyazine (Neuleptil)	15	Not used	5–60 mg daily	?	?	–	?	?	?	?
Pipotiazine palmitate (Piportil L4)[e]	0.85 (25 mg q 4 weeks)	20 mg q 4 weeks	25–250 mg q 3–4 weeks	?	–	p. 94	?	?	?	?
Thioridazine (Mellaril)[l]	100	Not recommended	Usual dose: Up to 400 mg daily; 200–800 mg daily in hospitalized patients	97–99%	10–60%	9–30	1A2, 2D6	2D6[p]	74–81% (100–400 mg; 620–900 nmol/L)	?

Drug	Comparable Daily Dose (mg) (based on D_2 affinity and pharmacokinetics)	Apparent Clinical Equivalence in Schizophrenia (mg)*	Monograph Doses for Psychosis	Protein Binding	Bioavail-ability	Elimi-nation Half-Life[h]	CYP-450 Metabol-izing Enzymes[j]	CYP-450 Inhibitor [k]	%D_2 Receptor Occupancy[a] (dose & plasma level)[b]	%5-HT_{2A} Occupancy (dose)
Thioxanthenes										
Flupenthixol (Fluanxol)	5	8	3–6 mg daily as maintenance dose; up to 12 mg daily used in some patients	99%	30–70%	26–36	?	2D6[w]	70–74% (6 mg; 2–5 nmol/L)	?
Flupenthixol decanoate (Fluanxol inj.)[e]	1.8 (50 mg q 4 weeks)	24 mg q 4 weeks	20–80 mg q 2–3 weeks	99%	–	p. 94	?	2D6[w]	81% (40 mg q 7 days; 19 nmol/L)	?
Thiothixene (Navane)	5	10	15–60 mg; greater than 60 mg daily rarely increases beneficial responses	90–99%	50%	34	1A2	2D6	?	?
Zuclopenthixol (Clopixol)[e]	12	40	10–50 mg to start; increase by 10– 20 mg every 2 to 3 days; usual daily dose: 20–60 mg; doses above 100 mg daily not recommended	98%	44% R	12–28	2D6	2D6	?	?
Zuclopenthixol acetate (Clopixol acuphase)[e]	30 mg q 2–3 days	15 mg q 3 days	Usual dose: 50–150 mg IM and repeated every 2–3 days as needed to a maximum of 4 injections (a second injection may need to be given 1–2 days after the first, in some patients)	98%	–	36	2D6	2D6	?	?
Zuclopenthixol decanoate (Clopixol depot)[e]	9 (120 mg q 2 weeks)	120 mg q 4 weeks	Usual maintenance dose: 150–300 mg q 2 to 4 weeks	98%	–	p. 94	2D6	2D6	81% (200 mg q 14 days; 50 nmol/L)	?

NOTE: Comparable doses are only approximations. Generally doses used are higher in the acute stage of the illness than in maintenance. Monograph doses are just a guideline, and each patient's medication must be individualized. Plasma levels are available for some antipsychotics but their clinical usefulness is limited. The use of conversion ratios from an oral to a depot preparation is appropriate as a starting point, but wide intra- and interindividual variations in pharmacokinetic parameters require careful clinical monitoring of the patient. It is recommended that the initially effective dose be reduced, or the injection interval increased, after 4–6 weeks to prevent possible accumulation of the drug as plasma concentrations approach steady-state.

* Views of Dr. Jeffries, based on clinical judgment.
** Based on clinical studies/APA Practice Guidelines 1997 (not on D_2 affinity).

(a) D_2 receptor occupancy appears to correlate with clinical efficacy in controlling positive symptoms of schizophrenia, (b) Approximate conversion: nmol/L = 3 × ng/ml, (c) Not marketed in Canada, (d) Monitor cardiac function in doses above 15 mg/day, (e) Not marketed in USA, (f) Half-life longer (mean 66–111 h) in children and adults with Tourette's syndrome, (g) Prescribing/monitoring restrictions in Canada and the USA, (h) Occupancy higher 2 h vs 12 h post dose, (j) Cytochrome P-450 isoenzymes involved in drug metabolism, (k) CYP-450 isoenzymes inhibited by drug, (l) indicated only for patients with schizophrenia who cannot tolerate other antipsychotic drugs or who fail to respond to them, (m) Main isoenzyme involved in metabolism, where known, (o) Specific to metabolite, (p) Potent inhibition of isoenzyme, (w) Weak inhibition of isoenzyme

Comparison of Depot Antipsychotics

	Flupenthixol decanoate (Fluanxol)	Fluphenazine enanthate (Moditen; Prolixin)	Fluphenazine decanoate (Modecate; Prolixin)	Haloperidol decanoate (Haldol LA)	Pipotiazine palmitate (Piportil L4)	Zuclopenthixol decanoate (Clopixol Depot)
Chemical class	Thioxanthene	Piperazine phenothiazine	Piperazine phenothiazine	Butyrophenone	Piperidine phenothiazine	Thioxanthene
Form	Esterified with decanoic acid (a 10-carbon chain fatty acid) and dissolved in vegetable oil; must be hydrolyzed to free flupenthixol; metabolites inactive	Esterified with a 7-carbon chain fatty acid and dissolved in sesame oil; must be hydrolyzed to free fluphenazine	Esterified with decanoic acid and dissolved in sesame oil; must be hydrolyzed to free fluphenazine	Esterified with decanoic acid and dissolved in sesame oil; must be hydrolyzed to free haloperidol	Esterified with palmitic acid in sesame oil; must be hydrolyzed to free pipotiazine	Esterified with decanoic acid in coconut oil; must be hydrolyzed to free zuclopenthixol
Strength supplied	(2%)–20 mg/ml (10%)–100 mg/ml	25 mg/ml	25 mg/ml 100 mg/ml	50 mg/ml 100 mg/ml	25 mg/ml 50 mg/ml	200 mg/ml
Usual dose range	20–100 mg	25–100 mg	12.5–100 mg	50–300 mg	50–250 mg	150–300 mg
Usual duration action	2–4 weeks	2 weeks	4 weeks	4 weeks	4 weeks	2–4 weeks
Dose comparative to 100 mg CPZ (approx.)	1.8 mg/day (50 mg q 4 weeks)	0.93 mg/day (13 mg q 2 weeks)	0.46 mg/day (13 mg q 4 weeks)	1.1 mg/day (30 mg q 4 weeks)	0.85 mg/day (24 mg q 4 weeks)	9 mg/day (120 mg q 2 weeks)
Clinical equivalence in schizophrenia[(a)]	24 mg q 4 weeks	16 mg q 4 weeks	15 mg q 4 weeks	40 mg q 4 weeks	20 mg q 4 weeks	120 mg q 4 weeks
Pharmacokinetics						
Peak plasma level*	4–7 days	2–5 days	First peak within 24 hours (due to presence of hydrolized "free" fluphenazine); level drops, then peaks again in 8–12 days	3–9 days	Approx. 4 days	3–7 days
Elimination half-life**	8 days (after single injection), 17 days (multiple dosing)	3.5–4 days (after single injection)	Over 14 days (single injection), up to 102 days (multiple dosing)	18–21 days	Approx. 15 days	19 days

(a) View of Dr Jeffries, based on clinical judgement
* Important as indicator when maximum side effects will occur
** Useful for determining dosing interval; steady state will be reached in approximately 5 half-lives

Comparison of Depot Antipsychotics (cont.)

	Flupenthixol decanoate (Fluanxol)	Fluphenazine enanthate (Moditen; Prolixin)	Fluphenazine decanoate (Modecate; Prolixin)	Haloperidol decanoate (Haldol LA)	Pipotiazine palmitate (Piportil L4)	Zuclopenthixol decanoate (Clopixol Depot)
Adverse Effects: Generally side effects are similar to oral drugs in same class	Flupenthixol	Fluphenazine	Fluphenazine	Haloperidol	Pericyazine	Zuclopenthixol
CNS	Both sedating and alerting effect reported; can cause excitation	Both drowsiness and insomnia reported	Both drowsiness and insomnia reported	Both drowsiness and insomnia reported	Low sedative potential Excitation reported in approx. 12% of patients	Both drowsiness and insomnia reported (less frequent than with oral zuclopenthixol)
Extrapyramidal	Frequent	More frequent than with decanoate (up to 50% of patients)	Frequent Note: increased frequency of dystonia noted with use of "older" multipunctured multidose vials due to presence of "free" fluphenazine	Frequent, however, reported less often than with oral haloperidol	Frequent, esp. if dose over 100 mg q 4 weeks	Reported in 5 – 15% of patients
Skin and local reactions	Indurations rarely seen (at high doses) Photosensitivity and hyperpigmentation very rare; dermatological reactions seen	No indurations reported; dermatological reactions have been reported	One case of induration seen at a high dose; dermatological reactions have been reported	Inflammation and nodules at injection site (may be more common with 100 mg/ml preparation) Less common if deltoid used One case of photosensitization reported; "tracking" reported	No indurations reported; dermatological changes reported	No indurations but local dermatological reactions reported
Laboratory changes	Within normal variation	No hepatotoxicity; hematological changes within normal variation; some ECG changes seen	One case of jaundice reported; hematological changes within normal variation; ECG changes seen in some patients	Within normal variation	Transient changes in liver function studies seen	Transient changes in liver function seen
Use in pregnancy	No evidence of teratogenicity in animals or humans	Single report of infant born with multiple anomalies (first trimester exposure also to doxylamine)	No evidence of teratogenicity; extrapyramidal disorder seen in infants after delivery	No evidence of teratogenicity	No teratogenicity and low toxicity seen in animals	No teratogenicity and low toxicity seen in animals

Extrapyramidal Side Effects of Antipsychotics

	Acute Extrapyramidal Effects	Tardive Syndromes
Onset	Acute or insidious (up to 30 days)	After months or years of treatment, especially if drug dose decreased or discontinued
Proposed mechanism	Most EPS symptoms are due to dopamine (D_2) blockade Akathisia may be mediated by different mechanisms and is therefore more responsive to other treatments (e.g., benzodiazepines, β-blockers – see page 97	Supersensitivity of postsynaptic dopamine receptors induced by long-term blockade
Treatment	Respond to antiparkinsonian drugs See p. 97	Antiparkinsonian drugs generally worsen tardive dyskinesia Most treatments unsatisfactory; some are aimed at balancing dopaminergic and cholinergic systems Can mask symptoms by further suppressing dopamine with antipsychotics Risperidone, quetiapine and olanzapine are less likely to induce tardive dyskinesia; clozapine has not been associated with tardive dyskinesia and may have antidyskinetic effects; antidyskinetic properties also reported with risperidone and olanzapine See p. 98

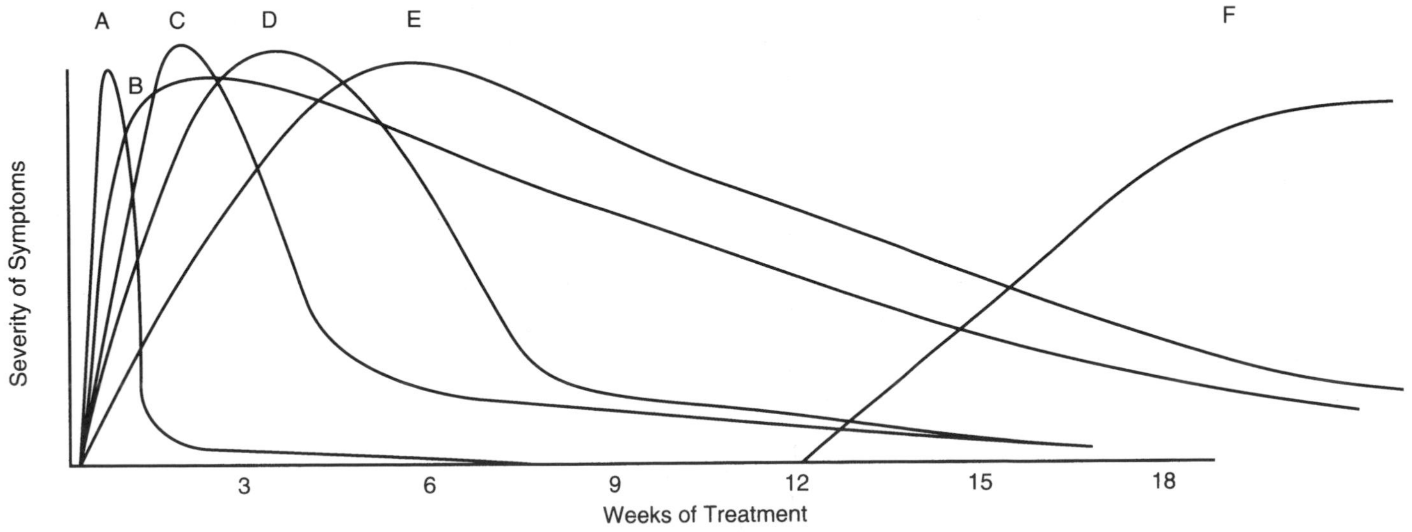

A: Dystonic reactions: uncoordinated spastic movements of muscle groups (e.g., trunk, tongue, face)
B: Akathisia: restlessness, pacing (may result in insomnia)
C: Akinesia: decreased muscular movements
D: Rigidity: coarse muscular movement; loss of facial expression
E: Tremors: fine movement (shaking) of the extremities ("pill-rolling")
Rabbit syndrome
Pisa syndrome: can either be acute or tardive in nature (rare; occurs more commonly in people with brain damage/abnormality)
F: Tardive syndromes

Type	Physical (motor) symptoms	Psychological symptoms	Onset	Risk Factors	Clinical Course	Treatment	Differential diagnosis
Dystonias	Torsions and spasms of muscle groups; muscle spasms, e.g., oculogyric crisis, trismus, laryngo-spasm, torti/retro/an-tero-collis tortipelvis, opisthotonus, blepharospasm	Anxiety, fear, panic Dysphoria Repetitive meaningless thoughts	Acute (usually within first 5 days)	Young males, children Neuroleptic naive High potency antipsychotics Rapid dose increase Lack of prophylactic antiparkinsonian medication Previous dystonic reaction Hypocalcemia, hyperthyroidism, hypoparathyroidism Recent cocaine use	Acute, painful, spasmodic; oculogyria may be recurrent Acute laryngeal/pharyngeal dystonia may be potentially life-threatening	Sublingual lorazepam, IM benztropine, IM diphenhydramine To prevent recurrence: prophylactic antiparkinsonian agents Reduce dose or change antipsychotic	Seizures Catatonia Hysteria Malingering Hypocalcemia
Akathisia	Motor restlessness, fidgeting, pacing, rocking, shifting from foot to foot Respiratory symptoms: dyspnea or breathing discomfort	Restlessness, irritability Agitation, violent outbursts Feeling "wound-up" or "antsy"	Acute to insidious (within hours to days)	Elderly female High caffeine intake High potency antipsychotics Anxiety Diagnosis of affective disorder(?) Microcytic anemia Low serum ferritin	May continue through entire treatment Suggested that may contribute to suicide and/or violence	Antiparkinsonian drugs not very effective Diazepam, clonazepam, lorazepam, β-blockers, cyproheptadine (preliminary reports) Reduce dose or change antipsychotic	Psychotic agitation/decompensation Severe agitation Anxiety Drug-seeking behavior/withdrawal
Pseudoparkinsonism	Stiffness, shuffling, mask-like face, "pill-rolling"-type tremor (4–8 cycles per second; greater at rest and bilateral), akinesia, rigidity, stooped posture, postural instability, micrographia, bradykinesia, drooling	Slowed thinking Fatigue, anergia Cognitive impairment Depression	Acute to insidious (within 30 days)	Elderly female High potency antipsychotics Increased dose Concurrent neurological disorder	May continue through entire treatment	Antiparkinsonian drug Reduce dose or change antipsychotic	Negative symptoms of schizophrenia Idiopathic Parkinson's disease Depression
Pisa Syndrome	Leaning to one side		Can be acute or tardive	Elderly patients Compromised brain function	Often ignored by patients	Antiparkinsonian drug (higher doses)	
Rabbit Syndrome	Fine tremor of lower lip		After months of therapy	Elderly patients		Antiparkinsonian drug	

Extrapyramidal Side Effects of Antipsychotics (cont.)

Type	Physical (motor) symptoms	Psychological symptoms	Onset	Risk Factors	Clinical Course	Treatment	Differential diagnosis
Tardive dyskinesia	Involuntary choreoathetoid movements of face (e.g., tics, frowning, grimacing), lips (pursing, puckering, smacking), jaw (chewing, clenching), tongue ("fly-catcher," rolling, dysarthria), eyes (blinking, spasms), limbs (tapping, twitching), trunk (rocking, twisting), neck (nodding), respiratory (dyspnea, gasping, sighing, grunting, forceful breathing) Often coexists with parkinsonism and akathisia Abnormal movements disappear during sleep	Cognitive impairment Distress (talking, swallowing, eating) and embarrassment Negative symptoms?	After 3 or more months of therapy Common early sign is "worm-like" movement of the tongue ("fly-catcher tongue")	Elderly female, children Previous acute EPS Chronic use of high doses of antiparkinsonian drugs Nonpsychotic diagnosis, affective disorder Diabetes Cognitive impairment/brain damage Alcohol/drug abuse May be associated with genetic variation of the D_3 receptor gene	Persistent – discontinuation of antipsychotic early increases chance of remission Spontaneous remission in 14–24% after 5 years	Switch to a second generation antipsychotic (clozapine reported to decrease blepharospasm) Suggestions for treatment include: Vitamin E up to 1600 IU (contradictory data) Pyridoxine 200 mg/day Clonazepam 0.5–6 mg/day Tetrabenazine 25–75 mg/day Clonidine .05–.2 mg/day	Spontaneous or withdrawal dyskinesia Stereotypic behavior Tourette's Syndrome Huntington's Chorea or other neurological conditions Movement disorder secondary to co-prescribed drug
Tardive dystonia	Sustained muscle contractions of face, eyes, neck, limbs, back, or trunk (craniocervical area involved most frequently), e.g., blepharospasm, laryngeal dystonia, dysarthria, retroflexed hands	Distress, embarrassment	After months or years of therapy	Young male Genetic predisposition (?) Neurological disorder, mental retardation Coexisting tardive dyskinesia Akathisia	Persistent; discontinuation of antipsychotic early increases chance of remission	Switch to a second generation antipsychotic (clozapine reported to decrease blepharospasm) Suggestions for treatment include: Tetrabenazine 25–75 mg; Higher doses of anticholinergics (e.g., trihexyphenidyl 40 mg/day); Botulinum toxin 25–50 mg/site (multiple sites used) Reserpine 1–5 mg/day Benzodiazepines	Myoclonus Motor tics Idiopathic dystonia Meige syndrome
Tardive akathisia	Persistent symptoms of akathisia	As for akathisia	After months of therapy; after drug withdrawal	As for akathisia Coexisting tardive dyskinesia and dystonia	Persistent, discontinuation of antipsychotic early increases chance of remission Fluctuating course	Switch to a second generation antipsychotic Suggested treatments include: Clonidine .05–.5 mg/day; Benzodiazepines; β-blockers	As for akathisia

Switching Antipsychotics

NEUROLEPTIC NON-RESPONSE

- Ascertain diagnosis is correct
- Ascertain patient is compliant with therapy
- Ensure there has been an adequate trial period
- Ensure dosage prescribed is therapeutic (too low or excessive doses should be re-evaluated); therapeutic range, for the average healthy adult, is considered to be between 2 and 20 mg haloperidol equivalents (less for first-episode schizophrenia)

Factors Complicating Response

- Concurrent drug abuse (alcohol, street drugs)
- Concomitant use of metabolic enhancers (e.g., carbamazepine, cigarette smoking – see Drug Interactions, p. 72)
- Psychosocial factors that hinder response

Switching Neuroleptics

- If side effects limit dose or contribute to non-compliance, switching between classes is appropriate
- Evidence does not suggest a differential response between "conventional" neuroleptics
- Switching from a "conventional" to a "second generation" agent may result in enhanced response
- Switching from "second generation" agents to clozapine may offer response in up to a further 50% of patients

REASONS FOR SWITCHING

- Persistent positive symptoms – switch to a "conventional" or a "second generation" antipsychotic
- Persistent negative symptoms – switch to a "second generation" antipsychotic or lower the dose
- Relapse despite compliance
- Non-compliance – consider a depot preparation
- Persistent extrapyramidal side effects (EPS) despite dosage decrease
- Tardive dyskinesia (TD) – clozapine offers least risk
- Persistent/chronic side effects, e.g., galactorrhea, impotence, weight gain (see chart pp. 88–89)

METHODS

- Four options:
  (1) Withdraw the first drug gradually and begin the second drug following a washout period – not clinically practical when patient is experiencing symptoms
  (2) Stop the first drug and start the second drug at its usual initial dose; increase the dose over a 2–4 week period – not usually recommended unless the patient has had a serious adverse reaction to the first drug, as may result in drug withdrawal symptoms
  (3) Maintain the first drug for 2–3 weeks while titrating the dose of the second drug; then withdraw the first drug over 1–2 weeks – may be suitable when initiating quetiapine
  (4) Decrease the dose of the first drug and start the second at a low dose; continue decreasing the dose of the first drug as the second one is increasing over a 2–4 week period (data suggest olanzapine can be started at 10 mg and maintained at this dose) – the preferred method of drug conversion. Be aware of additive or synergistic side effects of both drugs. Avoid, whenever possible, the ongoing use of two or more antipsychotics simultaneously
- Consider (1) rebound or withdrawal effects of discontinued medication (especially if the drug is withdrawn abruptly, e.g., clozapine, quetiapine), (2) risk of relapse, (3) need for auxiliary medication (e.g., antiparkinsonian drug) during the conversion process, and (4) additive or synergistic effects of both drugs

"Conventional" drug to "conventional" drug:

- For equivalent doses see table pp. 90–93
- Consider side effects of each drug and the need for auxiliary medication such as antiparkinsonian agents

Low potency to high potency:

- Rebound cholinergic and sedative effects are possible
- Taper first drug gradually as second drug is added

High potency to low potency:

- Continue antiparkinsonian drug, if currently prescribed, until the changeover is complete to prevent the emergence of EPS, then withdraw the antiparkinsonian drug gradually

Switching Antipsychotics (cont.)

"Conventional" drug to "second generation" drug:

- Gradual onset of action noted with some "second generation" agents; decrease the conventional agent gradually while increasing the "second generation" drug

"Second generation" drug to "conventional" drug:

- Taper first drug gradually as second drug is added
- Caution when switching from clozapine, as response to conventional and "second generation" agents seem to be less satisfactory following its use
- Clozapine and quetiapine withdrawal (especially abrupt withdrawal) has been associated with a high incidence of rebound psychosis – may need to be withdrawn over several weeks

Antipsychotic Augmentation Strategies

A. Refractory Positive Symptoms

ANTICONVULSANTS

- E.g., valproate, carbamazepine, lamotrigine
- May be useful in patients with excitation, aggressive or impulsive behavior or EEG abnormalities
- Carbamazepine can reduce antipsychotic plasma levels, while valproate can increase antipsychotic plasma levels (see Interactions, p. 70)
- Do not combine carbamazepine with clozapine (although this is not absolutely contraindicated – monitor especially closely for blood dyscrasias)

LITHIUM

- Plasma level: 0.9–1.2 mmol/L
- Contradictory data as to efficacy reported
- Can be of benefit in patients with concomitant mood symptoms (e.g., schizoaffective); however, affective symptoms need not be present for response
- Clinical improvement may be evident in the first week
- May also decrease the rate of relapse in chronic patients
- Monitor side effects, including neurotoxicity, especially if the antipsychotic is prescribed in higher dose

BENZODIAZEPINES

- Doses variable (e.g., diazepam 15–300 mg used in studies)
- Useful in agitated, anxious, acutely psychotic patients (e.g., lorazepam)
- Noted to decrease hallucinations and delusions
- Improvement may be modest and short-lived
- Some benefit reported with alprazolam in stable outpatients with predominant anxiety and negative symptoms

RESERPINE

- Dose: 1–12 mg/day
- Contradictory results reported as to benefit as augmentation strategy
- Symptoms that improve include: motor hyperactivity, agitation, assaultiveness, as well as disorientation, delusions and hallucinations
- Increased EPS, or depression, can occur; other side effects include hypotension and exacerbation of asthma or ulcers

2ND GENERATION + CONVENTIONAL ANTIPSYCHOTICS

- There are few controlled studies that evaluate the efficacy of combining two antipsychotics; some evidence supports adjunctive (low-dose) conventional agent augmentation of clozapine or olanzapine in treatment-refractory patients
- May instate risk of D_2-related side effects with such combinations, including acute EPS, elevated prolactin and tardive dyskinesia

ELECTROCONVULSIVE THERAPY

- Of benefit in acute schizophrenia, especially if catatonic or affective symptoms present
- Some reports suggest superiority with bilateral treatment; usually 12–20 treatments required
- Symptoms that improve include: delusions, hallucinations, agitation, hostility and depression
- Modest evidence of efficacy in treatment-refractory patients and benefits appear short-lived
- Lack of guidelines regarding maintenance ECT in those who have responded

B. Refractory Negative Symptoms

It is important to distinguish primary and secondary negative symptoms. Secondary negative symptoms should be treated, as necessary

DOPAMINE AGONISTS

- Short-term improvement only noted with use of D_2-agonists such as bromocriptine (see p. 212) and apomorphine

L-Dopa

- Dose: 300–2000 mg/day
- Response may not be evident for 7–8 weeks
- Best response in patients who have been ill for less than 5 years
- Increased agitation, hostility and exacerbation of positive symptoms can occur

Stimulants

- E.g., dextroamphetamine, methylphenidate
- Transient improvement in negative symptoms and cognitive function reported
- Exacerbation of positive symptoms can occur

ANTIDEPRESSANTS

- TCAs, SSRIs and MAOIs reported to decrease negative symptoms, poor social or work functioning in some patients

SELEGILINE

- Selective, irreversible MAO-B inhibitor
- Dose: 5 mg bid
- Reduction in negative symptoms, depressive symptoms and extrapyramidal symptoms reported (see p. 217)

Antiparkinsonian Agents

PRODUCT AVAILABILITY

Chemical Class	Generic Name	Trade Name[(A)]	Dosage Forms and Strengths
Dopamine agonists	Amantadine	Symmetrel	Capsules: 100 mg Oral syrup: 50 mg/5 ml
Antihistamine	Diphenhydramine	Benadryl	Capsules: 25 mg, 50 mg Chewable tablets: 12.5 mg Oral solution: 6.25 mg/5 ml, 12.5 mg/5 ml Injection: 50 mg/ml
	Orphenadrine	Disipal[(C)], Norflex	Tablets: 50 mg, 100 mg[(B)] Injection[(B)]: 30 mg/ml Extended-release tablets[(B)]: 100 mg
β-blockers	Propranolol	Inderal	Tablets: 10 mg, 20 mg, 40 mg, 60 mg[(B)], 80 mg, 120 mg[(C)] Injection: 1 mg/ml
		Inderal LA	Sustained-release capsules: 60 mg, 80 mg, 120 mg, 160 mg
Benzodiazepines	Diazepam	Valium	Tablets: 2 mg, 5 mg, 10 mg Oral solution: 5 mg/ml Injection: 5 mg/ml
		Diazepam Intensol[(B)]	Oral concentrate[(B)]: 5 mg/ml
		Diastat	Rectal gel: 5 mg/ml
		Diazemuls[(C)]	Emulsion injection (IV)[(C)]: 5 mg/ml
	Lorazepam	Ativan	Tablets: 0.5 mg, 1 mg, 2 mg Sublingual tablets[(C)]: 0.5 mg, 1 mg, 2 mg Injection: 2 mg/ml[(B)], 4 mg/ml
	Clonazepam	Rivotril[(C)], Klonopin[(B)]	Tablets: 0.5 mg, 1 mg, 2 mg
Anticholinergic agent	Benztropine	Cogentin	Tablets: 0.5 mg, 1 mg, 2 mg Injection: 1 mg/ml
	Biperiden	Akineton	Tablets: 2 mg Injection[(B)]: 5 mg/ml
	Ethopropazine	Parsitan	Tablets: 50 mg
	Procyclidine	Kemadrin	Tablets: 2.5 mg[(C)], 5 mg Oral solution[(C)]: 2.5 mg/5 ml
	Trihexyphenidyl	Artane	Tablets: 2 mg, 5 mg Oral solution[(B)]: 2 mg/5 ml

[(A)] Generic preparations may be available, [(B)] Not marketed in Canada, [(C)] Not marketed in USA

INDICATIONS*

To relieve the neurological (muscular) side effects induced by antipsychotics (see pp. 104–106 for comparison of drugs):

- ▲ Acute dyskinesias, dystonias
- ▲ Pseudoparkinsonian effects (tremor, rigidity, shuffling)
- ▲ Akathisia (restlessness)
- ▲ Akinesia (decreased muscle movement)
- ▲ "Rabbit syndrome," "Pisa syndrome"
- Neuroleptic-induced sexual dysfunction (amantadine)

GENERAL COMMENTS

- No clear evidence that one drug is more efficacious than another; individual patients may respond better, or tolerate one drug over another
- Controversy exists whether antiparkinsonian agents should be given prophylactically to patients at risk of developing EPS with antipsychotic drugs (see p. 97), or whether they should be used only when EPS develops
- Akathisia may only respond to treatment with anticholinergic agents when symptoms of parkinsonism are also present

PHARMACOLOGY

- Centrally-active anticholinergic drugs cross the blood-brain barrier, block excitatory cholinergic pathways in the basal ganglia, and restore the dopaminedopamine/acetylcholine balance disrupted by neuroleptic drugs, thus treating EPS
- Muscarinic receptors are subclassified into M_1 (predominate in the striatum) and M_2 (predominate in cardiac ventricles) subtypes. Antiparkinsonian drugs show a range of selectivity on M_1 vs M_2 as follows: biperiden > procyclidine > trihexyphenidyl > benztropine. M_1 selectivity predicts lower peripheral side effects
- Anticholinergic drugs also block presynaptic reuptake of dopamine (primarily benztropine), norepinephrine (primarily diphenhydramine), and serotonin (weakly)
- Amantadine has moderate NMDA (n-methyl-D-aspartate) receptor blocking properties and exerts its activity by increasing dopamine at the receptor

DOSING

- See chart pp. 107–108
- Dosage increases must be balanced against the risk of evoking anticholinergic side effects
- Plasma-level monitoring is not currently advocated

ADVERSE EFFECTS

1. CNS Effects

- CNS effects: seen primarily in the elderly and at high doses; include stimulation, disorientation, confusion, hallucinations, restlessness, weakness, incoherence, headache; cognitive impairment including decreased memory and distractibility
- Excess use/abuse of these drugs may lead to an anticholinergic (toxic) psychosis with symptoms of disorientation, confusion, euphoria (see Toxicity), in addition to physical signs such as dry mouth, blurred vision, dilated pupils, dry flushed skin
- dopamine-agonist activity of amantadine can occasionally cause worsening of psychotic symptoms, nightmares, insomnia, and mood disturbances

2. Anticholinergic Effects

- Related to anticholinergic potency: atropine > trihexyphenidyl > benztropine > biperiden > procyclidine > orphenadrine > diphenhydramine
- Common: dry mouth, blurred vision, constipation, dry eyes, flushed skin
- Occasional: delayed micturition, urinary retention, sexual dysfunction
- Excess doses can suppress sweating, resulting in hyperthermia

3. Cardiovascular

- Palpitations, tachycardia; high doses can cause arrhythmias

4. GI Effects

- Nausea, vomiting

PRECAUTIONS

- Use cautiously in patients with conditions in which excess anticholinergic activity could be harmful, e.g., prostatic hypertrophy, urinary retention, narrow-angle glaucoma

* ▲ Approved indications

Antiparkinsonian Agents (cont.)

- May decrease sweating; use cautiously in hot weather to prevent hyperthermia
- Use with caution in patients with respiratory difficulties, as antiparkinsonians can dry bronchial secretions and make breathing more difficult
- Caution when using amantadine in patients with peripheral edema or history of congestive heart failure
- If withdrawn abruptly may cause restlessness, anxiety, dyskinesia, dysphoria, sweating and diarrhea; akinetic depression reported
- Euphorigenic and hallucinogenic properties may lead to abuse of anticholinergic agents
- Use of antiparkinsonian agents in patients with existing TD can exacerbate the movement disorder and may unmask latent TD

TOXICITY

- Can occur following excessive doses, with combination therapy, in the elderly, or with drug abuse
- Autonomic signs: dilated pupils, dry flushed skin, thirst, tachycardia, urinary retention, constipation, paralytic ileus, anorexia, staggering gait
- Mental signs: clouded sensorium, dazed, perplexed or fearful countenance, insomnia, euphoria, irritability, excitation, disorientation in time and space, difficulties in thinking and concentration, exacerbation of psychotic behavior, visual hallucinations (grasping at air), and tactile hallucinations (picking objects from skin)

Management

- If toxicity is suspected, stop all drugs with anticholinergic activity; symptoms should abate within 24–48 h
- Physostigmine 1–3 mg IM has been used to reverse both central and peripheral effects; use of this drug is not currently recommended as it can cause seizures, cardiac effects, and excessive cholinergic effects

PEDIATRIC CONSIDERATIONS

- Doses up to 80 mg trihexyphenidyl have been employed in the treatment of dystonic movements in children; these were well tolerated with few side effects

GERIATRIC CONSIDERATIONS

- The elderly are very sensitive to anticholinergic drugs. Monitor for constipation, urinary retention as well as increased confusion, memory loss, and disorientation. Avoid drugs with potent central or peripheral anticholinergic activity (biperiden may be most appropriate agent)
- Caution when using two or more drugs with anticholinergic properties

USE IN PREGNANCY

- A possible association found between use of anticholinergic antiparkinsonian drugs and minor malformations; prophylactic use of these drugs during pregnancy is not recommended
- Avoid amantadine and diphenhydramine

Breast milk

- No specific data available; however, infants are sensitive to anticholinergic effects of drugs, therefore breastfeeding is discouraged
- Anticholinergic properties may inhibit lactation

NURSING IMPLICATIONS

- Antiparkinsonian drugs should be given only to relieve extrapyramidal side effects of neuroleptics; excess use or abuse can precipitate a toxic psychosis
- Some side effects of these drugs (i.e., anticholinergic) are additive to those of neuroleptics; observe patient for signs of side effects or toxicity
- Monitor patient's intake and output. Urinary retention can occur, especially in the elderly; bethanechol (Urecholine) can be used to reverse this problem
- To help prevent gastric irritation, administer drug after meals
- Relieve dry mouth by giving patient cool drinks, ice chips, sugarless chewing gum, or hard, sour candy. Suggest frequent rinsing of the mouth, and teeth should be brushed regularly. Patients should avoid calorie-laden beverages and sweet candy as they not only increase the likelihood of dental caries, but will also promote weight gain. Formerly well-fitting dentures may become ill-fitting, and

can cause rubbing and/or ulceration of the gums. May predispose patient to monilial infections. Products that promote or replace salivation (e.g., MoiStir, Saliment) may be of benefit

- Blurring of near vision is due to paresis of the ciliary muscle. This can be helped by wearing suitable glasses, reading by a bright light or, if severe, by the use of Pilocarpine eye drops 0.5%
- Dry eyes may be of particular difficulty to the elderly or those wearing contact lenses. Artificial tears or contact lens wetting solutions may be of benefit in dealing with this problem
- Anticholinergics reduce peristalsis and decrease intestinal secretions, leading to constipation. Increasing fluids and bulk (e.g., bran, salads) as well as fruit in the diet is beneficial. If necessary, bulk laxatives (e.g., Metamucil, Prodiem) or a stool softener (e.g., Surfak) can be used; lactulose may be used for chronic constipation
- Warn the patient not to drive a car or operate machinery until response to the drug has been determined
- Appropriate patient education regarding medication and side effects is necessary prior to discharge
- If akathisia does not respond to standard antiparkinsonian agents, diphenhydramine, propranolol, lorazepam, clonazepam, or diazepam can be tried

PATIENT INSTRUCTIONS

For detailed patient instructions on antiparkinsonian agents, see the Patient Information Sheet on p. 258

- Antiparkinsonian drugs are used *only* to relieve muscular side effects caused by neuroleptics; other side effects will not be helped
- Do not increase the dose without consulting your doctor
- Overuse will result in dry mouth, blurred vision, constipation; may cause confusion and memory impairment

DRUG INTERACTIONS

- Only clinically significant interactions are listed below

Class of Drug	Example	Interaction Effects
Adsorbent	Activated charcoal, antacids, kaolin-pectin (attapulgite), cholestyramine	Oral absorption decreased when used simultaneously
Anticholinergic	Antidepressants, antihistamines	Increased atropine-like effects causing dry mouth, blurred vision, constipation, etc. May produce inhibition of sweating and may lead to paralytic ileus High doses can bring on a toxic psychosis
Antidepressant		
SSRI	Paroxetine	Increased plasma level of procyclidine (by 40%)
NDRI	Bupropion	Case reports of neurotoxicity in elderly patients, in combination with amantadine
Antihypertensive	Hydrochlorothiazide, triamterene	Reduced renal clearance of amantadine resulting in drug accumulation and possible toxicity
Antipsychotic	Haloperidol, trifluoperazine	May aggravate tardive dyskinesia or unmask latent TD May decrease plasma level of neuroleptic Increased anticholinergic effects
Caffeine		May offset beneficial effects by increasing tremor and akathisia
Co-trimoxazole (Trimethoprim / Sulfamethoxazole)		Competition for renal clearance resulting in elevated plasma level of amantadine
Digoxin		Increased bioavailability of digoxin tablets (not capsules or liquids) Increased plasma level of digoxin due to decreased gastric motility
Quinidine		Inhibited renal clearance of amantadine (in males)
Quinine		Increased plasma level of amantadine due to inhibited renal clearance (by 27% in males)

Effects on Extrapyramidal Symptoms

Antiparkinsonian Agent	Tremor	Rigidity	Dystonia	Akinesia	Akathisia
Amantadine (Symmetrel)	++	++	+	+++	++
Benztropine (Cogentin)	++	+++	+++	++	++
Biperiden (Akineton)	++	++	++	+++	++
β-Blockers (e.g., propranolol, nadolol)	+	–	–	–	+++
Clonazepam (Rivotril, Klonopin)	–	+	+	–	+++
Diazepam (Valium)	+	++	++	+	+++
Diphenhydramine (Benadryl)	++	+	+++	–	+++
Ethopropazine (Parsitan)	+++	++	+	+	++
Lorazepam (Ativan)	+	+	+++	–	+++
Orphenadrine (Disipal, Norflex)	++	++	–	++	+
Procyclidine (Kemadrin)	++	++	++	++	++
Trihexyphenidyl (Artane)	++	++	++	+++	++

Based on literature and clinical observations: – effect not established, + some effect (20% response), ++ moderate effect (20–50% response), +++ good effect (> 50% response)

Comparison of Antiparkinsonian Agents

Antiparkinsonian Agents	Usual Dose (mg)	Therapeutic Effects	Adverse Effects	Dose	CYP-450 Metabolizing Enzymes [a]	CYP-450 Inhibition [b]
Amantadine (Symmetrel)	100	May improve akathisia, akinesia, rigidity, acute dystonia, parkinsonism, and tardive dyskinesia; may enhance the effects of other antiparkinsonian agents Tolerance to fixed dose may develop after 1–8 weeks May be useful in levodopa-induced movement disorder Found effective in treating neuroleptic and SSRI-induced sexual dysfunction Effective in treating neuroleptic-induced weight gain Early data suggest a possible role in ADHD, conduct disorder and in treating cocaine craving and use	Common: indigestion, excitement, difficulty in concentration, dizziness Less often: peripheral edema, skin rash, livido reticularis (mottled skin discoloration), tremors, slurred speech, ataxia, depression, insomnia, and lethargy (these are dose-related and disappear on drug withdrawal) Confusion, hallucinations and seizures reported in the elderly and in patients with renal insufficiency Less anticholinergic than other agents; safe to use low doses in glaucoma	Orally: 100–400 mg daily Children: 2.5 mg/kg per day	–[c]	–[c]
Antihistamines						
Diphenhydramine (Benadryl)	25	Has effect on tremor Sedative effect may benefit tension and excitation; may enhance the effects of other antiparkinsonian agents	Somnolence and confusion, especially in the elderly	IM/IV: 25–50 mg for dystonia Orally: 25–50 mg qid	2D6	2D6
Orphenadrine (Disipal, Norflex)	50	Some effect on rigidity Modest effect on sialorrhea Mild stimulant Beneficial effects tend to wear off in 2–6 months	Slight dryness of mouth, sedation, mild central excitation	Orally: 50 mg tid up to 400 mg/day	2D6, 3A4, 2C	2D6, 2B6
β-Blockers						
Propranolol (Inderal)	10	Very useful for akathisia and tremor	Monitor pulse and blood pressure; do not stop high dose abruptly due to rebound tachycardia	Orally: 10 mg tid to 120 mg daily	IA2, 2D6[w], 2C19	IA2, 3A4[w], 2D6[w]
Benzodiazepines						
Diazepam (Valium, etc.)	5	Beneficial effect on akathisia and acute dystonia Muscle relaxant	Drowsiness, lethargy (see p. 112)	Orally: up to 5 mg qid IV: 10 mg for acute dystonia by slow direct IV push (rate of 5 mg (1 ml)/ min)	3A4, 2C9, 2C19, 2B6	
Lorazepam (Ativan)	2	Beneficial effect on akathisia Excellent for acute dyskinesia (sublingual works quickest)	Drowsiness, lethargy (see p. 112)	Orally: up to 2 mg qid Sublingual: 1–2 mg up to tid IM: 1–2 mg for dystonia	–	–
Clonazepam (Rivotril, Klonopin)	0.5	Useful for akathisia	Drowsiness, lethargy (see p. 112)	Orally: 1–4 mg/day	2B4, 2E1, 3A4	2B4

Comparison of Antiparkinsonian Agents (cont.)

Antiparkinsonian Agents	Usual Dose (mg)	Therapeutic Effects	Adverse Effects	Dose	CYP-450 Metabolizing Enzymes [a]	CYP-450 Inhibition [b]
Benztropine (Cogentin)	2	Beneficial effect on rigidity Relieves sialorrhea and drooling Powerful muscle relaxant; sedative action Cumulative and long-acting; once-daily dosing can be used (preferably in the morning) IM/IV: dramatic effect on dystonic symptoms	Dry mouth, blurred vision, urinary retention, constipation Increases intraocular pressure Toxic psychosis when abused or overused	Orally: 1–2 mg bid up to 6 mg bid if needed IM/IV: 1–2 mg; may repeat in 30 min	2D6	
Biperiden (Akineton)	4	Has effect against rigidity and akinesia	Less likely to cause peripheral anticholinergic effects May cause euphoria and increased tremor	Orally: 2–8 mg daily; up to 16 mg per day	?	?
Ethopropazine (Parsitan, Parsidol)	100	Has effect against rigidity; improves posture, gait, and speech Specific for tremor	Dry mouth, postural dizziness, somnolence, and confusion can occur Low anticholinergic activity; safe to use in moderate doses in patients with glaucoma	Starting oral dose: 50 mg tid up to 400 mg per day; in major tremor start with 100 mg tid and may increase to 900 mg/day	?	?
Procyclidine (Kemadrin)	5	Similar to trihexyphenidyl Milder and questionable effect on tremor Useful agent to use in combination when muscle rigidity is severe	Less pronounced side effects than with trihexyphenidyl; slight blurring of vision Stimulation and giddiness in some patients Can be abused	Starting oral dose: 2.5 mg bid May need up to 30 mg/day	?	2D6
Trihexyphenidyl (Artane)	5	Mild to moderate effect against rigidity and spasm (occasionally get dramatic results) Tremor alleviated to a lesser degree; as a result of relaxing muscle spasm, more tremor activity may be noted Stimulating – can be used during the day for sluggish, lethargic, and akinetic patients	Dry mouth, blurred vision, GI distress Less sedating potential Severe and persistent mental confusion, cognitive impairment may occur, esp. in the elderly; must recognize this as a toxic state At toxic doses get restlessness, delirium, hallucinations; these disappear when the drug is discontinued (most anticholinergic of the antiparkinsonian agents – liable to be abused as a euphoriant)	Orally: 4–15 mg daily, up to 30 mg tolerated in younger patients	?	?

(a) Cytochrome P-450 isoenzymes involved in liver metabolism of drug, (b) CYP-450 isoenzymes inhibited by drug, (c) Undergoes little metabolism; 90% of dose recovered unchanged in the urine; does not affect the metabolism of other drugs

Anxiolytic Agents

GENERAL COMMENTS

- Anxiolytic agents can be classified as follows:

Chemical Class	Agent	Page
Antihistamine[(A)]	Example: Hydroxyzine[(A)] (Atarax, Vistaril)	See[(A)] below
Azaspirodecanedione (Azaspirone)	Buspirone	See p. 121
Barbiturates[(B)]	Examples: Amobarbital sodium[(C)] (Amytal) Phenobarbital[(D)] (Luminal)	See[(B)] below See[(B)] below
Benzodiazepines		See below

[(A)] CNS depressant with few side effects; used primarily for itching of psychogenic origin. Dose: 10–400 mg/day. Tolerance to sedative effects will develop over time. Has been used in children as anxiolytic, but clinical efficacy not substantiated and adverse effects may be troublesome (including drowsiness, affective and cognitive symptoms).
[(B)] Act as CNS depressants; seldom used as anxiolytics, because they are habit-forming, causing physical dependence; they can have severe withdrawal symptoms; tolerance develops quickly, requiring increased dosage; they have a low margin of safety (therapeutic dose close to toxic dose); they are involved in many drug interactions (induce metabolizing enzymes); they can evoke behavioral complications including hyperactivity and conduct disorders in children, and depression in adults
[(C)] Amobarbital sodium IV preparation useful for diagnosis, narcoanalysis (dose: 400–800 mg by slow IV push over minutes)
[(D)] Phenobarbital has been used as an anxiolytic for those unable to benefit from benzodiazepines or buspirone (dose: 30–90 mg/day)

Benzodiazepines

GENERAL COMMENTS

- Benzodiazepines can be categorized as follows:

		Anxiolytic	Sedative/Hypnotic	Anticonvulsant	Potency
Short-acting	Midazolam (Versed)[(A)]	+	+++		–
	Triazolam (Halcion)	+	+++		high
Intermediate	Alprazolam (Xanax)	++	+	+	high
	Bromazepam (Lectopam)[(C)]	++			high
	Estazolam (ProSom)[(B)]	+	+++	+	–
	Halazepam (Paxipam)[(B)]	++			medium
	Lorazepam (Ativan)	+++	++	++	high
	Oxazepam (Serax)	++	+		low
	Temazepam (Restoril)	+	+++	+	low
Long-acting	Chlordiazepoxide (Librium)	++			low
	Clonazepam (Rivotril, Klonopin)	++	+	+++	high
	Clorazepate (Tranxene, Tranxilene)	++			medium
	Diazepam (Valium)	+++	++	+	medium
	Flurazepam (Dalmane)	+	+++		medium
	Nitrazepam (Mogadon)[(C)]	+	+++	++	–
	Quazepam (Doral)[(B)]	+	+++	+	–

Activity: + weak, ++ moderate, +++ strong, [(A)] Acute use only, [(B)] Not marketed in Canada, [(C)] Not marketed in the USA

Benzodiazepines (cont.)

PRODUCT AVAILABILITY

Chemical Class	Generic Name	Trade Name[A]	Dosage Forms and Strengths
Benzodiazepine	Alprazolam	Xanax Xanax TS[C]	Tablets: 0.25 mg, 0.5 mg, 1 mg, 2 mg[B] Tablets: 2 mg
	Bromazepam[C]	Lectopam	Tablets: 1.5 mg, 3 mg, 6 mg
	Chlordiazepoxide	Librium Libritabs [B]	Capsules: 5 mg, 10 mg, 25 mg Injection[B]: 100 mg/ml Tablets: 5 mg, 25 mg
	Clonazepam	Rivotril, Klonopin[B]	Tablets: 0.5 mg, 1 mg, 2 mg
	Clorazepate	Tranxene[C], Tranxilene[B] Tranxene SD[B]	Tablets: 3.75 mg, 7.5 mg, 15 mg Tablets: 11.25 mg, 22.5 mg
	Diazepam	Valium Diazepam Intensol[B] Diastat Diazemuls[C]	Tablets: 2 mg, 5 mg, 10 mg Oral solution: 5 mg/ml Injection: 5 mg/ml Oral concentrate[B]: 5 mg/ml Rectal gel: 5 mg/ml Emulsion injection (IV)[C]: 5 mg/ml
	Estazolam[B]	ProSom	Capsules: 15 mg Tablets: 1 mg, 2 mg
	Flurazepam	Dalmane	Capsules: 15 mg, 30 mg
	Halazepam[B]	Paxipam	Tablets: 20 mg, 40 mg
	Lorazepam	Ativan	Tablets: 0.5 mg, 1 mg, 2 mg Sublingual tablets[C]: 0.5 mg, 1 mg, 2 mg Injection: 2 mg/ml[B], 4 mg/ml
	Midazolam	Versed	Syrup[B]: 2 mg/ml Injection: 1 mg/ml, 5 mg/ml
	Nitrazepam[C]	Mogadon	Tablets: 5 mg, 10 mg
	Oxazepam	Serax	Tablets: 10 mg[C], 15 mg, 30 mg[C] Capsules[B]: 10 mg, 15 mg, 30 mg
	Quazepam[B]	Doral	Tablets: 7.5 mg, 15 mg
	Temazepam	Restoril	Capsules: 7.5 mg[B], 15 mg, 30 mg
	Triazolam	Halcion	Tablets: 0.125 mg, 0.25 mg

[A] Generic preparations may be available, [B] Not marketed in Canada, [C] Not marketed in USA

INDICATIONS*

- ▲ • Management of mild to moderate anxiety, tension, excitation and agitation
- ▲ • Generalized anxiety disorder
- ▲ • Management of acute and chronic alcohol withdrawal syndromes

* ▲ Approved indications

- ▲ • Convulsions: status epilepticus, petit mal, infantile spasms, simple-partial and complex-partial seizures
- ▲ • Insomnia
- ▲ • Panic disorder with or without agoraphobia (alprazolam)
- ▲ • Muscle spasms, dystonia, "restless legs" syndrome
- ▲ • Other: cardioversion, endoscopy and bronchoscopy, enhancement of analgesia during labor and delivery, preoperative sedation
- Akathisia due to neuroleptic agents
- May reduce abnormal movements associated with tardive dyskinesia (clonazepam)
- Sedation in severe agitation (IV)
- In mania used concomitantly with neuroleptic or lithium to control agitation; may potentiate antipsychotics and decrease dosage requirements
- Depression (alprazolam)
- Mania and bipolar affective disorder prophylaxis (clonazepam); may prevent antidepressant-induced mania and decrease rate of cycling
- In schizophrenia used with neuroleptic to control agitation; may potentiate neuroleptics; diazepam used alone in high doses suggested to improve paranoia
- Social phobia (alprazolam, clonazepam, diazepam, lorazepam)
- Catatonia (parenteral and sublingual lorazepam; diazepam, clonazepam)
- Myoclonus, restless legs syndrome, Tourette's syndrome (clonazepam)
- Acute dystonia (SL or IM lorazepam)
- Delirium (lorazepam)
- Neuralgic pain (clonazepam)
- Premenstrual dysphoric disorder (alprazolam)
- Control of violent outbursts, assaultive behavior (clonazepam); used also in combination with lithium, antipsychotic or β-blocker
- Alprazolam withdrawal (clonazepam)

PHARMACOLOGY

- Depress the CNS at the levels of the limbic system, the brain-stem reticular formation, and the cortex
- Benzodiazepines bind to the "benzodiazepine"-GABA-chloride receptor complex, facilitating the action of GABA (an inhibitory neurotransmitter) on CNS excitability. Intensity of action depends on degree of receptor occupancy

GENERAL COMMENTS

- Clonazepam has 5HT potentiating properties

DOSING

- See pp. 117–120 for individual agents
- Following IV administration of diazepam or chlordiazepoxide, local pain and thrombophlebitis may occur due to precipitation of the drug, or due to an irritant effect of propylene glycol; IV diazepam emulsion (Diazemuls) is less likely to cause this problem
- IM use is discouraged with chlordiazepoxide and diazepam as absorption is slow, erratic, and possibly incomplete; local pain often occurs. Lorazepam IM is adequately absorbed

PHARMACOKINETICS

- See pp. 117–120 for individual agents
- Marked interindividual variation (up to 10-fold) is found in all pharmacokinetic parameters. Age, smoking, liver disease, physical disorders, as well as concurrent use of other drugs may influence parameters by changing the volume of distribution and elimination half-life of these drugs
- Well absorbed from GI tract after oral administration; food can delay the rate, but not the extent of absorption; onset of action is determined by rate of absorption and lipid solubility
- Lipid solubility denotes speed of entry into (lipid) brain tissue, followed by extensive redistribution to adipose tissue. Benzodiazepines have a high volume of distribution (i.e., the tissue drug concentration is much higher than the blood drug concentration)
- The duration of action is determined mainly by the distribution and not by elimination half-life (except for ultra-short half-life drugs like midazolam and triazolam)
- Differences in pharmacokinetics between the various benzodiazepines have been presumed to indicate clinical differences as well –

Benzodiazepines (cont.)

this is not necessarily so. However, present rationale for selection of a benzodiazepine remains the difference in pharmacokinetic profile. Generally, short-acting agents can be used as hypnotics and for acute problems relating to anxiety, while long-acting agents can be used for chronic conditions where a continuous drug effect is needed

- The potency of a benzodiazepine is the affinity of the parent drug, or its active metabolites, for benzodiazepine receptors, in vivo.
- It is suggested that the longer the half-life of a benzodiazepine, the greater the likelihood that the compound will have an adverse effect on daytime functioning (e.g., hangover). However, with shorter half-life benzodiazepines, withdrawal and anxiety between doses (rebound) and anterograde amnesia are seen more often
- The major pathways of metabolism are hepatic microsomal oxidation and demethylation. Conjugation to more polar (water-soluble) glucuronide derivatives allows for excretion. Biotransformation by oxidation can be impaired by disease states (e.g., hepatic cirrhosis), by age or by drugs that impair the metabolism. Drugs undergoing conjugation only (e.g., oxazepam) are not so affected

ONSET AND DURATION OF ACTION

- Benzodiazepines that undergo conjugation (e.g., temazepam, oxazepam) have longer elimination half-lives in women than in men

ADVERSE EFFECTS

- Are few, and often disappear with adjustment of dosage

1. CNS Effects

- Most common are extensions of the generalized sedative effect, e.g., fatigue, drowsiness
- Impaired mental speed, central cognitive processing ability, memory and perceptomotor performance (dose-related)
- Anterograde amnesia (more likely with high potency agents or higher doses); sexual dysmnesia (midazolam)
- Chronic use: decreased concentration, memory impairment and impaired cognitive processes
- Behavior dyscontrol with irritability and impulsivity; paradoxical agitation – insomnia, hallucinations, nightmares, euphoria; rage, violent behavior; most likely in patients with a history of aggressive behavior or unstable emotional behavior, e.g., borderline personality disorder (less likely with oxazepam)
- Confusion and disorientation – primarily in the elderly. Periods of blackouts or amnesia have been reported
- Treatment-emergent depression (13% incidence with clonazepam)
- Excessive doses (parenterally) can result in apnea and respiratory depression
- Dysarthria, muscle weakness, incoordination, ataxia (up to 22% with clonazepam at doses above 2 mg/day), nystagmus
- Headache

2. Other Adverse Effects

- Anticholinergic effects, e.g., blurred vision (mild), dry mouth
- Sexual dysfunction including decreased libido, erectile dysfunction, anorgasmia, ejaculatory disturbance and gynecomastia; abnormal size and shape of sperm reported
- Dizziness (up to 12% with higher doses of clonazepam)
- Increased salivation (clonazepam)
- Rare reports of purpura and thrombocytopenia with diazepam
- Few documented allergies to benzodiazepines; rarely reported skin reactions include rashes, fixed drug eruption, photosensitivity reactions, pigmentation, alopecia, bullous reactions, exfoliative dermatitis, vasculitis, erythema nodosum

WITHDRAWAL

- Benzodiazepines present different risks of physiological dependence at therapeutic doses, depending on the individual as well as the drug's potency and its elimination half-life
- Discontinuation of a benzodiazepine can produce:
  - Withdrawal: occurs 1–2 days (short-acting) to 5–10 days (long-acting) following any drug discontinuation. Common symptoms include insomnia, agitation, anxiety, perceptual changes, dysphoria, headache, muscle aches, twitches, tremors, loss of appetite and GI distress. Catatonia and depression have also been reported. Severe reactions can occur such as grand mal or petit mal seizures, coma, and psychotic states

- Rebound: occurs hours to days after drug withdrawal; symptoms (of anxiety) are similar but more intense than those reported originally
- Relapse: symptoms occur weeks to months after drug withdrawal and are similar to original symptoms of anxiety

Management

- To withdraw a patient from a benzodiazepine, an equivalent dose of diazepam should be substituted (see pp. 117–120) and withdrawal done according to the following protocol:
  - Reduce diazepam by 10 mg daily until a total daily dose of 20 mg is reached
  - Then reduce by 5 mg daily to an end point of total abstinence; propranolol may aid in withdrawal process

☞ **This protocol should not be used for alprazolam, which must be decreased by 0.5 mg weekly; quicker withdrawal may result in delirium and seizures**

- Carbamazepine (in therapeutic doses) may aid in the withdrawal process
- Alternatively, alprazolam may be substituted with an equal dose of clonazepam (in divided doses), then decreased by 1 mg daily

PRECAUTIONS

- Do not use in patients with sleep apnea
- Administer with caution to elderly or debilitated patients, those with liver disease, and to patients performing hazardous tasks requiring mental alertness or physical coordination
- Benzodiazepines may diminish the therapeutic efficacy of electroconvulsive therapy (ECT) by raising the seizure threshold
- Anxiolytics lower the tolerance to alcohol, and high doses may produce mental confusion similar to alcohol intoxication
- Can cause physical and psychological dependence, tolerance, and withdrawal symptoms – correlated to dose and duration of use
- Benzodiazepines are at risk of being abused by susceptible individuals (e.g., habitual polydrug users); they prefer agents with rapid peak drug effects (e.g., diazepam, lorazepam)
- Withdrawal symptoms resemble those of alcohol and barbiturates, e.g., tremor, agitation, headache, nausea, delirium, hallucinations, metallic taste. Abrupt withdrawal following prolonged use of high doses can produce grand-mal seizures (especially with alprazolam)

TOXICITY

- Rarely if ever fatal when taken alone; may be lethal when taken in combination with other drugs, such as alcohol and barbiturates
- Symptoms of overdose include hypotension, depressed respiration, and coma

Management

- Flumazenil injection (a benzodiazepine antagonist) reverses the hypnotic-sedative effects of benzodiazepines. Repeated doses may be required due to the short duration of action of flumazenil

PEDIATRIC CONSIDERATIONS

- Probable indications for anxiolytics include seizure disorder, generalized anxiety disorder, adjustment disorder, insomnia, night terrors, and somnabulism
- High potency benzodiazepines (clonazepam) useful for panic disorder/agoraphobia, social phobia and separation anxiety disorder
- Benzodiazepines are metabolized faster in children than in adults; may require small divided doses to maintain blood level
- Adverse effects include sedation, cognitive and motor effects; disinhibition with irritability and agitation reported in up to 30% of children – primarily in younger impulsive patients with mental retardation
- Midazolam has been given intranasally at a dose of 0.2 mg/kg for pre-operative sedation
- Chronic use in children should be carefully evaluated to prevent possible adverse effects on physical and mental development
- With clonazepam, troublesome hypersecretion in the upper respiratory tract can occur in children with chronic respiratory diseases

GERIATRIC CONSIDERATIONS

- Caution when using drugs that are metabolized by oxidation (e.g., diazepam, estazolam) as they can accumulate in the elderly or in persons with liver disease
- Caution when combining with other drugs with CNS effects; excessive sedation can cause confusion, disorientation
- Elderly are more vulnerable to adverse CNS effects, specifically as to balance (risk of falls), gait, memory, cognition, behavior
- Data indicates that benzodiazepine use increases risk of falls, leading to femur fractures, by about 60%; risk increased with dose and in females
- Higher risk of motor vehicle accidents documented in elderly taking long-acting benzodiazepines

Benzodiazepines (cont.)

USE IN PREGNANCY

- Benzodiazepines and metabolites freely cross the placenta and accumulate in fetal circulation
- Some studies suggest an association between benzodiazepine use in the first trimester and teratogenicity; data contradictory; 0.4–0.7% incidence of cleft palate – suggest ultrasound screening of fetus
- High doses or prolonged use by mother in third trimester may precipitate fetal benzodiazepine syndrome: including floppy infant syndrome, impaired temperature regulation and withdrawal symptoms in newborn

Breast milk

- Benzodiazepines are excreted into breast milk in levels sufficient to produce effects in the newborn, including sedation, e.g. infant can receive up to 13% of maternal dose of diazepam and 7% of lorazepam dose
- Metabolism of benzodiazepines in infants is slower; long-acting agents can accumulate
- American Academy of Pediatrics considers benzodiazepines as drugs "whose effect on nursing infants is unknown but may be of concern"

NURSING IMPLICATIONS

- Assess the anxiety level of patients on these drugs to determine if anxiety control has been accomplished or if over-sedation has occurred
- Inform patients that activities requiring mental alertness should not be performed after taking drug
- Caution patients not to use other CNS depressant drugs (e.g., antihistamines or alcohol) without consulting the doctor
- Excessive consumption of caffeinated beverages will counteract the effects of anxiolytics
- Tolerance and physical addiction can occur; withdrawal symptoms can be produced with abrupt discontinuation after prolonged use

PATIENT INSTRUCTIONS

For detailed patient instructions on anxiolytic drugs, see the Patient Information Sheet on p. 259.

- Do not stop drug abruptly (especially if on a high dose); withdrawal reactions may be severe
- Tolerance to effects may develop with chronic use; let your physician know if effectiveness of drug has decreased
- The dose should be maintained as prescribed; do not increase dose without consulting physician
- Take caution when driving a car or operating machinery until response to the drug is determined
- May enhance the effects of alcohol and other CNS drugs; do not self-medicate with over-the-counter medication without consultation
- Report any memory lapses or amnesia to your physician immediately
- Avoid excessive caffeine intake (coffee, tea, cola, chocolate) as effects of medication may be decreased
- Avoid ingestion of grapefruit juice while on alprazolam and triazolam as blood levels of these drugs can be elevated

DRUG INTERACTIONS

- Many interactions; only clinically significant ones listed below

Class of Drug	Example	Interaction Effects
Allopurinol		Decreased metabolism and increased half-life of benzodiazepines that are metabolized by oxidation (see charts pp. 117–120), leading to increased drug effect
Amiodarone		Reduced metabolism and increased plasma level of midazolam
Anesthetics	Ketamine Volatile (e.g., halothane)	Prolonged recovery with diazepam due to decreased metabolism Decreased protein binding of diazepam resulting in increased pharmacological effects

Class of Drug	Example	Interaction Effects
Antibiotic	Erythromycin, clarithromycin, troleandomycin Chloramphenicol Quinolones: ciprofloxacin, enoxacin	Decreased metabolism and increased plasma levels of midazolam and triazolam (by 54% and 52% respectively); no interaction with azithromycin Decreased metabolism of benzodiazepines that are metabolized by oxidation Decreased metabolism of diazepam
Anticoagulant	Warfarin	Decreased PT ratio or INR response with chlordiazepoxide
Anticonvulsant	Carbamazepine Phenobarbital Phenytoin Valproate	Increased metabolism and decreased plasma level of alprazolam (>50%) and clonazepam (19–37%) Increased metabolism of diazepam; additive CNS effects Decreased phenytoin plasma level reported with clonazepam Increased phenytoin level and toxicity reported with diazepam and chlordiazepoxide Displacement by diazepam from protein-binding resulting in increased plasma level Decreased metabolism and increased pharmacological effects of clonazepam and lorazepam
Antidepressant Cyclic SARI SSRI	 Desipramine, imipramine Nefazodone Fluoxetine, fluvoxamine, sertraline	 Increased plasma levels of desipramine and imipramine with alprazolam Increased plasma levels of alprazolam (by 200%) and triazolam (by 500%) due to inhibited metabolism via CYP3A4 Decreased metabolism and increased plasma level of alprazolam (by 100%) and diazepam with fluoxetine and fluvoxamine leading to increased drug effect; 13% decrease in clearance of diazepam with sertraline
Antifungal	Itraconazole, ketoconazole fluconazole	Decreased metabolism and increased half-life of chlordiazepoxide and midazolam; decreased metabolism of triazolam (6–7 fold); reduce dose by 50–75%
Antipsychotic	Clozapine	Marked sedation, increased salivation, hypotension (collapse), delirium, and respiratory arrest reported; more likely to occur early in treatment when clozapine is added to benzodiazepine regimen
Antituberculosis therapy	Isoniazid Rifampin	Decreased metabolism of benzodiazepines that are metabolized by oxidation (triazolam clearance decreased by 75%) Increased metabolism of benzodiazepines that are metabolized by oxidation due to enzyme induction of CYP3A4 (diazepam by 300%, midazolam by 83%)
β-blockers	Propranolol	Increased half-life and decreased clearance of diazepam (no interaction with alprazolam, lorazepam or oxazepam)
Caffeine		May counteract sedation and increase insomnia
Cimetidine		Decreased metabolism of benzodiazepines that are metabolized by oxidation (no effect with ranitidine, famotidine or nizatidine)
CNS depressant	Barbiturates, antihistamines Alcohol	Increased CNS depression; with high doses coma and respiratory depression can occur Alprazolam reported to increase aggression in moderate alcohol drinkers Brain concentrations of various benzodiazepines altered by ethanol: triazolam and estazolam concentrations decreased, diazepam concentration increased, no change with chlordiazepoxide

Benzodiazepines (cont.)

Class of Drug	Example	Interaction Effects
Digoxin		Decreased metabolism and elimination of digoxin
Diltiazem		Increased plasma level of triazolam (by 100%), and of midazolam, due to inhibited metabolism via CYP3A4
Disulfiram		Decreased metabolism of benzodiazepines that are metabolized by oxidation
Estrogen	Oral contraceptives	Decreased metabolism of benzodiazepines that are metabolized by oxidation
Grapefruit juice		Decreased metabolism of alprazolam, midazolam , diazepam and triazolam via CYP3A4 resulting in increased peak concentration and bioavailability
Kava Kava		May potentiate CNS effects causing increased side effects and toxicity
Lithium		Increased incidence of sexual dysfunction (up to 49%) when combined with clonazepam
L-Dopa		Benzodiazepines can reduce the efficacy of l-dopa secondary to the GABA-agonist effect
Omeprazole		Increased ataxia and sedation due to decreased metabolism of benzodiazepines metabolized by oxidation (no effect with lansoprazole)
Probenecid		Decreased clearance of lorazepam (by 50%)
Propoxyphene		Increased level of alprazolam due to inhibited hydroxylation
Protease inhibitor	Ritonavir, Indinavir	Increased plasma level of benzodiazepines that are metabolized by oxidation via CYP3A4 (e.g., triazolam, alprazolam)
Smoking – cigarettes		Increased clearance of diazepam and chlordiazepoxide due to enzyme induction

Comparison of the Benzodiazepines

Drug	Comparative Dose (mg)**	Peak Plasma Level PO	Lipid Solubility[c]	Elimination Half-life	Metabolites*** (m = main metabolite)	Comments	Clinical Considerations
Alprazolam	0.5	1–2 h	moderate	9–20 h	Metabolized by oxidation: 29 metabolites; principal ones are: α-hydroxyalprazolam (m) desmethylalprazolam 4-hydroxyalprazolam Metabolized by CYP3A4[p] and 1A2	Rapidly and completely absorbed 80% protein bound Well absorbed sublingually Plasma level of alprazolam may correlate with efficacy in panic disorder	Use: anxiolytic sedative alcohol withdrawal depression characterized by anxiety panic attack prophylaxis adjunct in depression tid dosing recommended Increases stage 2, and decreases stages 1 and 4 and REM sleep; caution on withdrawal (see p. 105) Low degree of sedation Case reports of behavioral side effects including mania
Bromazepam[b]	3.0	0.5–4 h	low	8–30 h	Metabolized by oxidation: 3-hydroxybromazepam Metabolized by CYP3A4	Metabolite reported to have anxiolytic activity; does not accumulate on chronic dosing	Use: anxiolytic
Chlordiaze-poxide	25.0	1–4 h	moderate	4–29 h (parent drug) 28–100 h (metabolites)	Metabolized by oxidation: desmethylchlordiazepoxide (m) oxazepam desmethyldiazepam	Onset of activity may be delayed; parent compound less potent than metabolites Metabolites accumulate on chronic dosing IM drug erratically absorbed	Use: anxiolytic sedative alcohol withdrawal 2- to 3-fold increase in half-life seen in patients with cirrhosis Antacids* decrease absorption in GI tract, but do not influence completeness of absorption Moderate degree of sedation
Clonazepam	0.25	1–4 h	low	19–60 h	Metabolized by oxidation: no active metabolite Metabolized primarily by CYP2B4, 2E1 and 3A4	Quickly and completely absorbed; slow onset of activity Dosage varies depending on usage Anxiety: 0.5–8 mg/day Panic disorder/agoraphobia: 2–8 mg/day Acute mania: 4–24 mg/day Aggression: 1–3 mg/day Adjunct in psychotic states: 2–10 mg/day	Use: anticonvulsant anxiolytic panic attack prophylaxis prophylaxis of BAD manic episode of BAD akathisia aggressive behavior Moderate degree of sedation

Comparison of the Benzodiazepines (cont.)

Drug	Comparative Dose (mg)**	Peak Plasma Level PO	Lipid Solubility[c]	Elimination Half-life	Metabolites*** (m = main metabolite)	Comments	Clinical Considerations
Clorazepate Dipotassium	10.0	0.5–2 h	high	1.3–120 h (metabolites)	Metabolized by oxidation: N-desmethyldiazepam	Hydrolyzed in the stomach to active metabolite (parent compound inactive) Rate of hydrolysis depends on gastric acidity, therefore absorption is unreliable (one study disputes this) Metabolite accumulates on chronic dosing	Use: anxiolytic alcohol withdrawal Antacids and sodium bicarbonate reduce the rate and extent of appearance of active metabolite in the blood Fast onset of action Moderate degree of sedation
Diazepam	5	1–2 h	high	14–70 h (parent drug) 30–200 h (metabolites)	Metabolized by oxidation: N-desmethyldiazepam (m) oxazepam 3-hydroxydiazepam temazepam Metabolized by CYP3A4, 2C9, 2C19 and 2B6	In males has shorter half-life and higher clearance rate than in females Less protein-bound in elderly, therefore attains higher serum levels Rapid onset of action followed by a redistribution into adipose tissue; accumulation on chronic dosing im drug erratically absorbed 2- to 3-fold increase in half-life seen in patients with cirrhosis Smoking: associated with higher diazepam clearance especially in young	Use: anxiolytic sedative anticonvulsant (status epilepticus) alcohol withdrawal akathisia muscle relaxant preoperative sedation Increases stage 2, and decreases stages 1 and 4 and REM sleep Fast onset of action High degree of sedation
Estazolam[a]	1	0.5–6 h	low	8–24 h	Metabolized by oxidation: 4-hydroxyestazolam 1-oxoestazolam Metabolized by CYP3A4	Metabolites inactive Metabolism impaired in the elderly and in hepatic disease	Use: hypnotic sedative Caution on withdrawal High doses can cause respiratory depression
Flurazepam	15	0.5–1 h	high	0.3–3 h (parent drug) 40–250 h (metabolites)	Metabolized by oxidation: N-desalkylflurazepam (m) OH-ethylflurazepam flurazepam aldehyde Metabolized by CYP2C and 2D6	Rapidly metabolized to active metabolite Elderly males accumulate metabolite more than young males on chronic dosing	Use: hypnotic Decreases stage 1 and increases stage 2 sleep; no effect on REM Increase in daytime sedation over time; hangover Fast onset of action
Halazepam[a]	40	1–3 h	low	14 h mean (parent) 30–96 h (metabolites)	Metabolized by oxidation: N-desmethyldiazepam (m) 3-hydroxyhalazepam	Metabolites active Adjust dose in the elderly	Use: anxiolytic Moderate degree of sedation

Drug	Comparative Dose (mg)**	Peak Plasma Level PO	Lipid Solubility(c)	Elimination Half-life	Metabolites*** (m = main metabolite)	Comments	Clinical Considerations
Lorazepam	1	Oral: 1–6 h IM: 45–75 min IV: 5–10 min SL: 60 min	low	8–24 h	Conjugated to form lorazepam glucuronide	Metabolite not pharmacologically active Slow onset of action Give at least twice daily to maintain steady state levels Well absorbed sublingually Half-life and Vd doubled in patients with cirrhosis Clearance reduced in elderly by 22% (one study) Not involved in metabolism interactions via CYP enzymes	Use: anxiolytic sedative preoperative sedation muscle relaxant catatonia manic phase of BAD akathisia acute dystonia Significant anterograde amnesia produced, which doesn't correlate directly to its sedative potency Blood levels fall quickly on discontinuation; withdrawal symptoms appear sooner than with long-acting drugs Decreases stage 1 and REM
Midazolam	Acute use only	0.5–1 min	high	1–4 h (parent) 1–20 h (metabolites)	Metabolized by oxidation: 1-OH-methylmidazolam 4-OH-midazolam Metabolized primarily by CYP3A4	Metabolites active Metabolism significantly impaired in patients with cirrhosis	Use: preoperative sedative, anxiolytic, IV induction of anesthesia (in 30–60 s) post-ECT agitation IV dose: 1–2.5 mg over at least 2 min May lower blood pressure Fast onset of action Produces anterograde amnesia; may induce false sexual beliefs
Nitrazepam(b)	2.5	0.5–7 h	low	15–48 h	Metabolized by nitroreduction by CYP2E1 No active metabolites	Excreted as amino and acetamide analogues Metabolism impaired in elderly and in hepatic disease Accumulates with chronic use	Use: sedative Decreases REM sleep
Oxazepam	15	1–4 h	low	3–25 h	Conjugated to oxazepam glucuronide	Metabolites not pharmacologically active Half-life and plasma clearance not affected much by age or sex or by liver disease Slow onset of action Give at least twice daily to maintain steady state No metabolism interactions	Use: anxiolytic sedative alcohol withdrawal muscle relaxant Can lower aggression levels in patients with a history of belligerence and assault without releasing paradoxical rage responses Can cause withdrawal insomnia Low sedative potential

Comparison of the Benzodiazepines (cont.)

Drug	Comparative Dose (mg)**	Peak Plasma Level PO	Lipid Solubility[c]	Elimination Half-life	Metabolites*** (m = main metabolite)	Comments	Clinical Considerations
Quazepam[a]	7.5	1.5 h	high	15–40 h (parent) 39–120 h (metabolites)	Metabolized by oxidation: 2-oxoquazepam Desalkylflurazepam Metabolized primarily by CYP2D6	Rapidly absorbed and metabolized Accumulation on chronic dosing – not associated with marked residual effects	Use: hypnotic anxiolytic Suppresses REM sleep, prolongs REM latency, increases stage 2 and decreases stages 1, 3, and 4 Rebound effects, anterograde amnesia and impaired performance not reported
Temazepam	10	2.5 h mean	moderate	3–25 h	Conjugated	Hard gelatin capsule; variable rate of absorption depending on formulation; 5% excreted as oxazepam in the urine; plasma concentration too low to detect No accumulation with chronic use; no metabolism interactions	Use: anxiolytic sedative On doses of 30 mg/day or more, may cause hangover, morning nausea, headache, drowsiness, and vivid dreaming Decreases sleep stages 3 & 4 Rebound insomnia has been reported
Triazolam	0.25	1–2 h	moderate	1.5–5 h	Metabolized by oxidation: 7-α-hydroxyderivative Metabolized by CYP3A4[p]	Metabolite inactive; negligible accumulation of drug due to high hepatic clearance (dependent on hepatic blood flow and microsomal oxidizing capacity) Although half-life is short, clinical effects have been observed up to 16 h after a single dose Well absorbed sublingually	Use: hypnotic Decreases stage 1, and increases stage 2 sleep; significantly increases latency to REM compared with baseline Rebound insomnia and anxiety reported Dose-related anterograde amnesia reported, especially in doses above 0.5 mg daily Reports of rage, automatism Report of hypothermia when combined with desipramine (neither drug causes this effect alone); potentiates anorexic effect of desipramine

* Apply to all benzodiazepines except where noted, ** Doses are approximate (alprazolam and clonazepam are relatively less potent, when dealing with anxiety, relatively more when dealing with panic); the doses used are substitute doses when switching among various benzodiazepines (they are approximately equal to phenobarbital 30 mg or pentobarbital 100 mg), *** See comments under Pharmacokinetics p. 104

(a) Not marketed in Canada, (b) Not marketed in USA, (c) High lipid solubility denotes fast entry into (lipid) brain tissue, (p) Primary route of metabolism, where known

Buspirone

PRODUCT AVAILABILITY

Chemical Class	Generic Name	Trade Name[A]	Dosage Forms and Strengths
Azaspirone	Buspirone	Buspar	Tablets: 5 mg[B], 10 mg

[A] Generic preparations may be available, [B] Not marketed in Canada

INDICATIONS*

- ▲ Anxiolytic, useful in:
  - chronic anxiety
  - situations where sedation or psychomotor impairment may be dangerous
  - patients with a history of substance abuse or alcohol abuse
- Treatment of obsessive compulsive disorder; may potentiate anti-obsessional effects of SSRIs or clomipramine
- Antidepressant effects reported in doses of 40–90 mg/day; useful in patients with concomitant anxiety; may augment effect of antidepressants in treatment-refractory depression
- Premenstrual dysphoric disorder
- Preliminary studies show some efficacy in insomnia with concomitant anxiety
- Preliminary reports show some efficacy in posttraumatic stress disorder and body dysmorphic disorder
- Preliminary reports show buspirone may aid in smoking cessation and alcohol withdrawal (primarily in patients with concomitant anxiety)
- Treatment of agitation, aggression/antisocial behavior, sexual preference disorders
- Preliminary data suggest efficacy in the treatment of anxiety and irritability in pervasive developmental disorders and ADHD
- Treatment of neuroleptic-induced akathisia; preliminary data suggest benefit in tardive dyskinesia (60–160 mg/day)
- May be useful in alleviating sexual side effects and bruxism caused by SSRI antidepressants
- Contradictory evidence as to efficacy in social phobia; may be useful as an augmenting agent in partial responders to SSRIs

GENERAL COMMENTS

- Buspirone (Buspar) is a selective anxiolytic of the azaspirone class; unlike the benzodiazepines, it has no anticonvulsant or muscle-relaxant properties
- Tolerance to effects of buspirone has not been reported
- Has a low potential for abuse or addiction
- Lack of effect on respiration may make it useful in patients with pulmonary disease or sleep apnea – may actually stimulate respiration
- Minimal effect on cognition, memory or driving performance

PHARMACOLOGY

- Unlike the benzodiazepines, buspirone does not bind to the GABA-"benzodiazepine" receptor complex, but has a marked effect on serotonin transmission and affects nonadrenergic and dopaminergic activity
- A 5-HT_{1A} agonist; chronic administration causes downregulation of 5-HT_2 receptors

DOSAGE

- 5–30 mg daily in divided doses
- A lag time of 1–2 weeks may be needed for the anxiolytic effect to occur; rarely doses up to 60 mg daily are required

☞ **Not effective on a prn basis**

* ▲ Approved indications

Buspirone (cont.)

PHARMACOKINETICS

- Absorption is virtually complete; first-pass effect reduces bioavailability to about 4%
- Food may reduce rate of absorption and decrease extent of first-pass effect
- Highly bound to plasma proteins
- Peak plasma level: 0.7–1.5 h. Onset of action takes days to weeks; maximum effect seen in 3–4 weeks
- Elimination half-life: 1–11 h. Metabolite: 1-(2-pyrimidinyl) piperazine (active); parent drug metabolized by CYP3A4 and 2C19; metabolite metabolized by 2D6

ADVERSE EFFECTS

- Causes little sedation; does not impair psychomotor or cognitive functions
- Headache (up to 6%), dizziness (up to 12%), lightheadedness (3%), nervousness (5%), excitement (2%), fatigue, paresthesia, numbness and GI upset seen in less than 10% of patients
- Withdrawal effects have not been reported
- Due to its effect on dopamine, the possible risk of neurological effects has been a concern; however, buspirone does not lead to postsynaptic dopamine receptor hypersensitivity since it binds only to presynaptic dopamine autoreceptors; when combined with neuroleptic, increases in extrapyramidal reactions (including dyskinesias) have been reported
- Can precipitate hypomania or mania (primarily in elderly); high doses may worsen psychosis
- Dose-dependent increase in prolactin and growth hormone levels reported

PRECAUTIONS

- Has no cross-tolerance with benzodiazepines and will not alleviate benzodiazepine withdrawal; when switching, taper benzodiazepine dose while adding buspirone to the regimen
- Caution in patients with seizure disorder as drug has no anticonvulsant activity

TOXICITY

- No deaths have been reported
- Excessive doses produce extension of pharmacological effects including dizziness, nausea, and vomiting; monitor respiration, BP, and pulse, and give symptomatic and supportive therapy

PEDIATRIC CONSIDERATIONS

- Buspirone used in aggression, autism, anxiety disorders, and to augment SSRIs in obsessive-compulsive disorder (10–30 mg/day)
- Behavior activation, euphoria, increased aggression and psychosis reported

GERIATRIC CONSIDERATIONS

- Buspirone does not cause sedation, cognitive impairment, disinhibition or motor impairment in the elderly
- Used in behavior disturbances of dementia at doses of 20–45 mg/day
- Dosage should be decreased in patients with reduced hepatic or renal function

USE IN PREGNANCY

- Safety in pregnancy has not yet been determined; no teratogenicity in animal studies

Breast milk

- Buspirone and metabolites are excreted in human milk; no data on safety

NURSING IMPLICATIONS

- The effect of buspirone is gradual; improvement may be seen 7–10 days after starting therapy
- As an immediate response does not occur, buspirone should be taken consistently, not on a prn basis

PATIENT INSTRUCTIONS

For detailed patient information on buspirone, see the Patient Information Sheet on p. 260.

- Expect a gradual improvement in anxiety over 2–4 weeks
- Do not increase the dose without prior consultation with the physician

DRUG INTERACTIONS

Class of Drug	Example	Interaction Effect
Antidepressant		
SARI	Trazodone	Case of serotonin syndrome with high dose of trazodone
Irreversible MAOI	Phenelzine, tranylcypromine	Elevated blood pressure reported
SSRI	Fluoxetine, fluvoxamine	May potentiate anti-obsessional effects of the antidepressants Increased plasma level of buspirone (3-fold) with fluvoxamine Case reports of serotonin syndrome, euphoria, seizures or dystonia with combination
Antifungal	Itraconazole	Increased plasma level of buspirone (13-fold) due to inhibited metabolism via CYP3A4
Antipsychotic	Haloperidol	Increased plasma level of haloperidol by 26% due to inhibited metabolism
Benzodiazepine	Diazepam	Increased serum level of benzodiazepine
Calcium-channel blocker	Verapamil, diltiazem	Increased peak plasma level of buspirone (3–4-fold) due to inhibited metabolism via CYP3A4
Cyclosporin A		Increased serum level of cyclosporin A with possible renal adverse effects
Digoxin		Effects of digoxin may be increased
Erythromycin		Increased plasma level of buspirone (5-fold) due to inhibited metabolism via CYP3A4
Grapefruit juice		Increased peak plasma level of buspirone (up to 15-fold), AUC (up to 20-fold) and half-life (1.5-fold) due to inhibited metabolism via CYP3A4
Rifampicin		Decreased peak plasma concentration and half-life of buspirone due to induced metabolism via CYP3A4

HYPNOTICS/SEDATIVES

PRODUCT AVAILABILITY

Chemical Class*	Generic Name	Trade Name[(A)]	Dosage Forms and Strengths
Antihistamines	Hydroxyzine	Atarax, Vistaril[(B)]	Capsules: 10 mg, 25 mg, 50 mg Oral syrup: 10 mg/5 ml Injection: 50 mg/ml
	Diphenhydramine	Benadryl	Capsules: 25 mg, 50 mg Chewable tablets: 12.5 mg Oral solution: 6.25 mg/5 ml, 12.5 mg/5 ml Injection: 50 mg/ml
	Doxylamine[(B)]	Unisom	Tablets: 25 mg
Barbiturate	Amobarbital	Amytal	Capsules: 60 mg, 200 mg Injection: 500 mg/vial
	Pentobarbital	Nembutal	Capsules: 50 mg[(B)], 100 mg Oral solution[(B)]: 18.2 mg/5 ml Injection: 50 mg/ml Suppositories[(B)]: 30 mg, 60 mg, 120 mg, 200 mg
	Secobarbital	Seconal	Capsules: 100 mg
Benzodiazepines			see pp. 109–120
Chloral derivative	Chloral hydrate	Noctec, Aquachloral[(B)]	Capsules: 500 mg Oral solution: 500 mg/5 ml
Acetaldehyde polymer	Paraldehyde		Injection: 5 ml
Amino acid	L-Tryptophan[(C)]	Tryptan	Tablets: 500 mg, 1 g Capsules: 500 mg
Tertiary acetylenic carbinol	Ethchlorvynol[(B)]	Placidyl	Capsules: 200 mg, 500 mg, 750 mg
Cyclopyrrolone	Zopiclone[(C)]	Imovane	Tablets: 5 mg, 7.5 mg
Imidazopyridine derivative	Zolpidem[(B)]	Ambien	Tablets: 5 mg, 10 mg
Pyrazolopyrimidine	Zaleplon	Sonata[(B)], Starnoc[(C)]	Capsules: 5 mg, 10 mg

[(A)] Generic preparations may be available, [(B)] Not marketed in Canada, [(C)] Not marketed in USA
* Many of these drugs are no longer recommended for use as hypnotics because of their low therapeutic index and high addiction liability. Drugs most commonly used today as hypnotics include the benzodiazepines, chloral hydrate, zopiclone, zaleplon, and zolpidem. See comparison chart, pp. 129–132

INDICATIONS*

- ▲ • Nocturnal sedation; short-term management of insomnia
- ▲ • Preoperative sedation

* ▲ Approved indications

GENERAL COMMENTS

- Prior to treatment of insomnia, determine if sleep disturbance is
  - due to a primary sleep disorder (e.g., sleep apnea, restless legs syndrome, narcolepsy)
  - due to psychiatric disorder (e.g., depression, mania)
  - drug-induced (e.g., theophylline, sympathomimetics)
  - due to medical disorder (e.g., thyroid, peptic ulcer)
  - due to use of excessive caffeine, alcohol
- Treat the primary cause, wherever possible
- Use of hypnotics is recommended for limited time periods; long-term, continuous treatment is not recommended (except L-tryptophan)

PHARMACOLOGY

- Hypnotics suppress the reticular formation of the midbrain to various degrees resulting in sedation, sleep, or anesthesia
- Benzodiazepines bind to the "benzodiazepine"-GABA-chloride receptor complex in the brain
- Zolpidem and zaleplon bind selectively to $GABA_{A1}$ receptors

DOSING

- See pp. 129–130 for individual agents
- Dosage should be adjusted in the elderly and in patients with hepatic impairment

PHARMACOKINETICS

- See pp. 129–130
- Zaleplon: absorption and peak plasma level decreased with high fat meal (C_{max} and T_{max} decreased by 35%). Japanese patients showed increased C_{max} and AUC by 37% and 64%, respectively
- Zolpidem: peak plasma level increased (by more than 50%) and half-life increased in female elderly patients and in cirrhosis
- Zopiclone: half life doubled in elderly patients

ONSET AND DURATION OF ACTION

- See table pp. 129–130
- Tolerance to effects of many hypnotics occurs after 2 weeks of continuous use

ADVERSE EFFECTS

- See chart pp. 131–132
- Day-time sedation; dependent on drug dosage, half-life, and patient tolerance
- Anterograde amnesia is dependent on drug potency and dose
- Rebound insomnia is dependent on drug dose, half-life, and duration of use
- High dose can impair respiration and blood pressure

WITHDRAWAL

- See chart pp. 131–132 for specific drugs
- Discontinuation of hypnotics can produce:
  - Withdrawal: occurs within 1–2 days (short-acting) to 3–7 days (long-acting) following discontinuation of regular use of most hypnotics (for more than 2 weeks) ; suggested to occur less frequently with zopiclone and zolpidem. Common symptoms include insomnia, agitation, anxiety, perceptual disturbances (e.g., photophobia), malaise and anorexia. Abrupt withdrawal of high doses may result in seizures and/or psychosis
  - Rebound: occurs hours to days after drug withdrawal; described as worsening of insomnia beyond pretreatment levels. More likely to occur with short-acting agents
  - Relapse: recurrence of the insomnia, to pretreatment levels, when the hypnotic is discontinued
- Can occur with chronic use of all hypnotics

Management

- Withdrawal of a hypnotic (after chronic use) should be tailored to each patient, with gradual tapering of the drug over several weeks

PRECAUTIONS

- Abrupt withdrawal of hypnotics (excluding antihistamines, zopiclone, and L-tryptophan) may produce anxiety, insomnia, dizziness, nausea, vomiting, twitching, hyperthermia, tremors, convulsions, and death; psychosis and delirium have been reported following abrupt withdrawal of ethchlorvynol

Hypnotics/Sedatives (cont.)

- Withdrawal should be accomplished by switching to a comparable dose of a long-acting barbiturate (e.g., phenobarbital) and tapering the dose gradually (by 30 mg/day). For benzodiazepines, see pp. 112–113
- Long-term administration of barbiturates has been associated with osteomalacia in adults, because of altered vitamin D metabolism
- Avoid use in addiction-prone individuals (except L-tryptophan)
- Abuse may result in clouding of consciousness and visual hallucinations
- Use in individuals with sleep apnea is contraindicated

TOXICITY

- Symptoms of overdose include: excitement, restlessness, delirium, nystagmus, ataxia, and stupor (does not apply to L-tryptophan); hypothermia has been reported with barbiturates
- Overdoses of ethchlorvynol are more difficult to treat than barbiturate overdose
- Lethal dose of chloral hydrate is approximately 10 times the therapeutic dose (5–10 g)

PEDIATRIC CONSIDERATIONS

- Barbiturates:
  - chronic use has been associated with hyperkinetic states with symptoms such as reduced attention span, and destructive or aggressive reactions; developmental delays reported with mental slowing
  - long-term administration associated with rickets due to altered vitamin D metabolism
- Chloral hydrate:
  - dosage: 50 mg/kg body weight is recommended; high doses can depress respiration and blood pressure
  - used as a sedative for non-invasive procedures (e.g., EEG, CT scan) and for sedation of neonates, infants, and children (under age of 6)
- Antihistamines:
  - paradoxical CNS excitation can occur

GERIATRIC CONSIDERATIONS

- As a rule, lower doses should be utilized in the elderly
- Caution when using drugs that are metabolized by oxidation (e.g., flurazepam), as they can accumulate in the elderly or in persons with liver disease
- Caution when combined with other drugs with CNS properties; additive effects can cause confusion, disorientation
- Anterograde amnesia reported with higher doses
- Diphenhydramine reported to decrease disturbed behavior in patients with dementia

USE IN PREGNANCY

See pp. 131–132 for individual agents. For benzodiazepines, see p. 114

Breast milk

- The American Academy of Pediatrics considers many hypnotics/sedatives compatible with breastfeeding – see table pp. 129–130

NURSING IMPLICATIONS

- Counsel patient regarding chronic use of hypnotic and loss of efficacy of drug over time (tolerance), L-tryptophan, zopiclone and zolpidem excepted
- Suggest that abrupt withdrawal after chronic use may result in serious side effects and rebound symptoms; drugs should be tapered over time
- Suggest alternative methods of treating insomnia (e.g., avoid caffeine, do relaxation exercises, avoid daytime naps)
- Assess personal sleep habits to determine causes or contributing factors to insomnia (e.g., alcohol, caffeine, etc.)

PATIENT INSTRUCTIONS

For detailed patient instructions on hypnotics/sedatives, see the Patient Information Sheet on p. 261.

- Continued regular use may result in loss of efficacy; sudden stoppage may cause worsening of sleep patterns and rebound anxiety
- Do not increase the dose without prior consultation with the physican

DRUG INTERACTIONS

- Only clinically significant interactions are listed below

Class of Drug	Example	Interaction Effect
Antibiotic	Erythromycin	*Zopiclone* increased plasma level of zopiclone due to decreased clearance
Anticoagulant	Dicumarol, warfarin	*Chloral hydrate* will displace drugs that are protein-bound and temporarily enhance hypoprothrombinemic response; increased or decreased PT ratio or INR response *Barbiturates* will induce metabolism and decrease the efficacy of anticoagulants; on withdrawal, excess bleeding can occur *Ethchlorvynol* may reduce the hypoprothrombinemic effect *Paraldehyde:* decreased PT ratio or INR response
Anticonvulsant	Carbamazepine, phenytoin	*Zopiclone:* decreased plasma level of zopiclone due to induced metabolism via CYP3A4
Antidepressant		
SSRI, RIMA, MAOI	Fluoxetine, moclobemide, phenelzine, tranylcypromine	*L-Tryptophan* combination may produce increased serotonin activity resulting in twitching, agitation ("serotonin syndrome") Additive antidepressant effect in treatment-resistant patients
SSRI	Fluoxetine, fluvoxamine	Increased sedation and side effects of *chloral hydrate* due to inhibited metabolism
SSRI/SNRI/NDRI	Sertraline, venlafaxine, bupropion	*Zolpidem:* case reports of hallucinations and delirium with sertraline, fluoxetine, paroxetine, venlafaxine and bupropion
Tricyclics	Imipramine Desipramine	*Zolpidem:* in one study 5/8 patients on combination experienced anterograde amnesia; case report of visual hallucinations with combination
Antihistamine	Terfenadine, astemizole	*Chloral hydrate:* potentiation of QT prolongation – AVOID
Caffeine	Tea, coffee, colas	May counteract sedation and increase insomnia
Cimetidine		*Zaleplon:* increased peak plasma level and AUC of zaleplon by 85% due to inhibition of metabolism via CYP3A4 and aldehyde oxidase
CNS depressant	Alcohol, neuroleptics	Increased CNS depression and psychomotor impairment; in "high" doses coma and respiratory depression can occur
Disulfiram		Avoid *paraldehyde;* since it is metabolized to acetaldehyde, an alcohol-like reaction will occur
Grapefruit juice		*Zaleplon:* increased plasma level of zaleplon due to inhibited metaboilsm via CYP3A4
Ketoconazole		*Zolpidem:* decreased oral clearance of zolpidem by 41%; half-life increased by 26% *Zopiclone:* increased AUC and elimination half-life due to decreased metabolism
Lithium		Increased efficacy and increased plasma level of lithium with *L-tryptophan*
Oral contraceptive		*Chloral hydrate:* decreased efficacy of the oral contraceptive due to induction of microsomal enzymes
Protease inhibitor	Ritonavir	*Zolpidem:* increased plasma level of zolpidem due to decreased metabolism via CYP3A4

Hypnotics/Sedatives (cont.)

Class of Drug	Example	Interaction Effect
Rifampin		*Zolpidem:* decreased peak plasma level of zolpidem by 60% and increased elimination half-life by 36% *Zaleplon:* decreased AUC of zaleplon by 80% *Zopiclone:* decreased plasma level of zopiclone due to induced metabolism
β-Blocker **Corticosteroid** **Estrogen** **Doxycycline** **Griseofulvin** **Theophylline** **Oxtriphylline** **Phenylbutazone** **Protease inhibitors** **Quinidine** **Valproate**	Propranolol Dexamethasone Oral contraceptives Ritonavir, sequinavir Divalproex, valproic acid	*Barbiturates* will induce the metabolism and reduce the efficacy of these drugs

For drugs interacting with benzodiazepines see pp. 114–116; for L-tryptophan also see p. 157

Comparison of Hypnotics/Sedatives

	Usual Oral Adult Dose	Onset of Action	Half-life	Efficacy/ Tolerance	CYP-450 Metabolizing Enzyme[c]	CYP-450 Effect[d]	Indications
ANTIHISTAMINES							
Diphenhydramine (Benadryl, Nytol)	25–300 mg		1–3 h	Lose efficacy with time	–	2D6 inhibitor	Sedation, insomnia
Hydroxyzine (Atarax)	10–400 mg	15–30 min	8–10 h		–	–	Anxiety
Doxylamine[a] (Unisom)	25–150 mg	2–3 h	10 h		–	–	Insomnia
BARBITURATES							
Amobarbital sodium (Amytal)	65–200 mg	30 min	14–42 h	Loses effect after 2 weeks	2C, 3A4	2B, 2C, 3A4 inducer	Diagnostic aid in hysteria and schizophrenia; acute convulsive episodes, status epilepticus
Pentobarbital (Nembutal)	50–200 mg	15 min	21–42 h	Loses effect after 2 weeks	2C, 3A4	2B, 2C, 3A4 inducer	Insomnia, daytime sedation for anxiety and tension, anesthesia
Secobarbital (Seconal)	50–200 mg	15 min	2–3 h	Loses effect after 2 weeks	–	–	Nocturnal and pre-operative sedation, dental procedures, sleep EEGs, acute convulsive disorders
Chloral Hydrate (Noctec)	0.5–2 g	30 min	4–8 h	Loses effect after 2 weeks	–	inducer	Nocturnal and pre-operative sedation; alcohol, barbiturate, and narcotic withdrawal; porphyria
Paraldehyde	10–30 ml (hypnotic) 5–10 ml (sedative)	10 min	4–8 h		–	–	Drug and alcohol withdrawal, excited psychiatric states, convulsive control in tetany and poisoning
L-Tryptophan[b] (Trofan, Tryptan)	1–5 g	variable	–	No tolerance reported	–	–	Insomnia, mood disorder prophylaxis
Ethchlorvynol (Placidyl)	0.5–1 g	15–30 min	5 h	Loses effect after 2 weeks	–	inducer	Insomnia
Zaleplon (Sonata, Starnoc)	5–10 mg (5 mg in elderly)	Rapid Peak level: 0.9–1.5 h	0.9–1.1 h	No tolerance after 4 weeks	3A4, aldehyde-oxidase	–	Insomnia
Zolpidem[a] (Ambien)	5–20 mg (5 mg in elderly)	30 min Peak level: 1.6 h	1.5–4.5 h	No tolerance after 50 weeks	3A4	–	Insomnia Early data suggest possible efficacy in treating Parkinson's disease

Comparison of Hypnotics/Sedatives (cont.)

	Usual Oral Adult Dose	Onset of Action	Half-life	Efficacy/ Tolerance	CYP-450 Metabolizing Enzyme[c]	CYP-450 Effect[d]	Indications
Zopiclone[b] (Imovane)	3.75–15 mg	30 min Peak level: 90 min	3.8–6.5 h (5–10 h in elderly)	No tolerance after 17 weeks	1A2, 2C9	?	Insomnia (increasing the dose above 15 mg may not produce increased efficacy)

(a) Not marketed in Canada, (b) Not marketed in USA, (c) Cytochrome P-450 isoenzymes involved in drug metabolism, (d) Effect of drug on cytochrome enzymes

	Effect on Sleep Architecture	Pregnancy/Lactation	Precautions	Main Side Effects
Antihistamine		In animals, teratogenicity seen in high doses; case reports in humans, but correlation not proven Excreted into human milk; newborn have increased sensitivity to antihistamines	Elderly patients more susceptible to adverse effects; may precipitate seizures in patients with focal lesions	Sedation, incoordination; anticholinergic effects at high doses (dry mouth, blurred vision, confusion, delirium etc.); GI disturbances; paradoxical CNS excitation can occur; tolerance to effects occurs within days or weeks
Barbiturate	Suppress REM sleep and delta sleep; REM rebound on withdrawal	Barbiturates cross the placenta; an increase in congenital defects and hemorrhagic disease of newborn reported Prolonged elimination of barbiturate reported in fetus Withdrawal symptoms seen in newborn Excreted in breast milk; American Academy of Pediatrics considers secobarbital compatible with breast-feeding	**AVOID** barbiturates in: severe hepatic impairment, porphyria, uncontrolled pain (delirium may result) pulmonary insufficiency, confused and restless elderly patients With low doses, patient may become euphoric, excited, restless, or violent; at high doses, can develop acute confusional state and respiratory depression Risk of suicide due to low lethal dose Risk of tolerance; high potential for abuse and dependence	CNS: confusion, hangover, drowsiness, weight gain, excitement if given to patients in severe pain skin rash (1–3%), nausea, vomiting Can cause severe depression (risk of suicide)
Chloral hydrate	REM sleep decreased in doses over 1 g	Crosses placenta; no reports of congenital defects in newborn Excreted in breast milk; one report of drowsiness in newborn; American Academy of Pediatrics considers drug compatible with breast-feeding	**CAUTION** in hepatic and renal impairment, gastritis, peptic ulcer, and cardiac distress Doses above 2 g can impair respiration and decrease blood pressure Tolerance can occur with chronic use; withdrawal reactions reported	Nausea, vomiting, hangover, skin rash Does not accumulate with chronic use Will induce hepatic enzymes and affect metabolism of other drugs; will displace other drugs from protein binding
Paraldehyde		Crosses placenta; fetal concentration equals that of maternal blood; respiratory depression seen in neonates	**AVOID** in gastroenteritis, liver damage, bronchopulmonary disease; may produce excitement or delirium in presence of pain Decomposed product should not be used (acetic acid odor). Do not give to persons receiving disulfiram Dissolves plastic; use glass container/ syringe; use product immediately after drawing up in syringe	Unpleasant taste, odor imparted into exhaled air; may irritate throat and mucous membranes if administered chronically – dilute liberally Injection can be painful if more than 5 ml injected; give deep im
L-Tryptophan (see pp. 156–157)	Decreased REM latency and REM sleep; increased non-REM and total sleep time	Contraindicated: **AVOID**	In combination with other serotonergic drugs can cause twitching or jerking, i.e., "serotonin syndrome." Eosinophilic myalgia reported with certain preparations made from impure raw material. Chronic use associated with niacin and pyridoxine deficiency	GI upset: nausea, vomiting
Ethchlorvynol	REM sleep decreased with 500 mg	Crosses placenta; no reports of congenital defects; withdrawal symptoms seen in neonates	**CAUTION** in hepatic and renal impairment, cardiac distress, porphyria Low lethal dose Risk of tolerance; withdrawal reactions reported	Nausea, hypotension, headache, dizziness, blurred vision, confusion, allergic reactions

Comparison of Hypnotics/Sedatives (cont.)

	Effect on Sleep Architecture	Pregnancy/Lactation	Precautions	Main Side Effects
Zaleplon	Sleep latency and short-wave sleep decreased	Safety in pregnancy not established Excreted in breast milk; not recommended for nursing mothers	Due to rapid onset of action, should be taken immediately before bedtime Rebound insomnia reported	Drowsiness, headache, GI upset, asthenia, myalgia, paresthesias, dry mouth, hangover, anterograde amnesia
Zolpidem	Decreased sleep latency Time spent in REM sleep decreased with higher doses No effect on stages 3 and 4	Not teratogenic in animal studies Total drug excreted in milk does not exceed 0.02% of administered dose Considered compatible with breast-feeding by the American Academy of Pediatrics	**CAUTION** in liver dysfunction, respiratory impairment; elderly more prone to confusion, falls Abuse reported Withdrawal reactions reported including GI symptoms, flushing, lightheadedness, panic attacks, nervousness, crying, confusion, disorientation, insomnia, suicidal ideation, tremors and seizures	Drowsiness, dizziness, ataxia, agitation, nightmares, diarrhea, nausea, headache, hangover, anterograde amnesia, sleep walking and sleep talking Dysphoria reported at high doses; rarely delirium and psychosis reported with perceptual distortions and hallucinations (case reports primarily in females)
Zopiclone	REM delayed but duration the same; stage 1 shortened; stage 2 increased	Not teratogenic in animal studies Crosses placenta; no congenital abnormalities reported in humans. Newborns have significantly lower birth weights and lower gestational age Excreted in breast milk; infant receives approx. 1% of administered dose – effect unknown	**CAUTION** in respiratory impairment, liver dysfunction and depression; elderly are more prone to adverse effects. Anticholinergic agents may decrease plasma level Not recommended in children Dependence rare and withdrawal effects are mild; rebound insomnia reported	Generally dose-related: bitter taste, dry mouth, GI distress, palpitations, dyspnea, tremor, rash, chills, sweating, agitation Severe drowsiness, confusion and incoordination are signs of drug intolerance or excessive dosage

Mood Stabilizers

GENERAL COMMENTS

- Mood stabilizers can be classified as follows:

Chemical Class	Agent	Page
Lithium	Example: Lithium carbonate	See p. 133
Anticonvulsant	Carbamazepine Gabapentin Clonazepam Lamotrigine Valproate	See p. 140
Tryptophan	L-Tryptophan	See p. 156

Lithium

PRODUCT AVAILABILITY

Chemical Class	Generic Name	Trade Name[A]	Dosage Forms and Strengths
Lithium salt	Lithium carbonate	Lithotabs Eskalith, Lithonate[B] Lithane[C], Carbolith[C] Lithobid, Eskalith CR Duralith[C]	Tablets: 300 mg Capsules: 150 mg, 300 mg, 600 mg Sustained-release tablets: 300 mg, 450 mg[B]
	Lithium citrate	Cibalith-S	Oral solution: 300 mg/5 ml

[A] Generic preparations may be available, [B] Not marketed in Canada, [C] Not marketed in USA

INDICATIONS*

- ▲ Long-term control or prophylaxis of manic depressive (bipolar affective) disorder
- ▲ Treatment of acute mania
- Prevention or diminution of the intensity of subsequent episodes of mania and depression
- May potentiate the action of antidepressants in depression and in obsessive-compulsive disorder
- Organic brain syndrome with secondary affective symptoms
- Treatment of chronic aggression/antisocial behavior/impulsivity; may be useful in patients with an affective component to symptoms
- May ameliorate restlessness and excitability in up to 50% of patients with schizophrenia
- Migraine, cluster headaches

* ▲ Approved indications

Lithium (cont.)

GENERAL COMMENTS

- "Classic" mania responds best (up to 80%). Other possible predictors of response include: family history of lithium response in a first degree relative and few prior episodes of mania or depression
- Less response noted in patients with dysphoric/psychotic mania or mixed states (30–40%), rapid-cycling BAD (20–30%), in patients with multiple prior episodes, in adolescents and in patients with substance abuse
- Suggested to be more effective in augmenting antidepressants in bipolar than in unipolar depression
- May be more effective in preventing manic or mixed episodes than depressive episodes
- As some rapid-cycling may be contributed to by lithium-induced hypothyroidism, it is important to regularly assess thyroid function

PHARMACOLOGY

- Exact mechanism of action unknown; postulated that lithium may stabilize catecholamine receptors, and may alter calcium-mediated intracellular functions and increase GABA activity. Lithium blocks the ability of neurons to restore normal levels of the second messenger system (phosphatidylinositol biphosphate), thereby reducing the responsiveness of neurons to muscarinic, cholinergic, α-adrenergic, etc., stimuli
- Research data suggest that chronic lithium use increases N-acetyl-aspartate levels in the brain, and may exert neuroprotective effects
- Lithium therapy requires reaching plasma concentrations that are relatively close to the toxic concentration
- Administration of lithium requires 10–14 days before the complete effect is observed, therefore acute mania is often treated with a neuroleptic; lithium is subsequently added to the treatment regimen

DOSING

- Dose is usually guided by plasma level; increase slowly to minimize side effects
  - Acute treatment: 900–2400 mg daily (0.8–1.2 mmol/L)
  - Maintenance: 400–1200 mg daily (0.6–1.0 mmol/L)
- Once patient is stabilized, once-daily dosing is preferable (if patient can tolerate)
- Patients sensitive to side effects that are related to high peak plasma levels, e.g., tremor, urinary frequency and GI effects (i.e., nausea), may respond to slow release preparations (e.g., Duralith)

PHARMACOKINETICS

- Peak plasma level: 1.5–2 h (slow release preparation = 4 h)
- Half-life: 8–35 h; once-daily dosing preferred (improved compliance and decreased urine volume and renal toxicity), half-life increases with duration of therapy (e.g., up to 58 h after 1 year's therapy)
- Patients in an acute manic episode appear to have an increased tolerance to lithium
- Excreted primarily by the kidney; therefore, adequate renal function is essential in order to avoid lithium accumulation and intoxication; clearance is significantly correlated with total body weight. Close relationship between level of dehydration and renal clearance
- Monitoring: measure first plasma level 5 days after starting therapy (unless toxicity is suspected). Measure once weekly for the first 2 weeks, thereafter at clinical discretion (at least every 6 months), or whenever a new drug is prescribed or if the dose is increased. Blood levels should be measured at TROUGH, i.e., 9–13 h after last dose
- Lithium is secreted in saliva reaching concentrations 3 times that seen in plasma – saliva composition is altered (see Adverse Effects/GI Effects below)

ADVERSE EFFECTS

1. CNS Effects

- General weakness (up to 33%), fatigue, dazed feeling and restlessness are usually transient and may coincide with peaks in lithium concentration
- Drowsiness, tiredness
- Cognitive blunting, memory difficulties (up to 28%), decreased speed of information processing, confusion, lack of drive, productivity or creativity [Management: assess lithium plasma level and thyroid function; slow-release preparation, a lower dose, or liothyronine may improve cognitive function]
- Slurred speech, ataxia – evaluate for lithium toxicity
- Neuromuscular: incoordination, muscle weakness, fine tremor/shakiness – up to 65% incidence; more frequent at higher doses and in combination with antidepressant or neuroleptic, with excessive caffeine use, or alcoholism. Frequency of tremor decreases with

time [Management: reduce dose, eliminate dietary caffeine; β-blocker (e.g., propranolol or atenolol) may be of benefit]. A coarse tremor may be a sign of lithium toxicity. Cogwheel rigidity and choreoathetosis reported
- Chronic treatment can affect the peripheral nervous system involving motor and sensory function
- Cases of tardive dyskinesia reported in patients on lithium who have not used neuroleptics for at least 6 months
- Seizures rare
- Headaches; rarely, papilledema/elevated intracranial pressure (pseudotumor cerebri) reported
- Case of somnambulism

2. GI Effects

- Usually coincide with peaks in lithium concentration and are probably due to rapid absorption of the lithium ion; most disappear after a few weeks; if occur late in therapy, evaluate for lithium toxicity
- Nausea – up to 50% incidence, abdominal pain [Management: administer with food, or use slow-release preparation]
- Vomiting – 20% incidence; higher with increased plasma level [Management: use multiple daily dosing, change to a slow-release preparation, or lower dose]
- Diarrhea, loose stools – up to 20% incidence. Slow release preparation may worsen this side effect in some patients [Management: if on a slow-release product, change to a regular lithium preparation; less problems noted with lithium citrate preparations; if all else fails and cannot decrease the lithium dose, loperamide prn]
- Metallic taste: composition of saliva altered (ions and proteins)
- Excessive thirst (up to 36% of incidence), dry mouth, mucosal ulceration (rare), hypersalivation occasionally reported
- Weight gain – up to 60% incidence (25% of patients gain excessive weight); may be related to increased appetite, fluid retention, altered carbohydrate and fat metabolism or to hypothyroidism [Management: reduce caloric intake]. Mean gain is 7.5 kg on lithium alone (may be higher with drug combinations) and may be related to dose

3. Cardiovascular Effects

- Bradycardia
- Dizziness and vertigo [Management: administer with food, use slow-release preparation to avoid peak lithium levels, or reduce dosage]
- ECG changes: 20–30% benign T-wave changes at therapeutic doses; use lithium cautiously in patients with pre-existing cardiac disease; arrhythmias and sinus node dysfunction occur less frequently (sinus node dysfunction reported with lithium-carbamazepine combination, with high plasma levels of lithium, in the elderly, and in patients taking other drugs that may affect conduction)
- Isolated cases of cardiac sinus node dysfunction [assess patient who has syncopal episode]

4. Renal Effects

- Usually seen after chronic use
- Polyuria and polydipsia – up to 40% risk (dose-related); monitor for fluid and electrolyte imbalance – usually reversible if lithium stopped; however, several cases of persistant diabetes insipidus reported up to 57 months after lithium stopped [potassium-sparing diuretic (amiloride 10–20 mg/day) or DDAVP (10 μg nasal spray or tablets 0.2 mg) may be useful]; sustained-release preparations may cause less impairment of urine concentrating function
- Changes in distal tubular function including impaired urine concentrating ability (not always reversible) and chronic focal interstitial nephritis
- Reduced glomerular filtration rates reported with chronic treatment (21% of patients after 15 years)
- Histological changes include: a) interstitial fibrosis, tubular atrophy and glomerulosclerosis, seen in 26% patients after treatment beyond two years – primarily those with impaired urine concentrating ability; b) distal tubular dilatation and macrocyst formation
- Rare cases of nephrotic syndrome with proteinuria, edema and hypoalbuminemia

5. Dermatological Effects

- Dry skin common
- Skin rash, pruritis, exacerbation of psoriasis [the latter may respond to inositol up to 6 g/day]
- Acne [may respond to: pyridoxine 50 mg bid, zinc sulfate 110 mg bid, or β-carotene 25,000 IU daily]
- Dryness and thinning of hair – may be related to hypothyroidism
- Folliculitis (may occur more frequently in the spring) [may respond to antihistamines]

6. Endocrine Effects

- Long-term effects: clinical hypothyroidism in up to 34% of patients – risk greater in women over age 40 and in rapid cyclers – may be more common in regions of high dietary iodine (monitor TSH level – may require levothyroxine therapy). Subclinical hypothyroidism (high TSN and normal free T_4) found in 25% of patients on lithium

Lithium (cont.)

- Goiter (not necessarily associated with hypothyroidism) – may be more common in regions of iodine deficiency
- Hyperparathyroidism with hypercalcemia reported in 10–40% of patients on maintenance therapy; may predispose to cardiac conduction disturbances; occasional reports of parathyroid adenoma and hyperplasia

7. Other Adverse Effects

- Blurred vision may be related to peak plasma levels; reduction in retinal light sensitivity
- Changes in sexual function – up to 10% risk; includes decreased libido, erectile dysfunction, priapism and decreased sperm motility; soreness and ulceration of genitalia (rare)
- Edema, swelling of extremities – evaluate for sodium retention [use diuretics with caution – see Interactions – spironolactone may be preferred]
- Anemia, leukocytosis (up to 18% of patients), leucopenia, albuminuria; rarely aplastic anemia, agranulocytosis, thrombocytopenia and thrombocytosis
- Rarely – can induce polyarthritis

WITHDRAWAL

- Rarely anxiety, instability, and emotional lability reported following abrupt withdrawal
- Rapid discontinuation may increase the risk of relapse
- 50% rate of manic or depressive recurrence within 3 to 5 months among previously stable patients reported with abrupt withdrawal

PRECAUTIONS

- Good kidney function, adequate salt and fluid intake are essential
- Excessive loss of sodium (due to vomiting, diarrhea, use of diuretics, etc.) causes increased lithium retention, possibly leading to toxicity; lower doses of lithium are necessary if the patient is on a salt-restricted diet (which includes most low-calorie diets)
- Heavy sweating can lead to diminished levels and efficacy of lithium
- Use cautiously and in reduced dosage in the elderly as the ability to excrete lithium decreases with age
- Some researchers suggest that concurrent ECT may increase the possibility of developing cerebral toxicity to lithium; discontinue during courses of ECT, if possible
- Do not rapidly increase lithium and neuroleptic dosage at the same time, due to risk of neurotoxicity

CONTRAINDICATIONS

- Brain damage
- Renal disease
- Cardiovascular disease
- Severe debilitation

TOXICITY

Mild Toxicity

- At lithium levels of 1.5–2 mmol/L; occasionally occurs with levels in the normal range
- Develops gradually over several days
- Side effects such as ataxia, coarse tremor, confusion, diarrhea, drowsiness, fasciculation, and slurred speech may occur

Management

- Stop lithium

Moderate/Severe Toxicity

- At lithium levels in excess of 2 mmol/L
- Severe poisoning may result in coma with hyperreflexia, muscle tremor, hyperextension of the limbs, pulse irregularities, hypertension or hypotension, ECG changes, peripheral circulatory failure, and epileptic seizures; acute tubular necrosis (renal failure) can occur
- Lithium toxicity may manifest as a catatonic stupor
- Deaths have been reported; when serum lithium level exceeds 4 mmol/L the prognosis is poor

Management

- Symptomatic: Reduce absorption, restore fluid and electrolyte balance, correct sodium depletion and remove drug from the body
- Blood lithium concentration may be reduced by forced alkaline diuresis or by prolonged peritoneal dialysis or hemodialysis
- Excretion may be facilitated by IV urea, sodium bicarbonate, acetazolamide, or aminophylline

- Convulsions may be controlled by a short-acting barbiturate (thiopental sodium)

PEDIATRIC CONSIDERATIONS

- Double blind controlled study suggests efficacy in children with chronic aggressive conduct disorders at doses of 900–2100 mg/day (0.78–1.55 mmol/L)
- Lithium has been used successfully in bipolar disorder, in periodic mood and behavior disorders and pervasive developmental disorder (autism)
- Half-life shorter and clearance is faster than seen in adults
- Maintain plasma level between 0.6 and 1.2 mmol/L
- Many children and adolescents with BAD present with mixed mood states or rapid cycling, and this often predicts diminished lithium response; other factors associated with non-response include: early onset ADHD and pre-pubertal onset of BAD symptoms
- Most common side effects in children include nausea, vomiting, tremor, polyuria, enuresis and ataxia; elevated TSH levels reported with combination of lithium and valproate
- Monitor thyroid, cardiac, and renal function every 6–12 months
- Lithium may decrease bone density by altering the concentration of parathyroid hormone

GERIATRIC CONSIDERATIONS

- Good kidney function, adequate salt and fluid intake are essential; ability to excrete lithium decreases with age, resulting in a longer elimination half-life
- Start therapy at lower doses and monitor serum level
- Incidence of side effects may be greater and occur at lower plasma levels, including tremor, GI disturbances, polyuria, ataxia, myoclonus and EPS
- Elderly are at increased risk for hyponatremia after an acute illness or if fluid intake is restricted
- Elderly are at higher risk for neurotoxicity and cognitive impairment, even at therapeutic plasma levels
- Slow release preparation may decrease side effects that occur as a result of peak plasma levels

USE IN PREGNANCY

- Avoid in pregnancy (especially first trimester), overall risk of fetal malformations is 4–12%; cardiovascular malformations can occur (0.05–0.1% risk of Ebstein's anomaly) – can be detected by fetal echocardiography and high resolution ultrasound at 16–18 weeks gestation
- Lithium clearance increased by 50–100% in pregnancy because of greater glomerular filtration rate; rate returns to pre-pregnancy levels after delivery
- Use of lithium near term may produce severe toxicity in the newborn, which is usually reversible, including nontoxic goiter, nephrogenic diabetes insipidus, floppy baby syndrome

Breast milk

- Present in breast milk at a concentration of 30–100% of mother's serum (infant's serum concentration is approximately equal to or less than that of the milk)
- The American Academy of Pediatrics considers lithium contraindicated during breastfeeding
- If breastfeeding is undertaken, the mother should be educated about signs and symptoms of lithium toxicity and risks of infant dehydration

NURSING IMPLICATIONS

- Accurate observation and assessment of patient's behavior before and after lithium therapy is initiated is important
- Be alert for, observe, and report any signs of side effects, or symptoms of toxicity; if toxic withhold the dose and call doctor immediately
- Check fluid intake and output; adjust fluid and salt ingestion to compensate if excessive loss occurs through vomiting or diarrhea
- May give lithium with meals to avoid GI disturbances
- Withhold morning dose of lithium until after the blood draw, on mornings when blood is drawn for a lithium level
- The patient and family should be educated regarding the drug's effects and toxicities
- Slow release preparations should not be broken or crushed. They may decrease side effects that occur as a result of high peak plasma levels (i.e., 1–2 h post dose), e.g., tremor

PATIENT INSTRUCTIONS

For detailed patient instructions on lithium, see the Patient Information Sheet on p. 263.

- Expect nausea, thirst, frequent urination, and generalized discomfort during the first few days

Lithium (cont.)

- Expect a lag of up to 3 weeks before the full beneficial effects of the drug are noticed
- Maintain adequate salt and fluid intake; do not go on any special diets without consulting the physician
- Avoid driving a car or operating hazardous machinery until response to the drug is determined
- Be aware of signs of early toxicity (diarrhea, vomiting, drowsiness, muscular weakness); if these occur, stop taking lithium and call the doctor immediately
- Carry an identification/instruction card with toxicity and emergency information, or wear a medic-alert bracelet
- Get lithium levels done regularly and have an outpatient follow-up of thyroid and renal functions every 12 months; do not take your lithium dose the morning of the blood test until after blood is drawn
- Do not alter your caffeine intake dramatically while taking lithium
- If you are taking a sustained-release preparation (e.g., Duralith), do not break or crush the tablet, but swallow it whole

LABORATORY TESTS

At beginning of treatment and at every admission:

1) serum electrolytes
2) Hb, Hct, WBC and differential, ESR
3) sensitive TSH, total T_4, T_4 uptake
4) BUN, creatinine
5) calcium
6) parathormone
7) ECG for patients over 45, or with a history of cardiac problems

On an out-patient basis, repeat tests (2) + (3) every 6 months; (4) every 12 months; (5) every 2 years; (6) every 5 years. As some rapid cycling may be due to lithium-induced hypothyroidism, it is important to regularly assess thyroid function

DRUG INTERACTIONS

- Only clinically significant interactions are listed below

Class of Drug	Example	Interaction Effects
Anesthetic	Ketamine	Increased lithium toxicity due to sodium depletion
Angiotensin-converting enzyme (ACE) inhibitor	Captopril, enalapril, lisinopril	Increased lithium toxicity due to sodium depletion; average increase in lithium level of 36% reported
Antibiotic/anti-infective	Ampicillin, doxycycline, tetracycline, spectinomycin, levofloxacin, metronidazole	Case reports of increased lithium effect and toxicity due to decreased renal clearance of lithium. Monitor lithium level if combination used
Anticonvulsant	Carbamazepine, phenytoin, valproate	Increased neurotoxicity of both drugs at therapeutic doses Synergistic mood-stabilizing effect with carbamazepine and valproate Valproate may aggravate action tremor
Antidepressant		
Cyclic, MAOIs, RIMA	Desipramine, tranylcypromine, moclobemide	Synergistic antidepressant effect in treatment-resistant patients May increase lithium tremor
SSRIs	Fluoxetine, fluvoxamine, sertraline	Elevated lithium serum level, with possible neurotoxicity and increased serotonergic effects (see p. 7) Synergistic effect in treatment-resistant depression and OCD

Class of Drug	Example	Interaction Effects
Antihistamine	Terfenadine, astemizole	Potentiation of QT prolongation – AVOID
Antihypertensive	Amiloride, spironolactone, thiazides, triamterene, methyldopa Acetazolamide, mannitol, urea β-blockers: propranolol, oxprenolol	Increased lithium effects and toxicity due to decreased renal clearance of lithium Increased renal excretion of lithium, decreasing its effect Beneficial effect in treatment of lithium tremor; propranolol lowers glomerular filtration rate and has been associated with a 19% reduction in lithium clearance
Antipsychotic	Molindone Haloperidol, perphenazine Clozapine	Increased plasma level of molindone reported; variable effects on plasma level of neuroleptics as well as lithium seen Increased neurotoxicity at therapeutic doses; may increase EPS Possible increased risk of agranulocytosis with clozapine; two cases of seizures reported with combination
Antiviral agent	Zidovudine	Reversal of zidovudine-induced neutropenia
Benzodiazepine	Clonazepam	Increased incidence of sexual dysfunction (up to 49%) reported with the combination
Ca-channel blocker	Verapamil, diltiazem	Increased neurotoxicity of both drugs; increased bradycardia and cardiotoxicity with verapamil due to combined calcium blockade
Caffeine		Increased renal excretion of lithium resulting in decreased plasma level May increase lithium tremor
Herbal diuretics	Agrimony, dandelion, juniper, licorice, horsetail, uva ursi Cola nut, guarana, maté	Elevated lithium level possible due to decreased renal clearance Increased excretion and decreased lithium level possible due to high content of caffeine in herbal preparations
Iodide salt	Calcium iodide	May act synergistically to produce hypothyroidism. AVOID
L-Tryptophan		Increased plasma level and increased efficacy and/or toxicity of lithium
Metronidazole		Decreased renal clearance of lithium resulting in elevated plasma levels. Monitor lithium level, creatinine and electrolyte levels and osmolality
NSAID	Ibuprofen, ketorolac, indomethacin, mefenamic acid, naproxen (no interaction with ASA); case reports with sulindac	Increased lithium level (by 12–66%) and possible toxicity due to decreased renal clearance of lithium. Monitor lithium level every 4–5 days until stable
Neuromuscular blocker	Succinylcholine, pancuronium	Potentiation of muscle relaxation
Psyllium	Metamucil, Prodiem	Decreased lithium level if drugs taken at the same time. Increased water drawn into the colon by the bulk laxatives would increase the amount of ionized lithium, which would remain unabsorbed
Sodium salt		Increased intake results in decreased lithium plasma level; decreased intake causes increased lithium plasma level
Theophylline	Aminophylline, oxtriphylline, theophylline	Enhanced renal lithium clearance and reduced plasma level (by approx. 20%) May increase lithium tremor
Trimethoprim/ Sulfamethoxazole		Case report of lithium toxicity within days of starting antimicrobial
Triptan	Sumatriptan, zolmitriptan	Increased serotonergic effects possible – monitor
Urinary alkalizer	Potassium citrate, sodium bicarbonate	Enhanced renal lithium clearance and reduced plasma level

Anticonvulsants

PRODUCT AVAILABILITY

Chemical Class	Generic Name	Trade Name[A]	Dosage Forms and Strengths
First generation	Clonazepam Phenytoin Phenobarbital Primidone	Rivotril[C], Klonopin[B] Dilantin Mysoline	See pp. 109–117 See p. 213 No longer used in psychiatry No longer used in psychiatry
Second generation	Carbamazepine Divalproex sodium Valproic acid	Tegretol Tegretol CR Depakote sprinkle[B] Depakote[B] Epival Depakene	Tablets: 200 mg Chewable tablets: 100 mg, 200 mg Oral suspension: 100 mg/5 mg Controlled-release tablets: 200 mg, 400 mg Capsules[B]: 125 mg Delayed-release tablets[B]: 125 mg, 250 mg, 500 mg Tablets: 125 mg, 250 mg, 500 mg Injection: 100 mg/ml[C] Capsules: 250 mg, 500 mg[C] Oral syrup: 250 mg/5 ml
Third generation	Gabapentin Lamotrigine Topiramate	Neurontin Lamictal Topamax	Capsules: 100 mg, 300 mg, 400 mg Tablets: 600 mg, 800 mg Tablets: 25 mg, 100 mg, 150 mg Chewable tablets: 2 mg[B], 5 mg See p. 214

[A] Generic preparations may be available, [B] Not marketed in Canada, [C] Not marketed in USA

INDICATIONS

	Carbamazepine	Valproate	Gabapentin	Lamotrigine
Acute mania/hypomania	▲ (Canada) **	▲	+/– (Bipolar II) (adjunctive drug – data contradictory)	+/– (data contradictory)
Prophylaxis of BAD	▲	+/– (data contradictory)	+ (open trials, adjunctive drug)	+/– (data contradictory)
Rapid-cycling BAD	+/–	+	+ (open trials, adjunctive drug)	+ (Bipolar II)
Mixed states	+	+	+ (open trials, adjunctive drug)	+

	Carbamazepine	Valproate	Gabapentin	Lamotrigine
Depression	+	+	–	+ (Bipolar I)
Anticonvulsant	▲Complex partial and limbic region seizures	▲Simple and complex partial seizures	▲Adjunctive in refractory epilepsy	▲Adjunctive or sole therapy in refractory epilepsy
Paroxysmal pain syndromes	▲	+	+	+ (preliminary data)
Migraine headaches	–	▲	+ (preliminary data)	–
Behavior disturbances (in dementia, explosive disorder, mental retardation, brain damage, autism spectrum disorders)	+ (alone or in combination with lithium, antipsychotics or β-blockers)	+	+ (preliminary data)	–
Panic disorder	+	+	+ (severe panic only; preliminary data)	–
Social phobia, generalized anxiety disorder	–	–	+	–
Posttraumatic stress disorder	+ (open trials)	+ (open trials)	–	+ (open trials)
Obsessive compulsive disorder	–	–	+ (adjunctive to SSRIs)	–
Borderline personality disorder	–	+ (preliminary data)	–	+ (preliminary data)
Paranoid ideation, hallucinations and negative symptoms of schizophrenia	+ (adjunctive drug)	+ (adjunctive drug)	–	+ (adjunctive drug – open trials)
Movement disorders	Dystonic disorder in children	–	Management of tardive dyskinesia in psychotic patients with affective features (preliminary data)	–
Drug dependence	Aid in alcohol or sedative/hypnotic withdrawal; may play a role in cocaine dependence	Aid in alcohol withdrawal (open trials)	May reduce craving for cocaine as well as its usage Aid in alcohol withdrawal (open trials)	–
Diabetes Insipidus	+	–	–	–

▲ Approved indications, **Not an approved indication in the USA

Anticonvulsants (cont.)

GENERAL COMMENTS

- For optimal response, in treatment-refractory patients, combination therapy may be required: e.g., with another mood stabilizer, an antipsychotic, antidepressant, or ECT

Carbamazepine

- Positive predictors of response include: dysphoric mania, an early age at onset and a negative family history of mood disorder and patients with neurological abnormalities
- Less response noted in patients with severe mania and rapid cycling

Valproate

- Positive predictors of response include: pure mania, mixed or dysphoric mania and rapid cycling; some response in mania with comorbid substance use disorder
- Less response noted in patients with comorbid personality disorder and severe mania
- May be more effective in treating and preventing manic and mixed episodes, than depressive episodes

Gabapentin

- May be more effective as an adjunctive medication in both Bipolar I and Bipolar II disorders (evidence limited to open trials)

Lamotrigine

- More effective in Bipolar I disorder against depression; suggested to have antidepressant properties
- Prophylaxis of rapid cycling and Bipolar II BAD

PHARMACOLOGY

- Anticonvulsant, antikindling, and GABAergic activity (carbamazepine, valproate, lamotrigine); lamotrigine and gabapentin inhibit excitatory amino acids (e.g., glutamate); gabapentin modulates calcium current and reduces NE and DA release
- Effective in inhibiting seizures kindled from repeated stimulation of limbic structures
- Block voltage-dependent sodium channels, stabilize neuronal membranes and inhibit release of excitatory amino acids
- Valproate increases serotonergic function

DOSING

- See p. 143 for specific agents
- Plasma level monitoring for carbamazepine and valproate (measured at trough) can help guide dosing
- Reduced dosages recommended in the elderly and in hepatic or renal disorders

PHARMACOKINETICS

- See p. 143 for specific agents
- With valproate, pharmacokinetics show significant variation with changes in body weight. Valproate exhibits concentration-dependent protein binding, therefore at high doses and plasma concentrations a larger proportion may exist in unbound (free) form
- Gabapentin shows dose-dependent bioavailability as a result of a saturable transport mechanism (better bioavailabilty with more frequent dosing; plasma level is proportional to the dose). Elimination is reduced in patients with renal dysfunction; adjust dose if creatinine clearance is < 60 ml/min

ADVERSE EFFECTS

- See pp. 144–146 for specific agents
- Common (for all anticonvulsants):
  - GI complaints, e.g., nausea [Management: take with food, change to an enteric-coated preparation, use ranitidine 150 mg/day or famotidine 20 mg/day]
  - dose-related lethargy, sedation, behavior changes/deterioration, reversible dementia/encephalopathy
  - dose-related tremor; tends to be rhythmic, rapid, symmetrical and most prominent in upper extremities [reduce dose if possible; responds to propranolol]
  - ataxia
  - changes in appetite, weight gain (except lamotrigine – more common in females; may be associated with features of insulin resistance. Weight increases with duration of treatment. Obesity may increase risk of hyperandrogenism in females
  - menstrual disturbances (except gabapentin), including: prolonged cycles, oligomenorrhea, amenorrhea, polycystic ovaries; elevated testosterone – rates may be higher in younger females

- Occasional (for all anticonvulsants):
  - dysarthia, incoordination
  - diplopia, nystagmus
- Rare – Anticonvulsant hypersensitivity syndrome with fever, rash and internal organ involvement; cross-sensitivity reported between carbamazepine and lamotrigine

Comparison of Anticonvulsants

	Carbamazepine	Valproate	Gabapentin	Lamotrigine
Dosing	Begin at 200 mg daily and increase by 100 mg twice weekly, until either side effects limit dose, or reach therapeutic plasma level Dose range: 300–1600 mg/day in single or divided dose	Begin at 250 mg bid and increase dose gradually, until either side effects limit dose, or reach therapeutic plasma level Once daily dosing has been used Loading dose strategy: – Oral – give stat dose of 20 mg/kg, then 12 h later initiate bid dosing at 10 mg/kg bid – IV: 1200–1800 mg/day over 3 days Dose range: 750–3000 mg/day in single or divided dose Maximum: 60 mg/kg/day	Begin at 300–400 mg/day and increase by 300–400 mg a day BAD range 900–4000 mg/day Usual dose: 900–1800 mg/day Anxiety: up to 3600 mg/day Dose range: 900–3600 mg/day given as tid dosing	Begin at 50 mg/day and increase by 12.5–25 mg per week up to 250 mg bid (lower if co-prescribed with valproate) Antidepressant dose: 200 mg/day Dose range: 100–500 mg/day given in single or divided dose
Recommended plasma level	17–54 μmol/L (4–12 μg/ml)	350–800 μmol/L (50–115 μg/ml)	No correlation	–
Pharmacokinetics				
Oral bioavailability	75–85%	78%	Dose-dependent (better bioavailability with qid dosing)	100%
Peak plasma level	1–6 h	1–4 h (may be delayed by food)	2–3 h	1–5 h (rate may be reduced by food)
Protein binding	75%	60–95% (concentration dependent)	Minimal	55%
Half-life	15–35 h (acute use); 10–20 h (chronic use) – stimulates own metabolism	5–20 h	5–7 h	33 h mean (acute dosing) 26 h mean (chronic dosing)
CYP-450 metabolizing enzymes	1A2, 3A4[m], 2C8, 2C9	2C9, UGT	Not metabolized – eliminated by renal excretion	Metabolized by glucuronic acid conjugation
CYP-450 effect	Inducer of CYP1A2, 3A4[p], 2C9, 2B6	Inhibitor of CYP2D6[w], 2C9, 2C19, UGT[p]	–	Weak inducer of UGT Inhibitor of CYP3A4, 2C19

[m] Main isoenzyme involved in metabolism, [p] Potent effect on isoenzyme, [w] Weak effect on isoenzyme, UGT = Uridine diphosphate glucuronosyltransferase

Comparison of Anticonvulsants (cont.)

	Carbamazepine	Valproate	Gabapentin	Lamotrigine
Adverse effects CNS	Sedation (11%), cognitive blunting, confusion (higher doses) Agitation, restlessness, irritability, insomnia Headache Tremors, ataxia (up to 50%), paresthesias (3%), acute dystonic reactions, chronic dyskinesias May exacerbate schizophrenia on withdrawal	Sedation, lethargy, behavior changes/deterioration, cognitive blunting, encephalopathy Activation, aggression Headache (3%) Tremors (10% adults; 15% children – tend to be rhythmic, rapid, symmetrical and most prominent in the upper extremities), ataxia, dysarthria, incoordination Rare cases of psychosis	Sedation (19%), fatigue, abnormal thinking, amnesia Nervousness, anxiety, hostility Rare switches to hypomania/mania Tremors (7%), ataxia, incoordination, dysarthria, myalgia Cases of depression	Sedation, asthenia, cognitive blunting, "spaced-out" feeling Agitation, activation, irritability, insomnia Switches to hypomania/mania Headache Tremors, ataxia (22%), incoordination, myalgia, arthralgia Myoclonic jerks with high serum levels
Anticholinergic	Blurred vision (6%), mydriasis, cycloplegia, ophthalmoplegia Dry mouth, slurred speech Constipation	–	Dry mouth or throat (2%) Constipation	Blurred vision, Constipation
GI	Nausea (4%) Weight gain minimal– may be secondary to peripheral edema Occasional weight loss	Nausea common, vomiting Weight gain (59%); mean gain of 8–21 kg reported; more common in females and high plasma levels; may be associated with features of insulin resistance Weight loss (5%)	Nausea Weight gain (dose-dependent)	Nausea, vomiting, diarrhea Rarely esophagitis No weight gain
Cardiovascular	Dizziness Vasculitis	Rarely dizziness Vasculitis	Dizziness (17%), hypotension Occasionally hypertension	Breathlessness, dizziness (38%) Conduction changes (prolongation of PR interval)

	Carbamazepine	Valproate	Gabapentin	Lamotrigine
Dermatological	Rash (10–15%) – severe dermatological reactions may signify impending blood dyscrasias Unusual bruising Hair loss (6%) Photosensitivity reactions Rarely: fixed drug eruptions, lichenoid-like reactions, bullous reactions, exfoliative dermatitis, Stevens-Johnson syndrome Hypersensitivity syndrome – rare; with fever, malaise, pharyngitis, skin eruptions and internal organ involvement	Rash Diaphoresis Hair loss (up to 12%); changes in texture or colour of hair Rare cases of Stevens-Johnson syndrome, toxic epidermal necrolysis, lupus, erythema multiforme or skin pigmentation	Pruritis	Rash (25%); in 2–3% require drug discontinuation – risk increased with higher doses, in females and in children, in combination with valproate Stevens-Johnson syndrome in 1–2% children and 0.1% of adults Rarely, erythema multiforme, toxic epidermal necrolysis and hypersensitivity syndrome (0.1%)
Hematologic	Transitory leukopenia (10%), persistent leukopenia (2%) Rarely, eosinophilia, aplastic anemia, thrombocytopenia, purpura and agranulocytosis	Reversible thrombocytopenia – may be related to high plasma levels; rare episodes of bleeding Macrocytic anemia, leucopenia, coagulopathies	Leukopenia (1%), purpura	Rarely, hematemesis, hemolytic anemia, pancytopenia
Hepatic	Transient enzyme elevation (5–15%) – evaluate for hepatotoxicity if elevation > 3 times normal Rarely, hepatocellular and cholestatic jaundice, granulomatous hepatitis and severe hepatic necrosis	Asymptomatic hepatic transaminase elevation (44%) Cases of severe liver toxicity (all patients were also taking lamotrigine)	–	Cases of severe liver toxicity (all patients also taking valproate)
Endocrine	Menstrual disturbances in females (19%) Decreased libido in males Elevation of total cholesterol (primarily HDL) Can lower thyroxine levels and TSH response to TRH	Menstrual disturbances (up to 45%) including prolonged cycles, oligomenorrhea, amenorrhea, polycystic ovaries (43%) In females: hyperandrogenism (increased testosterone in 33%), android obesity, hyper-insulinemia Flushing Decreased levels of HDL, low HDL/cholesterol ratio, increased triglyceride levels	–	Menstrual disturbances, dysmenorrhea, vaginitis

Comparison of Anticonvulsants (cont.)

	Carbamazepine	Valproate	Gabapentin	Lamotrigine
Ocular	Diplopia (16%), nystagmus (up to 50%), visual hallucinations, lens abnormalities; 2 cases of pigmentary retinopathy	Diplopia, nystagmus, asterixis (spots before the eyes)	Diplopia (6%), nystagmus, amblyopia	Diplopia (28%)
Other	Hyponatremia and water intoxication (4–12%) – more common with higher plasma levels Rarely: acute renal failure, osteomalacia, splenomegaly, lymphadenopathy, systemic lupus erythematosus, pancreatitis and serum sickness	Gingival hyperplasia Hyperammonia (up to 50%); usually asymptomatic but may cause increased sedation, confusion, stupor and/or coma Increased bone resorption with osteoporosis, osteopenia Rarely: osteomalacia, cholecystitis, pancreatitis, serum sickness	Rhinitis, pharyngitis	Rhinitis, pharyngitis Rarely, apnea, pancreatitis
Chronic or serious conditions	Bone marrow suppression, ocular effects, SIADH (hyponatremia), hypersensitivity syndrome (0.1%)	Endocrine (females), thrombocytopenia, leukopenia, hyperammonemia, hepatic toxicity, Stevens-Johnson syndrome	None known	Rash, Stevens-Johnson syndrome, toxic epidermal necrolysis, hypersensitivity syndrome (0.1%) PR prolongation

WITHDRAWAL

- No evidence of psychological or physical dependence to anticonvulsants
- Myoclonic jerks have been reported following the tapering of carbamazepine or valproate
- Abrupt discontinuation (especially in patients with a seizure disorder) may provoke rebound seizures – taper
- Rare reports of psychiatric symptoms on withdrawal, including psychosis (exacerbation of schizophrenia)

PRECAUTIONS

- Prior to treatment laboratory investigations should be performed (see p. 150)

Carbamazepine

- Carbamazepine induces its own hepatic metabolism; therefore, weekly determinations of serum carbamazepine should be done for the first 2 months, monthly for 6 months, then at clinical discretion (at least every 6 months) or when there is a change in drug regimen
- Carbamazepine induces the metabolism of drugs metabolized by the cytochrome P-450 system (see Interactions pp. 151–153)
- Because of its anticholinergic action, give cautiously to patients with increased intraocular pressure or urinary retention
- Orientals may need lower doses
- Tolerance to effects has been reported; efficacy not improved with dose increase
- Any cutaneous eruption, with fever, should be investigated for internal organ involvement. Check blood if patient reports fever, sore throat, petechiae or bruising. Mild degree of blood cell suppression can occur; stop therapy if levels drop below 3,000 white cells/mm^3; erythrocytes less than 4×10^6 mm^3; platelets less than 100,000 mm^3; hemoglobin less than 11 g/dl; reticulocyte count below 3%; or if serum iron rises above 150 mg/dl

- Patients who develop cutaneous reactions to carbamazepine should avoid the use of amitriptyline (as carbamazepine is a metabolite)
- Do not administer carbamazepine suspension together with any other liquid preparation as formation of an insoluble precipitate can occur
- A hypersensitivity syndrome with fever, skin eruptions and internal organ involvement occurs rarely – cross-sensitivity with other anticonvulsants suggested

Valproate

- Hepatic toxicity may show no relation to hepatic enzyme levels. Monitor liver function prior to therapy. Caution in patients with history of hepatic disease. In high-risk patients, monitor serum fibrinogen and albumin for decreases in concentration, and ammonia for increases. Stop drug if hepatic transaminase 2–3 times the upper limit of normal
- Platelet counts and bleeding time determinations are recommended prior to therapy and at periodic intervals; withdraw if hemorrhage, bruising, or coagulation disorder is detected
- Diabetic patients on valproic acid may show false-positive ketone results
- In patients with decreased or altered protain binding it may be more useful to monitor unbound (free) valproate concentrations rather than total concentrations
- Valproate will inhibit the metabolism of a number of drugs metabolized by cytochrome P-450 (see Interactions pp. 154–155)

Gabapentin

- An increased incidence of acinar cell adenomas and carcinomas was noted in the pancreas of male rats given high doses – the relevance to humans is unknown

Lamotrigine

- Severe, potentially life-threatening rashes have been reported – higher incidence in children, rapid dosage titration and in combination with valproate. Most occur within first 8 weeks of starting lamotrigine. Patient should be educated to report any rash, to the physician, immediately
- Use cautiously in patients with renal dysfunction as elimination half-life of lamotrigine is increased
- Due to potential of PR prolongation, lamotrigine should be used cautiously in patients with conduction abnormalities

CONTRAINDICATIONS

- Patients with a history of hepatic or cardiovascular disease or with a blood dyscrasia
- Hypersensitivity to any tricyclic compound (carbamazepine), and demonstrated hypersensitivity to any of the other agents
- Patients prescribed clozapine due to increased risk of agranulocytosis (carbamazepine)

TOXICITY

Carbamazepine

- Usually occurs with plasma levels above 50 μmol/L; children may be at risk for toxicity at lower serum concentrations due to increased production of toxic epoxide metabolite. Measurement of epoxide level may be beneficial in patients who develop clinical signs of carbamazepine toxicity at therapeutic concentrations of the parent drug
- The maximum plasma concentration may be delayed for up to 70 h after an overdose
- Signs:
  - dizziness, blood pressure changes, sinus tachycardia, ECG changes
  - drowsiness, stupor, agitation, disorientation, EEG changes, seizures and coma
  - nausea, vomiting, decreased intestinal motility, urinary retention
  - tremor, involuntary movements, opisthotonos, abnormal reflexes, myoclonus, ataxia
  - mydriasis, nystagmus
  - flushing, respiratory depression, cyanosis
- No known antidote, treat symptomatically

Valproate

- Maximum plasma concentration may not occur for up to 18 h following an overdose, and serum half-life may be prolonged
- Onset of CNS depression may be rapid (within 3 h); enteric-coated preparations may delay onset of symptoms
- Signs/symptoms: severe dizziness, hypotension, supraventricular tachycardia, bradycardia; severe drowsiness; trembling; irregular, slow or shallow breathing, apnea, respiratory depression and coma; loss of tendon reflexes, generalized myoclonus, seizures; cerebral edema – evident 2 to 3 days after overdose and may last up to 15 days; hematological changes, metabolic abnormalities; optic nerve damage

Anticonvulsants (cont.)

- Overdose can result in coma and death; naloxone may reverse the CNS depressant effects, and may also reverse anti-epileptic effects
- Supportive treatment

Gabapentin

- Signs and symptoms: double vision, slurred speech, drowsiness, lethargy and diarrhea – all patients recovered
- Gabapentin can be removed by hemodialysis

Lamotrigine

- Overdose can result in coma
- No known antidote – treat symptomatically

PEDIATRIC CONSIDERA TIONS

Carbamazepine

- Used in episodic dyscontrol and assaultive behavior disorder
- Start dose at 100 mg daily in divided doses and increase gradually; do not exceed 1000 mg/day and monitor plasma level; children have higher reported clearances than adults
- May be superior to lithium in the treatment of mania in adolescent bipolar disorder
- Children may be at risk for major toxicities at lower serum concentrations due to increased production of toxic metabolite; case reports of behavior disturbances, mania and worsening of tics
- Common side effects include: unsteadiness, dizziness, diplopia, drowsiness, nausea and vomiting
- Moderate to marked leukopenia reported
- Reported to elevate total cholesterol, low-density lipoproteins, ratio of total cholesterol to low-density lipoproteins, and gamma glutamyl transferase (GGT) levels in children

Valproate

- Efficacy reported in treatment of bipolar disorder, acute mania, migraine prophylaxis as well as temper/aggressive outbursts in adolescents and young adults
- Children under age 2 with other medical conditions are at risk of developing fatal hepatotoxicity
- Children ages 3–10 taking other anticonvulsants are at high risk for developing fatal hepatotoxicity
- Dose-related reversible thrombocytopenia reported – monitor
- Behavior deterioration seen (up to 2.4% risk)
- Use in children and adolescents may result in increased risk of hyperandrogenism and polycystic ovarian syndrome, delayed or prolonged puberty; excessive weight gain, hyperinsulinemia and dyslipidemia; decreased bone mineral density reported (in up to 14%) – may conduce to osteoporosis

Gabapentin

- Incidence of side effects in children reported to be similar to that in adults
- Case reports of behavioral problems, including aggression and irritability

Lamotrigine

- Has been used in adolescents as add-on therapy in refractory bipolar depression. Common side effects included headache, tremor, somnolence, and dizziness
- Risk of severe, life-threatening rash increased in children

GERIATRIC CONSIDERATIONS

- Dosing should be instituted more gradually in the elderly and those with liver impairment
- May cause confusion, cognitive impairment, ataxia (may lead to falls)
- Early data suggest efficacy in treating behavior disturbances in dementia
- Caution when combining with other drugs with CNS or anticholinergic properties; additive effects can result in confusion, disorientation, delirium

- Due to reduced protein binding and hepatic oxidation, elderly may have a higher proportion of unbound (free) valproate and a reduced clearance, resulting in elevated levels of unbound valproate (within therapeutic plasma levels of total drug)
- May have an increased risk for thrombocytopenia with valproate
- Elderly with pre-existing cardiac disease should have a thorough cardiac evaluation prior to carbamazepine use
- Higher risk of hyponatremia with carbamazepine
- Reduce dose of gabapentin if creatinine clearance < 60 ml/min

USE IN PREGNANCY

Carbamazepine

- Caution in pregnancy; 5.7% risk of teratogenic effects, lower birth rates and developmental delays in infants reported; up to 1% risk of spina bifida and 2.9% risk of congenital heart defects
- Clearance of carbamazepine can increase two-fold during pregnancy; dose requirement may need to be 100% higher

Breast milk

- The American Academy of Pediatrics considers carbamazepine compatible with breast-feeding
- Breast milk reported to contain 7–95% of maternal carbamazepine concentration; infant serum level is between 6–65% of maternal serum level
- Mother should be educated about the signs and symptoms of hepatic dysfunction and the CNS effects of carbamazepine on the infant

Valproate

- Avoid use in pregnancy; 11.1% risk of malformations – related to dose and drug plasma level (1.2% risk of spina bifida and up to 5% risk of neural tube defects)
- Neurological dysfunction and developmental deficits reported in some children exposed to valproate *in utero*
- Other problems attributed solely to valproate exposure include: musculoskeletal, cardiovascular, pulmonary, and genital abnormalities, and skin defects
- Fetal serum concentrations are 1.4 times maternal serum levels and half-life is longer than in the mother
- Total plasma valproate concentration decreases during pregnancy as a result of increased volume of distribution and clearance; plasma protein binding decreases

Breast milk

- No reports link the use of valproic acid with adverse effects in nursing infants; the American Academy of Pediatricians considers valproic acid compatible with breastfeeding
- Plasma level of infant reported to have up to 12% of maternal valproate serum concentration; half-life of valproate in neonates and infants is significantly longer than in adults
- Mother should be educated about the signs and symptoms of hepatic dysfunction and the hematological abnormalities of valproate in the infant

Gabapentin

- No evidence of impaired fertility or teratogenicity reported in animal studies. Risk to humans is currently unknown

Breast milk

- Unknown if gabapentin is excreted in breast milk

Lamotrigine

- Crosses the placenta; placenta levels low and comparable to levels in maternal plasma. Half-life of lamotrigine in infant is increased
- Lamotrigine metabolism appears to be induced during pregnancy and plasma levels increase rapidly after delivery

Breast milk

- Excreted in breast milk; the milk/plasma ratio of lamotrigine is about 0.6. Breastfeeding is not recommended

NURSING IMPLICATIONS

- Watch out for signs of fever, sore throat, and bruising or bleeding
- Close clinical and laboratory supervision should be maintained (see Adverse Effects and Monitoring) throughout treatment to detect signs of possible blood dyscrasia or liver involvement
- A rash, especially with carbamazepine or lamotrigine, may signal incipient blood dyscrasia; advise the physician
- Anorexia, nausea, vomiting, edema, malaise and lethargy may signify hepatic toxicity
- Check for urinary retention and constipation with carbamazepine; increase fluids to lessen constipation
- Liquid carbamazepine should not be mixed or taken at the same time as any other liquid medication

Anticonvulsants (cont.)

- Liquid valproate should not be administered with carbonated beverages
- Controlled-release tablets should not be crushed
- In females (particularly on valproate), monitor for menstrual disturbances, hirsutism, obesity, alopecia and infertility – two or more of these symptoms may be associated with polycystic ovaries
- Monitor patient's height, weight, and body mass index
- In the elderly, monitor for ataxia, confusion and cognitive impairment

PATIENT INSTRUCTIONS

For detailed patient instructions on Anticonvulsant Mood Stabilizers, see the Patient Information Sheet on p. 265

- Since drowsiness can occur, exercise caution when performing tasks that require alertness; will enhance the effects of alcohol and other CNS drugs
- Store your medication away from humidity (e.g., washroom cupboards) as drug may lose potency
- Report any symptoms such as malaise, weakness, lethargy, fever, sore throat, vomiting, bruising, bleeding or rash **immediately** to your physician
- Do not chew capsules as they can cause local irritation of mouth and throat; enteric-coated (controlled-release) tablets should not be broken or crushed, but should be swallowed whole
- Take your medication with food if gastric irritation (nausea) occurs
- Avoid drinking grapefruit juice while taking carbamazepine as it can elevate the blood level of carbamazepine
- If you are taking liquid carbamazepine, do not take it simultaneously with any other liquid preparation
- Do not take liquid valproate with carbonated beverages as the combination may result in irritation of the mouth
- To treat occasional pain avoid the use of acetylsalicylic acid (ASA or aspirin) as it can affect the blood level of valproate – acetaminophen or ibuprofen (and related drugs) are safer alternatives

MONITORING RECOMMENDATIONS

	Carbamazepine	**Valproate**	**Gabapentin**	**Lamotrigine**
Biochemical work-up	1) CBC including platelets and differential 2) Serum electrolytes 3) Liver function 4) ECG (in patients over age 45 or with a cardiac history)	1) CBC including platelets and differential 2) Liver function 3) total and HDL cholesterol and triglycerides	None required	None required
Follow-up	Repeat CBC after the first month, then 2–3 times a year Serum electrolytes every 6 months	Repeat test #1 and #2 monthly for 2 months, then 2–3 times a year Test #3 annually	None required	None required
Plasma level monitoring	Measure drug level 5 days after start of therapy and 5 days after change in dose or addition/deletion of any other drug (see Interactions pp. 151–153)	Measure drug level 5 days after start of therapy and 5 days after change in dose or addition/deletion of any other drug (see Interactions pp. 154–155 and Precautions p. 147)	None required	None required

DRUG INTERACTIONS • Clinically significant interactions are listed below

DRUGS INTERACTING WITH CARBAMAZEPINE

Class of Drug	Example	Interaction Effects
Acetazolamide		Increased plasma level of carbamazepine due to inhibited metabolism
Anesthetic	Halothane Methoxyflurane, isoflurane, sevoflurane	Enzyme induction may result in hepatocellular damage Enzyme induction may result in renal damage
Anthelminthic	Mebendazole	Decreased plasma level of mebendazole
Antibiotic	Erythromycin, troleandomycin, clarithromycin Doxycycline (no interaction with other tetracyclines)	Increased plasma levels of carbamazepine due to reduced clearance (by 5–41%) Decreased serum level and half-life of doxycycline due to enhanced metabolism (Alternatively, tetracycline can be used or doxycycline can be dosed q 12 h)
Anticoagulant	Dicumarol, warfarin	Enhanced metabolism of anticoagulant and impaired hypoprothombinemic response; decreased PT ratio or INR response
Anticonvulsant	Felbamate Phenytoin, primidone, phenobarbital Clonazepam, clobazam, ethosuximide, topiramate, oxycarbazine Valproate, valproic acid Lamotrigine Topiramate	Decreased carbamazepine level by 50%, but increased level of epoxide metabolite Decreased felbamate level Decreased carbamazepine level due to increased metabolism via CYP3A4, but ratio of epoxide metabolite increased Altered plasma level of co-prescribed anticonvulsant Clearance of the anticonvulsants is increased by carbamazepine, with possible decrease in efficacy (40% decrease in concentration of topiramate and of oxcarbazine metabolite) Increased plasma level of epoxide metabolite of carbamazepine; may result in toxicity even at therapeutic carbamazepine concentrations Decreased valproate level due to enzyme induction Synergistic mood stabilizing effect reported Increased plasma level of epoxide metabolite of carbamazepine by 10–45% with resultant increased side effects Increased metabolism of lamotrigine; half-life and plasma level decreased by approximately 40% Increased plasma level of carbamazepine by 20%
Antidepressant SSRI Cyclic (non-selective) SARI MAOI	 Fluoxetine, fluvoxamine Imipramine, doxepin, amitriptyline Nefazodone, trazodone Phenelzine	 Increased plasma level of carbamazepine and its active metabolite with fluoxetine; increased nausea with fluvoxamine Decreased plasma level of antidepressant by up to 46% due to enzyme induction Decreased plasma level of trazodone Increased plasma level of carbamazepine with nefazodone due to decreased metabolism via CYP3A4 Possible decrease in metabolism and increased plasma level of carbamazepine
Antifungal	Ketoconazole, fluconazole Fluconazole, itraconazole, ketoconazole	Increased plasma level of carbamazepine with ketoconazole (by 29%) due to inhibited metabolism via CYP3A4; clearance decreased by 50% with fluconazole Decreased plasma levels of antifungals

Anticonvulsants (cont.)

Class of Drug	Example	Interaction Effects
Antipsychotic	Phenothiazines, haloperidol, risperidone, thiothixene, olanzapine, zuclopenthixol, flupenthixol	Decreased plasma level of antipsychotic (up to 100% with haloperidol, 44% with olanzapine) Increased akathisia Increased neurotoxicity of both neuroleptic and carbamazepine at therapeutic doses
	Clozapine	Avoid combination due to possible potentiation of bone marrow suppression Decreased plasma level of clozapine by up to 63%
	Loxapine, haloperidol	Increased plasma level of carbamazepine and metabolite
	Chlorpromazine liquid, thioridazine liquid	Precipitation of a "rubbery mass" when carbamazepine suspension is combined with neuroleptic liquid preparations
Benzodiazepine	Alprazolam, clonazepam	Decreased plasma level of alprazolam (>50%) and clonazepam (19–37%) due to enzyme induction
β-Blocker	Propranolol	Decreased plasma level of β-blocker due to enzyme induction
Calcium-channel blocker	Diltiazem, verapamil (no interaction with nifedipine)	Increased plasma levels of carbamazepine due to decreased metabolism (total carbamazepine increased 46%, free carbamazepine increased 33%)
Cimetidine		Transient increase in carbamazepine levels and possible toxicity due to inhibited metabolism (no interaction with ranitidine, famotidine and nizatidine)
Corticosteroids		Decreased plasma level of corticosteroid due to enzyme induction
Cyclosporin		Decreased plasma level and efficacy of cyclosporin due to enzyme induction via CYP3A4
Danazol		Plasma levels of carbamazepine increased by 50–100%; half-life is doubled and clearance reduced by half
Desmopressin (DDAVP)		Concurrent use may increase antidiuretic effect, resulting in decreased sodium concentration with resultant seizures
Diclofenac		Increased plasma level of carbamazepine due to decreased metabolism
Disopyramide		Increased metabolism and decreased plasma level of disopyramide
Etretinate		Therapeutic failure with etretinate due to decreased plasma level
Folic acid		Decreased plasma level of folic acid
Grapefruit juice		Decreased metabolism of carbamazepine resulting in increased plasma level by up to 40%
Influenza vaccine		Decreased elimination and increased half-life of carbamazepine
Isoniazid		Increased plasma level of carbamazepine; clearance reduced by up to 45%
Isotretinoin		Decreased plasma level of carbamazepine and its metabolite
Lithium		Increased neurotoxicity of both drugs; sinus node dysfunction reported with combination Synergistic mood-stabilizing effect; may potentiate antidepressant or antimanic effect
Methadone		Decreased effect of methadone (up to 60%) due to enhanced metabolism
Methylphenidate		Decreased plasma level of methylphenidate and its metabolite
Modafinil		Decreased plasma level of modafinil due to enhanced metabolism

Class of Drug	Example	Interaction Effects
Metronidazole		Increased plasma level of carbamazepine due to inhibited metabolism
Muscle relaxant (non-depolarizing)	Gallamine, pancuronium	Decreased duration of action and efficacy of muscle relaxant
Oral contraceptive		Increased metabolism of oral contraceptive and increased binding of progestin and ethinyl estradiol to sex hormone binding globulin, may result in decreased contraceptive efficacy
Propoxyphene		Increased plasma level of carbamazepine due to reduced metabolism
Protease inhibitor	Ritonavir, saquinavir, indinavir, nelfinavir	Increased metabolism and decreased plasma level of ritonavir and saquinavir with possible loss of efficacy Increased plasma level of carbamazepine due to inhibited metabolism via CYP3A4
Quinine		Increased plasma level of carbamazepine (by 37%) and AUC (by 51%) due to inhibited metabolism
Rifampin		Decreased plasma level of carbamazepine
Terfenadine		Increased free carbamazepine level by 300% due to displacement from protein binding
Theophylline		Decreased theophylline level due to enzyme induction by carbamazepine; decreased carbamazepine level by up to 50%
Thyroid hormone		Decreased plasma level of thyroid hormone due to enzyme induction

DRUGS INTERACTING WITH VALPROATE

Class of Drug	Example	Interaction Effects
Antibiotic	Erythromycin	Increased valproate plasma level due to decreased metabolism
Anticoagulant	Warfarin	Inhibition of secondary phase of platelet aggregation by valproate, thus affecting coagulation; increased PT ratio or INR response Displacement of protein binding of warfarin (free fraction increased by 33%)
Anticonvulsant	Phenobarbital, primidone	Increased level of anticonvulsant (by 30–50%) due to decreased metabolism caused by valproate
	Carbamazepine	Decreased valproate levels due to increased clearance and displacement for protein binding Effects on carbamazepine levels are variable and inconsistent Synergistic mood-stabilizing effect in treatment-resistant patients
	Phenytoin, mephenytoin	Enhanced anticonvulsant effect due to displacement from protein binding (free fraction increased by 60%) and inhibited clearance (by 25%); toxicity can occur at therapeutic levels
	Felbamate	Increased plasma level of valproate (by 31–51%) due to decreased metabolism
	Lamotrigine	Increased lamotrigine plasma level (by up to 200%), half-life (by up to 50%) and decreased clearance (by 21%) Decreased plasma level of valproate with combination. This combination may be dangerous due to high incidence of Stevens-Johnson syndrome and toxic epidermal necrolysis
	Ethosuximide	Increased half-life of ethosuximide (by 25%)
	Topiramate	Case reports of delirium and elevated ammonia levels

Anticonvulsants (cont.)

Class of Drug	Example	Interaction Effects
Antidepressant		
Tricyclic	Amitriptyline, nortriptyline	Increased plasma level and adverse effects of antidepressant
SSRI	Fluoxetine	Increased plasma level of valproate (up to 50%)
Antipsychotic	Phenothiazines	Increased neurotoxicity, sedation, and extrapyramidal side effects due to decreased clearance of valproate (by 14%)
	Clozapine	Both increased and decreased clozapine levels reported; changes in clozapine/norclozapine ratio Case report of hepatic encephalopathy
	Haloperidol	Increased plasma level of haloperidol by an average of 32%
	Olanzapine	Combination associated with high incidence of weight gain
Antiviral agent	Zidovudine	Increased level of zidovudine (by 38%) due to decreased clearance
	Acyclovir	Decreased level of valproate
Anxiolytic	Clonazepam, chlordiazepoxide, lorazepam	Decreased metabolism and increased pharmacological effects of benzodiazepines resulting in increased sedation, disorientation (lorazepam clearance reduced by 41%)
	Clonazepam	Concomitant use may induce absence status in patients with a history of absence type seizures
	Diazepam	Increased plasma level of diazepam due to displacement from protein binding (free fraction increased by 90%)
Cimetidine		Decreased metabolism and increased half-life of valproate
CNS depressant	Alcohol	Increased sedation, disorientation Valproate displaces alcohol from protein binding and potentiates intoxicating effect
Isoniazid		Increased plasma level of valproate due to inhibited metabolism
Lithium		Synergistic mood-stabilizing effect in treatment-resistant patients Valproate may aggravate action tremor
Rifampin		Increased clearance of valproate (by 40%)
Salicylate	Acetylsalicylic acid, bismuth subsalicylate	Displacement of valproate from protein binding and decreased clearance, leading to increased level of free drug (4-fold), with possible toxicity
Thiopental		Displacement of thiopental from protein binding resulting in an increased hypnotic/anesthetic effect
Tolbutamide		Increase in free fraction of tolbutamide from 20 to 50% due to displacement from protein binding

DRUGS INTERACTING WITH GABAPENTIN

Class of Drug	Example	Interaction Effects
Antacid	Al/Mg containing antacids	Co-administration reduces gabapentin bioavailability by up to 24%

DRUGS INTERACTING WITH LAMOTRIGINE

Class of Drug	Example	Interaction Effects
Acetaminophen		Decreased half-life of lamotrigine by 15% and decreased AUC by 20% with chronic use of acetaminophen
Anticonvulsant	Carbamazepine, phenytoin, phenobarbital, primidone	Decreased plasma level and decreased half-life of lamotrigine due to increased clearance Increased plasma level of epoxide metabolite of carbamazepine by 10–45%; increased nausea, ataxia and nystagmus reported
	Valproate	Increased plasma level of lamotrigine (up to 200%) due to decreased metabolism; slight decrease in valproate levels Increased risk of life-threatening rash with combination

L-Tryptophan

PRODUCT AVAILABILITY

Chemical Class	Generic Name	Trade Name(A)	Dosage Forms and Strengths
Tryptophan	L-Tryptophan(C)	Tryptan	Capsules: 250 mg, 500 mg, 750 mg Tablets: 1 g

(A) Generic preparations may be available, (C) Not marketed in USA

INDICATIONS*

- ▲ Adjunct in the treatment of bipolar affective disorder; may potentiate the effects of lithium and neuroleptics in acute mania; some efficacy if used alone
- ▲ Potentiates the effects of lithium in prophylaxis
- Seasonal affective disorder
- Potentiates the effects of antidepressants in depression and obsessive compulsive disorder
- Sedative; will reduce sleep latency without distorting usual stages of sleep
- Decrease aggression and antisocial behavior
- May reduce neuroleptic-induced akathisia
- Preliminary data suggest possible usefulness in treatment of seasonal affective disorder and premenstrual dysphoric disorder

PHARMACOLOGY

- An amino acid that acts as a precursor for the synthesis of serotonin
- Reported to increase melatonin levels

DOSING

- Depression: 8–16 g/day
- Mania: 8–12 g/day
- Aggression: up to 16 g/day
- Sedation: up to 5 g at bedtime

PHARMACOKINETICS

- Half-life = 15.8 h
- Highly bound to plasma protein (80–90%)
- There is no correlation between dose and plasma level

ADVERSE EFFECTS

1. CNS Effects

- Drowsiness
- Headache
- Euphoria, disinhibition of mood and sexual behavior reported
- Tremors

2. GI Effects

- GI upset
- Anorexia

3. Anticholinergic Effects

- Constipation
- Dry mouth

4. Cardiovascular Effects

- Dizziness

PRECAUTIONS

- Protein-reduced diets can cause an amino acid imbalance when using L-tryptophan
- When used with lithium, lithium dose should be decreased and plasma levels monitored for toxicity
- A number of cases of eosinophilia-myalgia syndrome reported (cause traced to impurity in raw material); symptoms include fatigue,

* ▲ Approved indications

myalgia, shortness of breath, rash, swelling of extremities, congestive heart failure, and death
- Use with caution in patients with cataracts, as they seem to be related to metabolites of tryptophan (e.g., kynurenine)
- Caution in patients with a family history of diabetes as diabetogenic effect reported
- Vitamin B_6 (pyridoxine) deficiency can predispose to elevated levels of tryptophan metabolites which have been associated with bladder cancer

CONTRAINDICATIONS

- Irritation of urinary bladder (cystitis)
- Diabetes
- Patients with malabsorption in upper bowel
- Achlorhydric states

TOXICITY

- High doses cause vomiting and "serotonin" overdrive including shivering, diaphoresis, hypomania, and ataxia

PEDIATRIC CONSIDERATIONS

- Use contraindicated in children

GERIATRIC CONSIDERATIONS

- Used in agitation, aggression, and behavior problems in elderly demented patients
- Sedation is primary side effect

USE IN PREGNANCY

- Contraindicated
- Pregnancy has been associated with the accumulation of L-tryptophan metabolites (e.g., xanthurenic acid, kynurenine) due to inhibited metabolism

Breast milk

- Unknown

NURSING IMPLICATIONS

- Give drug with meals or snacks to reduce nausea
- When used with lithium, monitor for signs of toxicity including tremor, ataxia, and confusion; dermatological side effects may be exacerbated

PATIENT INSTRUCTIONS

For detailed patient instructions on L-tryptophan, see the Patient Information Sheet on p. 267.
- Do not begin a protein-reduced diet without consulting your physician
- Take with food or snacks to reduce nausea

DRUG INTERACTIONS

- Only clinically significant interactions are listed below

Class of Drug	Example	Interaction Effects
Antidepressant Tricyclic MAOI – Irreversible, RIMA, SSRI	 Amitriptyline Tranylcypromine, moclobemide, fluvoxamine	 Additive effects in treatment-resistant patients Additive effects in treatment-resistant patients; monitor for increased serotonergic effects
Estrogen/progestogen	Oral contraceptives, estradiol, diethylstilboestrol	Increased levels of metabolites, xanthurenic acid, kynurenine, due to inhibited metabolism
Lithium		Increased lithium level and possible toxicity Enhanced therapeutic effect for mania and prophylaxis of bipolar affective disorder in treatment-resistant patients

Psychostimulants

PRODUCT AVAILABILITY

Chemical Class	Generic Name	Trade Name[(A)]	Dosage Forms and Strengths
	Dextroamphetamine	Dexedrine	Tablets: 5 mg, 10 mg Spansules: 5 mg, 10 mg, 15 mg
	Methamphetamine[(B)]	Desoxyn	Tablets: 5 mg Sustained-release tablets: 5 mg, 10 mg, 15 mg
	Amphetamine resin complex[(B)]	Biphetamine	Capsules: 6.25 mg, 10 mg
	Dextroamphetamine/Amphetamine salts[(B)]	Adderall Adderall XR	Tablets: 5 mg, 7.5 mg, 10 mg, 12.5 mg, 15 mg, 20 mg, 30 mg Capsules: 10 mg, 20 mg, 30 mg
	Methylphenidate	Ritalin Ritalin SR, Metadate ER[(B)] Metadate CD[(B)] Concerta[(B)]	Tablets: 5 mg[(B)], 10 mg, 20 mg Sustained-release tablets: 10 mg[(B)], 20 mg Extended-release capsule: 20 mg Extended-release tablets: 18 mg, 36 mg, 54 mg
	Magnesium pemoline[(B)]	Cylert	Tablets: 18.75 mg, 37.5 mg, 75 mg

(A) Generic preparations may be available, (B) Not marketed in Canada

INDICATIONS*

- ▲ Attention-deficit/hyperactivity disorder (ADHD), primarily inattentive, combined or hyperactive-impulsive subtypes
- ▲ Parkinson's disease
- ▲ Narcolepsy
- ▲ Obesity (dextroamphetamine – USA only)
- Treatment-resistant depression
- Major depression in medically or surgically ill patients, or in elderly
- Augmentation of cyclic antidepressants, SSRIs, and RIMA
- Attention-deficit/hyperactivity disorder – in partial remission (ADHD-PR) adults
- Chronic fatigue and neurasthenia
- Diagnostic test for tricyclic use (i.e., a methylphenidate challenge test predicts positive response to imipramine or desipramine)
- Diagnostic test (0.5 mg/kg IV) to assess antipsychotic dose reduction (methylphenidate)
- Negative symptoms of schizophrenia; some improvement noted in cognitive deficits, mood, and concentration with low doses of dextroamphetamine
- Low doses of dextroamphetamine (up to 15 mg/day) produce temporary improvement in mania; high doses can induce manic behavior
- Improves fatigue and cognition in AIDS-related neuropsychiatric impairment
- Positive results with methylphenidate in decreasing anger, irritability and aggression in brain-injured patients, oppositional defiant disorder and ADHD
- Data suggests that dextroamphetamine and pemoline may treat antidepressant-induced sexual dysfunction
- Adjuvants in pain management
- Early data suggest benefit of methylphenidate (15–60 mg/day) as a treatment of cocaine abuse

* ▲ Approved indications

- Open label studies and case reports suggest cautious use of psychostimulants may augment the effects of SSRI in treatment-refractory paraphilias or paraphilia-related disorders

GENERAL COMMENTS

- General response occurs within the first week; response seen in up to 70% of children and 25–78% of adults with ADHD
- Psychostimulants suggested to suppress physical and verbal aggression and reduce negative or antisocial interactions
- Increasingly, literature suggests a role for these drugs in some adults that have residual symptoms of ADHD; however, use in adults should be with caution; stimulants may increase anxiety in ADHD, primarily inattentive subtype; the physician may need regulatory approval for the use of dextroamphetamine
- Use with caution and careful monitoring in patients with current abuse of drugs or alcohol (except for pemoline, which is not a controlled substance)
- Pemoline is not recommended as first-line therapy due to reports of late-onset hepatotoxicity that can progress to acute liver failure

PHARMACOLOGY

- Sympathomimetic amines – act as dopamine agonists
- Promote release of catecholamine neurotransmitters at synaptic junction, block the reuptake of catecholamines, prevent their breakdown by monoamine oxidase, and exert a direct effect on noradrenergic receptors; inhibit dopamine transporter protein resulting in potentiation of dopaminergic neurotransmission

DOSING

- See chart p. 163
- Treatment is started at low dose and gradually increased over several days; initial improvement noted may plateau after two weeks of continuous use (i.e., a decreased "energizing" feeling) – this does not imply tolerance. Patients should compare the plateau to their baseline, not to the peak effect seen in the first week, as otherwise there will be an urge to increase the dose
- Doses above 1.0 mg/kg/day have been suggested to treat ADHD-PR; this, however, has not been substantiated
- To minimize anorexia, give drug with or after meals; with Metadate CD food delays C_{max} by 1 h and a high-fat meal increases C_{max} by 30%
- Divided doses required with regular preparations of methylphenidate (dose every 2 to 6 h)
- Though controversial, as some data suggest continued activation, administration of a small dose (e.g., 5 mg) ½ hour before bedtime can sometimes help to calm the child so as to permit him to go to sleep
- Methylphenidate SR has a smoother onset, but no advantage in duration over regular tablets
- The sustained-release (SR) and extended-release formulations may decrease inter-dose dysphoria or "wear off" phenomenon. Dose 20 mg SR = 10 mg bid of regular formulation
- Combination of amphetamine and dextroamphetamine salts in Adderall provide a graded onset and duration of action; this may offer a "smoother" delivery of drug effect
- When switching to extended-release products from 20 mg of regular formulation of methylphenidate, substitute one 18–20 mg extended-release tablet in the morning

PHARMACOKINETICS

- Large interindividual variation in absorption and bioavailability
- Low protein binding
- Extended-release methylphenidate tablets are formulated with different cores which release the active drug at different times, into the body
- See chart, p. 163

ONSET AND DURATION OF ACTION

- See chart, p. 163

ADVERSE EFFECTS

- See chart, p. 164
- Effects on growth appear to be small and related to dose and duration of drug use [drug holidays used to minimize this – evidence is contradictory]

Psychostimulants (cont.)

- Heart rate and blood pressure should be monitored after every dose increase in patients with risk factors
- Drug-induced insomnia can be managed by changing the timing of the dose [clonidine 0.05–0.4 mg, melatonin, L-tryptophan, antihistamines or trazodone at bedtime may be useful]
- Anorexia, GI distress and weight loss [can be minimized by taking medication with meals, eating smaller meals more frequently or drinking high-calorie fluids]; if loss of weight exceeds 10% of body weight, consider switching to another agent
- Behavior rebound can occur in the late afternoon or evening; an afternoon dose, or the use of slow-release preparation can be tried
- Common adverse effects at any age can manifest as sadness, irritability, clinging behavior, insomnia or anorexia
- Dysphoria or sadness reported – may be related to withdrawal effects; use of sustained-release product or addition of a noradrenergic antidepressant may be helpful
- Chronic use may cause exacerbation of OCD symptoms
- Rare hepatotoxic effects have been associated with use of pemoline, sometimes occurring months after drug initiation; deaths have been reported. Stop drug if liver enzymes are elevated. Risk increased in patients with preexisting hepatic disease and in patients receiving concomitant methylphenidate
- Rare reports of psychotic reactions, primarily if high doses used, or in children with a genetic predisposition to psychosis

WITHDRAWAL

- Abrupt withdrawal after prolonged use may result in dysphoria, rebound insomnia, or a rebound in symptoms of ADHD

PRECAUTIONS

- Use cautiously in patients with anxiety, tension, agitation, restlessness
- Use with caution in patients with cardiovascular disease, including hypertension and tachyarrhythmias
- May lower the seizure threshold
- Use cautiously in hyperthyroidism as use may cause hypothyroidism
- May cause an idiopathic hypothyroidism, though patient euthyroid
- Monitor hepatic function (magnesium pemoline) every 2–4 weeks for 3 months, then every 6 months due to reports of hepatotoxicity (more frequent monitoring recommended by some clinicians); unknown if withdrawal of drug at first sign of toxicity will prevent liver failure
- Do periodic CBC (methylphenidate, dextroamphetamine) due to rare reports of leukopenia and nutrition-based anemia
- Chronic abuse in patients can lead to tolerance and psychic dependence; drug dependence in children is rare; however, it may be of concern in adolescents. Amphetamine used as a drug of abuse orally, intravenously, or nasally
- Tics or dyskinesias can be unmasked in children with ADHD with a genetic predisposition
- In patients with Tourette's syndrome there may be an initial worsening of tics; dose may need to be adjusted [clonidine may be effective]
- Tolerance to effects occurs in about 15% of patients; dose adjustment may be required

CONTRAINDICATIONS

- Use with caution and with careful monitoring in patients with a recent history of alcohol and/or drug abuse
- Do not use in patients with a history of functional psychosis
- Do not use pemoline in patients with liver disease
- Use cautiously if there is a positive family history of Tourette's syndrome (tic incidence 20–50% in this population)
- Anorexia nervosa
- Anxiety, tension, agitation
- Thyrotoxicosis, glaucoma
- Tachyarrhythmias, severe angina pectoris, severe hypertension

TOXICITY

- See p. 164

PEDIATRIC CONSIDERATIONS

- ADHD is the primary indication in children and adolescents; the robustness of effect is not as evident in adolescents
- May exacerbate symptoms in children with autism, schizophrenia, and other psychotic conditions
- Monitor height and weight (children); if constitutional small stature, drug holidays may help minimize growth suppression
- In preschoolers, clinical effects are more variable and adverse effects more common; reserve for more serious cases
- Rare reports of exacerbation of OCD symptoms in children on high doses

USE IN PREGNANCY

- See p. 164

GERIATRIC CONSIDERATIONS

- Useful in the treatment of elderly or medically ill patients with major depression
- Dosing before breakfast and lunch may facilitate daytime activity
- Initiate dosage gradually, e.g., 2.5 mg to start, increased by 2.5–5.0 mg every 2–3 days, as tolerated

NURSING IMPLICATIONS

- While medication has demonstrated superiority, a multimodal approach to treatment of ADHD is necessary in order to increase the probability of a positive outcome for the child; some non-pharmacological approaches include behavior modification, individual and family psychotherapy, as well as special education for the child
- Monitor therapy by watching for adverse side effects, mood, and activity level changes
- ADHD: monitor height and weight in children; drug-free periods are advocated
- Caution patients not to stop drug abruptly
- Doses in latter part of day may cause insomnia
- To minimize anorexia, give drug with or after meals
- Heart rate and blood pressure should be monitored after every dose increase

PATIENT INSTRUCTIONS

For detailed patient instructions on psychostimulants, see the Patient Information Sheet on p. 269.

- Take drug as prescribed; do not increase dose without physician's knowledge
- Report any changes in sleeping or eating habits or any changes in behavior
- Pemoline should be taken once daily in the morning; do not take psychostimulants in the evening unless specifically so directed, as they can cause initial insomnia
- Clinical improvement may be gradual (pemoline) and benefits may not be evident for up to 4 weeks
- Use caution when driving or performing tasks requiring alertness: these drugs can mask symptoms of fatigue and impair coordination
- Do not chew or crush long-acting/slow-release tablets or capsules; chewing regular methylphenidate tablets can result in earlier and higher plasma levels and increased adverse effects
- Take medication with or after meals to minimize a decrease in appetite

DRUG INTERACTIONS

- Clinically significant interactions are listed below

DRUGS INTERACTING WITH METHYLPHENIDATE

Class of Drug	Example	Interaction Effects
Anticonvulsant	Carbamazepine	Decreased plasma level of methylphenidate and its metabolite
	Phenytoin, phenobarbital, primidone	Increased phenytoin level due to inhibited metabolism

Psychostimulants (cont.)

Class of Drug	Example	Interaction Effects
Antidepressant		
MAOI (Irreversible)	Phenelzine, tranylcypromine, pargyline	Release of large amount of norepinephrine with hypertensive reaction; combination used RARELY to augment antidepressant therapy with strict monitoring
RIMA	Moclobemide	Increased blood pressure and enhanced effect if used over prolonged period or in high doses
Tricyclic	Amitriptyline, etc.	Used together to augment antidepressant effect Plasma level of antidepressant may be increased Cardiovascular effects increased, with combination, in children; monitor Case reports of neurotoxic effects with imipramine, but considered rare; monitor
SSRI		Additive effects in depression, dysthymia and OCD in patients with ADHD; may improve response in refractory paraphilias and paraphilia-related disorders Plasma level of antidepressant may be increased
Antipsychotic		Early data suggest that methylphenidate may exacerbate or prolong withdrawal dyskinesia following antipsychotic discontinuation
Clonidine		Additive effect on sleep, hyperactivity and aggression associated with ADHD
Guanethidine		Decreased hypotensive effect; may be dose dependent
Warfarin		Decreased metabolism of anticoagulant Increased PT ratio or INR response

DRUGS INTERACTING WITH DEXTROAMPHETAMINE

Class of Drug	Example	Interaction Effects
Acidifying agent	Ammonium chloride, fruit juices, ascorbic acid	Decreased absorption, increased elimination and decreased plasma level of dextroamphetamine
Alkalinizing agent	Potassium citrate, sodium bicarbonate	Increased absorption, prolonged half-life and decreased elimination of amphetamines
Antidepressant		
MAOI (Irreversible)	Phenelzine, tranylcypromine	Hypertensive crisis due to increased norepinephrine release; AVOID
RIMA	Moclobemide	Slightly enhanced effect if used over prolonged period or in high doses
SSRIs	Sertraline	Additive effects in depression, dysthymia and OCD in patients with ADHD Paroxetine may increase plasma level of dextroamphetamine due to inhibited metabolism via CYP2D6
Antipsychotic	Haloperidol, chlorpromazine	Antagonize stimulant and toxic effects of dextroamphetamine
Barbiturate	Phenobarbital, amobarbital	Antagonize pharmacological effects of amphetamines
Guanethidine		Decreased hypotensive effect; may be dose-dependent

Comparison of Psychostimulants

	Methylphenidate	Dextroamphetamine/Adderall	Magnesium Pemoline
Dosing			
ADHD	5–60 mg/day; 0.25–1.0 mg/kg body weight (divided doses); up to 3 mg/kg has been used in children Up to 120 mg/day used in adults with ADHD Extended-release: 18–20 mg qam; can increase by 18–20 mg weekly to a maximum of 60 mg/day	Dextroamphetamine: 2.5–40 mg/day; 0.1–0.8 mg/kg (divided doses); Spansules can be sprinkled on food Adderall: 2.5–5 mg to start and increase by 2.5–5 mg every 3–7 days up to 25 mg/day (given every 4–7 h). In adults up to 40 mg/day (in divided doses)	37.5–112.5 mg/day; 1–2 mg/kg/day; dose dependent on age (single morning dose) Up to 150 mg/day used in adults with ADHD
Depression	10–30 mg/day	Adduall XR: 10–30 mg qam Dextroamphetamine: 5–60 mg/day	– –
Narcolepsy	10–60 mg/day	Dextroamphetamine: 5–60 mg/day	
Pharmacokinetics			
Bioavailability	> 90%	> 90%	> 90%
Peak plasma level	Tabs: 0.3–4 h Slow release: 1–8 h Metadate CD: 1.5 h first peak and 4.5 h second peak Concerta: 1 h first peak and 6.8 h second peak	Dextroamphetamine: Tablets 1–4 h Spansules: 6–10 h Adderall: Tablets 1–2 h XR: 7 h	2 4 h
Protein binding	8–15%	12–15%	50%
Onset of effects	0.5–2 h	0.5–2 h Adderall: saccharate and aspartate salts have a delayed onset	Delayed; up to 3 weeks, though some response evident in first 3 days
Plasma half-life	Regular tabs: 2.9 h mean SR and Concerta: 3.4 h mean Metadate CD: 6.8 h mean	Dextroamphetamine: 6.5 h mean	Children: 7.2 h Adults: 12 h
Duration of action	Regular tabs: 3–5 h Slow release – theoretically 5–8 h, but 3–5 h practically Extended release: 12 h	Dextroamphetamine: Tabs 4–5 h Spansules: 7–8 h Adderall: Tabs 5–7 h XR: 12 h	Over 12 h
Metabolism	Inhibits CYP2D6 and 2C9 enzymes	Metabolized by CYP2D6	?

Comparison of Psychostimulants (cont.)

	Methylphenidate	Dextroamphetamine/Adderall	Magnesium Pemoline
Adverse Effects*			
CNS	Nervousness, insomnia (up to 28%), activation, irritability (up to 26%), headache (up to 14%), rebound depression, rarely psychosis Tourette's syndrome, tics (up to 10%)	Nervousness, insomnia, activation, anxiety, mania (with high doses), dysphoria, irritability, headache, confusion, delusions, rebound depression, psychosis Headache Tremor, Tourette's syndrome, tics	Insomnia, drowsiness, dizziness, hallucinations, headache, irritability, seizures, Dyskinetic movements of face and extremities
GI	GI irritability (up to 23%), anorexia (up to 41% dose-related), weight loss	GI irritability, anorexia, weight loss	GI irritability, anorexia, weight loss, stomach ache
Cardiovascular	Increased heart rate and blood pressure, at start of therapy, dizziness	Increased heart rate and blood pressure, at start of therapy, dizziness	Increased heart rate during chronic treatment
Anticholinergic	Dry mouth, blurred vision	Dry mouth, dysgeusia, blurred vision	–
Endocrine	Growth delay (height and weight); may be related to dose and length of use	Growth delay (height and weight); may be related to dose, length of use and multiple administration schedule Impotence, changes in libido	Growth delay (transient), weight loss
Allergic	Upper respiratory infections: pharyngitis (4%), sinusitis (3%), cough (4%) Leukopenia, blood dyscrasias, anemia, hair loss	Urticaria, anemia	Hepatotoxicity, jaundice, skin rash
Toxicity	CNS overstimulation with vomiting, agitation, tremors, hyperreflexia, convulsions, confusion, hallucinations, delirium, cardiovascular effects e.g., hypertension, tachycardia Supportive therapy should be given	Restlessness, dizziness, increased reflexes, tremor, insomnia, irritability, assaultiveness, hallucinations, panic, cardiovascular effects, circulatory collapse, convulsions, and coma Supportive therapy should be given	CNS overstimulation with agitation, euphoria; restlessness, hallucinations, dyskinetic movements, hyperreflexia, tachycardia, hypertension May lead to convulsions and coma Supportive therapy should be given Cases of hepatic toxicity (deaths reported) occurring after months of use
Use in Pregnancy	No evidence of teratogenicity reported	High doses have embryotoxic and teratogenic potential; use of amphetamine in pregnant animals has been associated with permanent alterations in the central noradrenergic system of the neonate Increased risk of premature delivery and low birth weight; withdrawal reactions in newborn reported	Safety not established
Breastfeeding	No data	Excreted into breast milk; recommended not to breastfeed	No data

* Dose related

COGNITION ENHANCERS

PRODUCT AVAILABILITY

Chemical Class	Generic Name	Trade Name[A]	Dosage Forms and Strengths
Piperidine	Donepezil	Aricept	Tablets: 5 mg, 10 mg
Acridine	Tacrine[B]	Cognex	Tablets: 10 mg, 20 mg, 30 mg, 40 mg
Carbamate	Rivastigmine	Exelon	Capsules: 1.5 mg, 3 mg, 4.5 mg, 6 mg
Phenanthrene alkaloid	Galantamine	Reminyl	Tablets: 4 mg, 8 mg, 12 mg Liquid: 2 mg/ml

[A] Generic preparations may be available, [B] Not marketed in Canada

INDICATIONS*

- ▲ Symptomatic treatment of mild to moderate Alzheimer's dementia (AD); no effect on the underlying dementing process
- Data suggest efficacy in treatment of memory dysfunction following brain injury and in dementia of Parkinson's disease
- Early data suggest benefit for hallucinations and behavioral disturbances of Lewy body dementia (donepezil, rivastigmine) – some worsening of parkinsonism with donepezil
- Early data suggest benefit of donepezil in treatment-refractory bipolar disorder and for visual hallucinations
- Open trials suggest that augmentation with donepezil may improve organization, mental efficiency and attention in treatment-refractory children and adolescents with ADHD
- Preliminary data suggest improvement, with donepezil, on neuropsychological tests of verbal fluency and attention in patients with schizophrenia; improved cognition reported in patients with schizoaffective disorder
- Galantamine suggested to improve cognition and behaviors related to depression and anxiety
- Open trials suggest benefit of donepezil in treating tardive dyskinesia; case reports of benefit with tacrine

GENERAL COMMENTS

- Double-blind placebo-controlled studies involving patients with mild to moderate Alzheimer's disease showed improvement in cognitive ability. Approximately 25% of patients had significantly improved attention, interest, orientation, communication and memory
- These drugs are suggested to ameliorate behavioral disturbances (such as apathy, depression, anxiety, disinhibition, aberrant motor behavior, delusions and hallucinations) as well as enhance cognition. Benefits are lost 6 weeks after drug withdrawal
- The improvement is often modest and benefits may not be evident until 6–12 weeks of continuous treatment. In long-term studies patients receiving treatment with cholinesterase inhibitors cross their baseline cognitive ability at week 40 to 50 and continue to decline thereafter. Discontinuation of therapy after 6 months has been recommended if treatment benefits cannot be documented by any of the appropriate scales (e.g., Mini Mental Status Examination)
- Economic analyses (from USA, UK and Canada) suggest that donepezil initiated in early stages of Alzheimer's disease may be cost neutral as a result of patients remaining in a less severe state of disease for a longer time
- Increasing evidence suggests these drugs alter the course of the disease and slow the rate of decline. Therapeutic response following re-initiation of therapy shown to be less than that obtained with initial therapy
- Patients with AD complicated with vascular risk factors did better on rivastigmine than on placebo; also these patients did better on rivastigmine than AD patients without vascular risk factors

* ▲ Approved indications

Cognition Enhancers (cont.)

- Failure to respond to one agent does not preclude response to another

PHARMACOLOGY

- It is postulated that these compounds increase acetylcholine levels in the brain (in preclinical studies they increased extracellular acetylcholine levels in the hippocampus and cerebral cortex); nicotinic cholinergic receptors may regulate cognitive functions, such as attention, and may increase the release of neurotransmitters throughout the brain
- Cholinesterase inhibitors with dual inhibitory action (BuChE – butyrylcholinesterase; AChE – acetylcholinesterase) may reduce plaque formation

DOSING

- See chart on p. 170
- Treatment is started at lower doses to minimize side effects
- Higher doses of tacrine have been associated with a better outcome
- Tacrine dose escalation is guided by transaminase (ALT/SGPT) levels expressed as × ULN (upper level of normal) and measured bi-weekly for 16 weeks (see product monograph for details)
- Patients who discontinued tacrine because of ALT/SGPT elevation may be rechallenged upon return to normal limits; if rechallenged, AST/SGPT should be monitored weekly for 16 weeks; the initial dose is 40 mg/day
- Patients who discontinue rivastigmine for longer than several days should be re-started at the lowest daily dose (1.5 mg od or bid) to reduce the possibility of severe vomiting; dosage should be titrated gradually to the maintenance dose

PHARMACOKINETICS

- See chart, p. 170
- Duration of cholinesterase inhibition does not reflect plasma half-life of drug (e.g., rivastigmine half-life is 1–2 h, but cholinesterase inhibition lasts up to 10 h
- Plasma rivastigmine levels are approximately 30% higher in elderly male patients than in young adults

ADVERSE EFFECTS

- See chart on pp. 171–172
- Most adverse effects are due to cholinomimetic activity: nausea, vomiting, diarrhea, constipation and anorexia
- Occur more often in patients over 85 years of age and in females
- Generally are mild and transient and resolve during drug administration
- Adverse effects are more frequent at higher doses; these can be minimized by administering the drug at the starting dose for 4–6 weeks prior to switching to a higher dose
- Gastrointestinal symptoms (e.g., cramping, nausea, vomiting) reported to respond to propantheline (7.5–15 mg); caution as to anticholinergic effects

Tacrine

- Elevating of liver transaminases is seen in approximately 50% of patients using dose of 160 mg/day; seen within the first 12 weeks of treatment. It returns to normal within 4–6 weeks after the discontinuation of tacrine; may not recur on drug rechallenge. Liver biopsy is not indicated in cases of uncomplicated ALT/SGPT elevation. Tacrine must be discontinued if transaminase levels rise to over 5 times the upper limit of normal

WITHDRAWAL

- Sudden worsening of cognitive function and behavior reported following drug withdrawal – suggest that dose be reduced by 50% every 2 weeks, with close monitoring

PRECAUTIONS

- Caution should be exercised if any of the following exists:
  - Known hypersensitivity to above compounds
  - History of syncope, bradycardia, bradyarrhythmia, sick sinus syndrome, conduction disturbances, congestive heart failure, coro-

nary artery disease, asthma, COPD, ulcers or increased risk for ulcers or GI bleeding (concomitant use of NSAIDS or higher doses of ASA)
- Patient with low body weight, over 85 years of age and/or female, or with a comorbid disease

CONTRAINDICATIONS

- Anesthesia: possible exaggeration of muscle relaxation induced by succinylcholine-type drugs
- Epilepsy: reduction of seizure threshold
- Parkinson's or severe Alzheimer's disease: safety and efficacy unknown
- Tacrine is contraindicated in patients who were previously treated with the drug and developed treatment-associated jaundice confirmed by elevated total bilirubin > 3.0 mg/dl
- Tacrine is contraindicated if there is known hypersensitivity to tacrine or acridine derivatives
- Galantamine is contraindicated in patients with severe hepatic and/or renal impairment (creatinine clearance < 9 ml/min)

TOXICITY

- Overdose can result in cholinergic crisis characterized by severe nausea, vomiting, salivation, sweating, bradycardia, hypotension followed by increasing muscle weakness, respiratory depression and convulsions

Management

- Institute general supportive measures
- Treatment: atropine sulfate 1 mg to 2 mg IV with subsequent doses depending on clinical response. The value of dialysis in over-dosage is not known
- In asymptomatic rivastigmine overdose – hold drug for 24 h, then resume treatment. Because of the short half-life of rivastigmine, the value of dialysis in treatment of cholinergic crisis is unknown

PEDIATRIC CONSIDERATIONS

- Not recommended for use in children

GERIATRIC CONSIDERATIONS

- Caution should be exercised and adverse events closely monitored when using donepezil in doses over 5 mg a day in this patient population
- Women, over age 85, with low body weights are at high risk for adverse effects
- Use caution in patients with comorbid disease
- Galantamine plasma concentrations are 30–40% higher in the elderly than in healthy young subjects

USE IN PREGNANCY

- Not recommended for women of childbearing potential, pregnant or nursing women

Breast milk

- Effect unknown

NURSING IMPLICATIONS

- Liver function should be monitored regularly in patients taking tacrine (i.e., every 2 weeks for the first 16 weeks, then monthly for two months, thereafter every 3 months)
- Anticholinergic agents (e.g., antinauseants) will antagonize the effects of these drugs and should be avoided

PATIENT INSTRUCTIONS

For detailed patient instructions on cognition enhancers, see the Patient Information Sheet on p. 271.

- The effectiveness of this medication depends upon its administration at regular intervals, as directed by the physician
- Report any new or unusual side effects to the physician
- Do not stop the medication abruptly, as changes in behavior and/or concentration can occur
- Do not self-administer over-the-counter preparations (e.g., antihistamines, antinauseants) without consultation with the physician or pharmacist

Cognition Enhancers (cont.)

DRUG INTERACTIONS

DRUGS INTERACTING WITH DONEPEZIL

Class of Drug	Example	Interaction Effects
Anticholinergic	Benztropine, diphenhydramine	Antagonism of effects
Anticonvulsant	Carbamazepine, phenytoin, phenobarbital	Increased metabolism of donepezil resulting in decreased efficacy
Antifungal	Ketoconazole	Inhibited metabolism of donepezil via CYP3A4
Antipsychotic	Risperidone	Exacerbation of EPS
β-Blocker	Propranolol	May potentiate bradycardia
Bethanechol		Synergistic effects: increased nausea, vomiting and diarrhea
Dexamethasone		Increased metabolism of donepezil resulting in decreased efficacy
Neuromuscular blocker	Succinylcholine, suxamethonium	Prolonged neuromuscular blockade
Quinidine		Inhibited metabolism of donepezil via CYP2D6
Rifampin		Increased metabolism of donepezil resulting in decreased efficacy

DRUGS INTERACTING WITH TACRINE

Class of Drug	Example	Interaction Effects
Antidepressant	SSRI – fluvoxamine	Increased plasma level of tacrine; peak plasma level increased 5-fold and clearance decreased by 88% due to inhibited metabolism via CYP1A2
Anticholinergic	Benztropine, chlorpheniramine	Antagonism of effects
Antipsychotic	Haloperidol	Exacerbation of EPS
β-Blockers	Propranolol	May potentiate bradycardia
Bethanechol		Synergistic effects: increased nausea, vomiting and diarrhea
Cimetidine		Increased effects of tacrine (peak level by 54%)
Neuromuscular blocker	Succinylcholine, suxamethonium	Prolonged neuromuscular blockade
NSAID	Ibuprofen	Reports of delirium (with delusions, hallucinations and insomnia)
Riluzole		Elevated plasma level of both agents
Smoking		Decreased plasma level of tacrine due to induction of metabolism via CYP1A2
Theophylline		Increased plasma level of theophylline (2-fold)

DRUGS INTERACTING WITH RIVASTIGMINE

Class of Drug	Example	Interaction Effects
Anticholinergic	Benztropine, diphenhydramine	Antagonism of effects
β-Blocker	Propranolol	May potentiate bradycardia
Neuromuscular blocker	Succinylcholine, suxamethonium	Prolonged neuromuscular blockade
Nicotine		Increased clearance of rivastigmine by 23%

DRUGS INTERACTING WITH GALANTAMINE

Class of Drug	Example	Interaction Effects
Anticholinergic	Benztropine, chlorpheniramine	Antagonism of effects
β-Blocker	Propranolol	May potentiate bradycardia
Antifungal	Ketoconazole	Increased AUC of galantamine by 30% due to inhibited metabolism via CYP3A4
Antibiotic	Erythromycin	Increased AUC of galantamine by 10% due to inhibited metabolism via CYP3A4
Antidepressant	Amitriptyline, fluoxetine, fluvoxamine	Decreased clearance of galantamine by 25–30% due to inhibited metabolism via CYP2D6
	Paroxetine	Increased AUC of galantamine by 40% due to inhibited metabolism via CYP2D6
Quinidine		Decreased clearance of galantamine by 25–30% due to inhibited metabolism via CYP2D6
Cimetidine		Increased AUC of galantamine by 16%

Comparison of Acetylcholinesterase Inhibitors

	Donepezil hydrochloride	Tacrine	Rivastigmine	Galantamine
Chemistry	Piperidine-based Reversible inhibitor of AChE and BuChE Binds preferentially to acetylcholinesterase in the brain and has little effect on cholinesterase in serum, heart or small intestine	Acridine derivative Reversible inhibitor of AChE and BuChE Binds non-selectively to all cholinesterases	Carbamate derivative Reversible inhibitor of AChE and BuChE May be more selective for AChE present in hippocampal neurons	Phenanthrene alkaloid AChE > BuChE Allosteric modulator of central nicotinic receptors
Dosing	Initial dose is 5 mg/day taken once daily; could be increased to 10 mg a day if no improvement is seen after 4–6 weeks of therapy. The maximum dose is 10 mg/day	Initial dose is 40 mg/day (10 mg qid) taken at regular intervals at least 1 h before meals for 6 weeks; ALT/SGPT must be monitored bi-weekly If there is no significant transaminase elevation, the dose can be increased to 80 mg/day (20 mg qid) The dose can be further increased to 120–160 mg/day at 6 week intervals if patient is tolerating treatment Dose titration and monitoring sequence should be repeated if patient suspends treatment for more than 4 weeks	Initial dose is 1.5 mg bid, given with meals; increase by 3 mg every 4 weeks Usual maintenance dose: 3–6 mg bid (with meals)	4 mg bid with food for 4 weeks; increase to 8 mg bid for 4 weeks; can increase dose to 12 mg bid In moderate hepatic impairment: 4 mg od
Pharmacokinetics Bioavailability	100% and is independent of food or time of day	17–33%; food reduces bioavailability by 30–40%	36%; food delays absorption, lowers C_{max}, and increases AUC by 25%	90%; food lowers C_{max} by 25% and delays T_{max} by 1.5 h
Peak plasma level	3–4 h	1–2 h	1.4–2.6 h	1 h
Plasma half-life	70–80 h in healthy adults; increases after multiple dose administration Clearance decreased by 20% in patients with liver cirrhosis Renal impairment has no effect on clearance	2 to 4 hours (independent of dose or plasma concentration) Clearance decreased with liver disease Renal impairment has no effect on clearance	1–2 h (in both young and elderly) Clearance decreased in patients with liver disease Renal impairment may increase plasma level	5–7 h Clearance decreased by 25% with liver disease In moderate and severe renal impairment AUC increased by 37% and 67%, respectively Clearance about 20% lower in females

	Donepezil hydrochloride	Tacrine	Rivastigmine	Galantamine
Plasma protein binding	96%, predominantly to albumin	55–75%	40%	18%
Metabolism	via CYP2D6 and 3A4 Four major metabolites, of which 2 are active	via CYP1A2 and 2D6 Has active metabolites	Metabolized by esterase enzymes – low risk of drug interactions Phenolic metabolite has approximately 10% of the activity of parent drug	via CYP2D6 and 3A4
Adverse effects				
GI	5–10%: nausea, vomiting, diarrhea, gastric upset, constipation; > 2%: anorexia	10–30%: nausea, vomiting, diarrhea, gastric upset; 5–10%: anorexia, flatulence, constipation	10–30% nausea, vomiting, diarrhea, abdominal pain > 30% anorexia (with weight loss, especially in females)	10–30% nausea, vomiting 5–10% diarrhea 5–10% anorexia > 1% flatulence
CNS	5–10%: insomnia, fatigue, headache; 2–5%: abnormal dreams, somnolence, agitation, activation, depression; < 2%: restlessness, aggression, irritability; < 1%: transient ischemic attack, hypokinesia, seizures Nightmares reported; manageable by switching from nighttime to morning dosing Rapid onset of manic symptoms in patients with a history of bipolar disorder reported Worsening of parkinsonism	2–10%: headache; 2–5%: nervousness, agitation, irritability, aggression, transient dysphoria, confusion, insomnia, somnolence, fatigue, depression, hallucinations, ataxia, tremor; < 2%: vertigo, paresthesias, seizures; < 1%: cerebrovascular accident, transient ischemic attack	2–10% headache > 5% sedation, asthenia > 2% anxiety, insomnia, aggression, hallucinations > 1% tremor, ataxia, abnormal gait cases of seizures	5–10% insomnia, headache, depression, fatigue, agitation 2–5% sedation, tremor < 1 % paranoia, delirium, ataxia, vertigo, hypertonia, seizures
Cardiovascular	2–10%: dizziness < 2%: syncope, atrial fibrillation, hypotension; < 1%: arrhythmia, first degree AV block, congestive heart failure, symptomatic sinus bradycardia, supraventricular tachycardia, deep vein thromboses	> 10–20%: dizziness; < 2%: hypertension, hypotension; < 1%: heart failure, myocardial infarction, angina, atrial fibrillation, palpitations, tachycardia, bradycardia	10–20% dizziness 2–5% syncope	5–10% dizziness 2% bradycardia, syncope >1% chest pain <1% edema, atrial fibrillation
Respiratory	> 5%: nasal congestion; < 2%: dyspnea; < 1%: pulmonary congestion, pneumonia, sleep apnea	> 5%: nasal congestion; < 2%: pharyngitis, sinusitis, bronchitis, pneumonia, dyspnea	> 2% nasal congestion < 2% dyspnea < 1% upper respiratory tract infections	>2% nasal congestion
Special senses	< 2%: blurred vision; < 1%: dry eyes, glaucoma	< 2%: conjunctivitis < 1%: dry eyes, glaucoma	> 2% tinnitus	–

Comparison of Acetylcholinesterase Inhibitors (cont.)

	Donepezil hydrochloride	**Tacrine**	**Rivastigmine**	**Galantamine**
Skin	2–10% flushing; < 2%: pruritis and urticaria	2–10%: hot flushes, rash < 2%: increased sweating	> 5% increased sweating Flushing	–
Urogenital	< 2%: frequent urination, nocturia; < 1%: prostatic hypertrophy; > 5%: incontinence	> 2%: frequent urination, incontinence, urinary tract infection; < 1%: haematuria, urinary retention	> 5% urinary tract infection > 2% frequent urination, incontinence	>5% urinary tract infection >2% hematuria >1% incontinence <1% urinary retention
Musculoskeletal	5–10%: muscle cramps, pain < 2% arthritis Case reports of Pisa syndrome	> 5%: myalgia < 2%: arthralgia, arthritis	< 1% arthralgia, myalgia, pain Case report of Pisa syndrome	5–10% muscle cramps
Liver	–	up to 50%: elevated ALT/SGPT	–	–
Other	< 2%: dehydration; < 1%: blood dyscrasias, jaundice, renal failure	< 2%: chills, fever, malaise, peripheral edema; < 1%: blood dyscrasias	< 1% dehydration, hypokalemia < 1% nose bleeds	2–5% anemia <1% blood dyscrasias

SEX-DRIVE DEPRESSANTS

PRODUCT AVAILABILITY

Chemical Class	Generic Name	Trade Name[(A)]	Dosage Forms and Strengths
Antiandrogen/Progestogen	Cyproterone	Androcur Androcur Depot	Tablets: 50 mg Injection (depot): 100 mg/ml
Progestogen	Medroxyprogesterone	Provera DepoProvera	Tablets: 100 mg Injection (depot): 50 mg/ml, 150 mg/ml
Luteinizing hormone-releasing hormone (LHRH) agonist	Leuprolide	Lupron Lupron Depot	Injection: 5 mg/ml Injection (depot): 1 mg/0.2 ml[(B)], 3.75 mg/ vial, 7.5 mg/vial, 11.25 mg/vial, 15 mg/vial[(B)], 22.5 mg/vial, 30 mg/vial
	Goserelin	Zoladex LA Zoladex	Implant (depot): 10.8 mg/vial Implant (depot): 3.6 mg/vial

[(A)] Generic preparations may be available, [(B)] Not marketed in Canada

INDICATIONS*

- Reduction of sexual arousal and libido (usually for sexual offenders)
- Inappropriate or disruptive sexual behavior in patients with dementia

GENERAL COMMENTS

- Efficacy: 35–95%, depending on type of sexual problem and motivation of patient
- Medroxyprogesterone and cyproterone are not effective in some patients despite high doses and over 90% reduction of testosterone levels
- Leuprolide and goserelin may cause a transient increase in leuteinizing hormone and testosterone, followed by a dramatic decrease and suppression of the hormones
- Seek consultation with an internist/endocrinologist prior to initiation of therapy, and yearly thereafter
- Longer acting depot injections (e.g., leuprolide 30 mg q 4 months) have been found of benefit in high risk sex offenders

PHARMACOLOGY

- Interfere with synthesis of testosterone
- Lower plasma testosterone levels; androgen levels decline over 2 to 4 weeks; with medroxyprogesterone and cyproterone androgen levels may subsequently rise, without necessarily a parallel increase in sexual drive

DOSING

- See p. 174
- Depot injections of medroxyprogesterone and cyproterone may initially be prescribed every 2 weeks with monitoring of serum testosterone and sexual self-report. Often, weekly injection schedule is necessary to achieve good behavioral control and testosterone suppression
- Anaphylaxis, while reported in the literature with leuprolide, has rarely been observed in clinical practice; however, some clinicians feel that one dose of short-acting leuprolide acetate is indicated

* not approved

Sex-Drive Depressants (cont.)

ADVERSE EFFECTS

- See p. 175
- The main serious long-term side effects of LHRH is decreased bone density [Treatment with alendronate, calcium, vitamin D and low-dose progesterone has been found to arrest or even reverse this side effect]

NURSING IMPLICATIONS

- Leuprolide: reconstitute drug only with 1 ml of diluent provided. Shake well. Suspension is stable for 24 h and can be stored at room temperature. Inject using 22 gauge needle (or larger). Injection may rarely cause irritation (burning, itching, and swelling)
- Goserelin pellet is injected subcutaneously into the anterior abdominal wall

PATIENT INSTRUCTIONS

For detailed patient instructions on sex-drive-depressants, see the Patient Information Sheet on p. 273.

- Drug must be taken consistently to maintain effect; report any changes in mood or behavior while on the drug

MEDICOLEGAL ISSUES

- As sex drive reduction is not an approved indication, patient consent should be sought
- Use of these drugs involves complex issues in regard to consent, as the patients are often under the legal system

DRUG INTERACTIONS

- Only clinically significant interactions are listed below

Class of Drug	Example	Interaction Effects
		INTERACTIONS WITH MEDROXYPROGESTERONE
Aminoglutethimide		Decreased plasma level of medroxyprogesterone
Rifampin		Decreased plasma level of medroxyprogesterone due to increased metabolism
		INTERACTIONS WITH CYPROTERONE
Alcohol		Alcohol may reduce the antiandrogenic effect of cyproterone when used for hypersexuality

Comparison of Sex-Drive Depressants

	Cyproterone	Medroxyprogesterone	Leuprolide	Goserelin
Dosing	Oral: 100–500 mg/day Depot: 100–600 mg/week	Oral: 100–600 mg/day Depot: 100–700 mg/week	Acetate (test dose): 1 mg* Depot: 3.75 – 7.5 mg/month; 11.25 or 22.5 mg q 3 months; 30 mg q 4 months	3.6 mg/month; or 10.8 mg q 3 months
Pharmacokinetics				
Peak plasma level	Oral: 3–4 h Depot: 3.4 h	Oral: not established Depot: few days	Not established	Not established
Half-life	Oral: 33–42 h Depot: 4 days	Oral: 30 h Depot: not established Metabolized via CYP3A4		4.2 h (males); 2–3 h (females) half-life increased to 12 h in renal impairment

* Test dose recommended by some clinicians

	Cyproterone	Medroxyprogesterone	Leuprolide	Goserelin
Monitoring Pretreatment	Serum testosterone, prolactin, LH, FSH, liver function, Hb, WBC, glucose blood pressure, weight	Serum testosterone, prolactin, LH, FSH, liver function, Hb, WBC, glucose blood pressure, weight	Serum testosterone, LH, FSH, ECG, BUN, creatinine, CBC, bone density	Serum testosterone, LH, FSH, ECG, BUN, creatinine, CBC, bone density
Chronic	Testosterone: q 6 months LH: q 6 months Prolactin: q 6 months Blood pressure, weight	Testosterone: q 6 months LH: q 6 months Prolactin: q 6 months Blood pressure, weight	Testosterone: q 1 month, for 4 months, then q 6 months BUN, creatinine: q 6 months; LH and prolactin: q 6 months Bone density: q 1 year	Testosterone: q 1 month for 4 months, then q 6 months BUN, creatinine: q 6 months LH and prolactin: q 6 months Bone density: q 1 year
Precautions	May impair carbohydrate metabolism, fasting blood glucose, and glucose tolerance test Hypercalcemia and changes in plasma lipids can occur Alcohol use may reduce the antiandrogenic effect Deep vein thrombosis and thromboembolism (smoking may increase risk)	May decrease glucose tolerance Monitor patients with conditions aggravated by fluid retention, e.g., asthma, migraine Deep vein thrombosis and thromboembolism (smoking may increase risk)		Transient elevation of BUN, creatinine, testosterone, and acid phosphatase reported
Adverse Effects	Atrophy of seminiferous tubules with chronic use (possibly reversible if drug stopped) Gynecomastia: 15–20%; [report that pretreatment with irradiation therapy will prevent this side effect] Decrease in body hair and sebum production Depression: 5–10%	Decreased sperm count, hot flashes, impotence, fatigue, hypertension, edema Increased appetite and weight gain Mild depression, lethargy, nervousness, insomnia, nightmares, headaches	Decreased sperm count, atrophy of seminiferous tubules, impotence Hot flashes Sweating, rash, edema (3%), nausea, other GI effects, loss of body hair, myalgia, spasms, lethargy, dyspnea Decreased bone density	Decreased sperm count, atrophy of seminiferous tubules, impotence Hot flashes Sweating, rash, edema (3%), nausea, other GI effects, loss of body hair, myalgia, spasms, lethargy, dyspnea Decreased bone density
Contraindications	Liver disease, thromboembolic disorders	Liver disease; thromboembolic disorders	Hypersensitivity to drug	Hypersensitivity to drug
Toxicity	No reports	No reports	No reports	No reports

Drugs of Abuse

GENERAL COMMENTS

- This chapter gives a general overview of common drugs of abuse and is not intended to deal in detail with all agents, or be a complete guide to treatment
- Slang names of street drugs change rapidly and vary with country, region, and drug subculture
- Drugs of abuse can be classified as follows:

Chemical Class	Agents[(A)]	Page
Alcohol	Alcohol	See p. 179
Hallucinogens	Examples: Lysergic acid diethylamide Cannabis Phencyclidine	See p. 182
Stimulants	Examples: Amphetamine Cocaine Sympathomimetics (incl. caffeine)	See p. 187
Opiates/Narcotics	Examples: Morphine Heroin Pentazocine	See p. 190
Inhalants/Aerosols	Examples: Glue Paint thinner	See p. 194
Gamma hydroxy butyrate		See p. 195
Sedative/Hypnotics*	Examples: Flunitrazepam Barbiturates Benzodiazepines Hypnotics	See p. 197 See p. 109 See p. 109 See p. 124
Nicotine*	Examples: Cigarettes, cigars	

(A) Only includes examples of most commonly used substances
* Not dealt with specifically in this chapter

DEFINITIONS

Drug Abuse

- Acute or chronic intake of any substance that: (a) has no recognized medical use, (b) is used inappropriately in terms of its medical indications or its dose

Drug Dependence

A. Psychological

- Craving or desire for continuous administration of a drug to provide a desired effect or to avoid discomfort

B. Physical

- A physiological state of adaptation to a drug which usually results in development of tolerance to drug effects and withdrawal symptoms when the drug is stopped – also called addiction

Tolerance

- Phenomenon in which increasing doses of a drug are needed to produce a desired effect

PHARMACOLOGY

- Research data have demonstrated that every drug of abuse increases dopamine activity in the nucleus accumbens of the brain; the increased dopamine is suggested to be associated with the pleasurable effects produced by the drug

GENERAL COMMENTS

- The effect which any drug of abuse has on an individual depends on a number of variables:
  1) dose (amount ingested, injected, sniffed, etc.)
  2) potency and purity of drug
  3) route of administration
  4) past experience of the user (this will predispose to selective behavioral response either on a pharmacologic or conditioning basis)
  5) present circumstances, i.e., environment, other people present, whether other drugs are taken concurrently
  6) personality and genetic predisposition of user
  7) age of user
  8) clinical status of user, i.e., type of psychiatric illness, degree of recent stress or loss, occurrence of a vulnerable phase of a circadian or ultradian rhythm, user's expectations, and present feelings
- Some users may have different experiences with the same drug on different occasions. They may encounter both pleasant and unpleasant effects during the same drug experience
- Many street drugs are adulterated with other chemicals, and may not be what the individual thinks they are; potency and purity of street drugs vary greatly
- It is questionable whether drugs of abuse can cause persistent psychiatric disorders in otherwise healthy individuals, or whether they precipitate latent psychiatric illness in predisposed individuals who already have significant premorbid psychopathology. Many abusers tend to be multiple drug users, therefore to say that a specific drug was implicated in a psychiatric disorder is difficult. Overall, in non-treatment community samples, it is estimated over 50% of drug users have at least one other psychiatric disorder
- Substance abuse has been associated with earlier onset of schizophrenia, decreased treatment responsiveness of positive symptoms and poor clinical functioning; similarly decreased treatment responsiveness in bipolar disorder can occur

ADVERSE EFFECTS

- See pharmacological/psychiatric effects under specific drugs
- Reactions are unpredictable and depend on the potency and purity of drug taken
- Psychiatric reactions secondary to drug abuse may occur more readily in individuals already at risk
- Renal, hepatic, cardiorespiratory, neurological, and gastrointestinal complications as well as encephalopathies can occur with chronic abuse of specific agents
- Intravenous drug users are at risk for infection, including cellulitis, hepatitis and AIDS
- Impurities in street drugs (especially if inhaled or injected) can cause tissue and organ damage (blood vessels, kidney, lungs, and liver)
- Psychological dependence can occur; the drug becomes central to a person's thoughts, emotions, and activities, resulting in craving
- Physical dependence can occur; the body adapts to the presence of the drug and withdrawal symptoms occur when the drug is stopped, resulting in addiction

TREATMENT

- See specific agents
- The diagnosis of the type of substance abused can be difficult in an Emergency Room when a patient presents as floridly psychotic, intoxicated or delirious. Blood and urine screens take time, therefore diagnosis must include mental status, physical and neurological examination, as well as a drug history, whenever possible; collateral history should be sought
- In severe cases, monitor vitals and fluid intake
- Agitation can be treated conservatively by talking with the patient and providing reassurance until the drug wears off (i.e., "talking down"). When conservative approaches are inadequate or if symptoms persist, pharmacological intervention should be considered
- Avoid low-potency neuroleptics due to anticholinergic effects, hypotension, and tachycardia

WITHDRAWAL

- See specific agents
- Identification of drug(s) abused is important; toxicology may help in identification whenever multiple or combination drug use is suspected
- If 2 or more drugs have been chronically abused, withdraw one drug at a time, starting with the one that potentially represents the greatest problem: e.g., in alcohol/sedative abuse, withdraw the alcohol first

LONG-TERM TREATMENT

- The presence of comorbid psychiatric disorders in substance abusers can adversely influence outcome in treatment of the substance abuse as well as the psychiatric disorder

Alcohol

SLANG

- Booze, hooch, juice, brew

PHARMACOLOGICAL/ PSYCHIATRIC EFFECTS

- Signs and symptoms are associated with blood alcohol level of approximately 34 mmol/L (higher in chronic users; 60–70 mmol/L)
- Effects of a single drink occur within 15 min and last approximately 60 min, depending on amount taken; renal elimination is about 10 g alcohol per hour (about 30 ml (1 oz) whiskey or 1 bottle of regular beer). Blood alcohol level declines by 4–7 mmol per hour.
- Tolerance decreases with age and with compromised brain function

Acute

- Disinhibition, relaxation, euphoria, agitation, drowsiness, impaired cognition, judgement, and memory, perceptual and motor dysfunction

☞ **Acute alcohol intake decreases hepatic metabolism of co-administered drugs by competition for microsomal enzymes**

Chronic

- Chronic use results in an increased capacity to metabolize alcohol and a concurrent CNS tolerance; psychological as well as physical dependence may occur; hepatic metabolism decreases with liver cirrhosis

☞ **Chronic alcohol use increases hepatic metabolism of co-administered drugs**

Physical

- Hand tremor, dyspepsia, diarrhea, morning nausea and vomiting, polyuria, impotence, pancreatitis, headache, hepatomegaly, peripheral neuropathy

Mental

- Memory blackouts, nightmares, insomnia, hallucinations, paranoia, intellectual impairment, dementia, Wernicke-Korsakoff syndrome, and other organic mental disorders
- Chronic alcohol use by patients with schizophrenia suggested to be associated with more florid symptoms, more re-hospitalizations, poorer long-term outcome and increased risk of tardive dyskinesia

RELATED PROBLEMS

- Up to 50% of alcoholics meet the criteria for lifetime diagnosis of major depression
- Withdrawal symptoms, physical violence, loss of control when drinking, surreptitious drinking, change in tolerance to alcohol, deteriorating job performance, change in social interactions, increased risk for stroke, and death from motor vehicle accidents

TOXICITY

- Hazardous alcohol consumption: greater than 80 g ethanol per day (approx. 6 bottles of regular beer, 270 ml (9 oz) spirits, or 720 ml (24 oz) wine)
- Risk increases when combined with drugs with CNS depressant activity

WITHDRAWAL

- Occurs after chronic use (i.e., drinking for more than 3 days, more than 500 ml of spirits or equivalent per day)
- Most effects seen within 5 days after stopping

Mild Withdrawal

- Insomnia, irritability, headache
- Usually transient and self-limiting

Severe Reactions

- Phase I: begins within hours of cessation and lasts 3–5 days. Symptoms: tremor, tachycardia, diaphoresis, labile BP, nausea, vomiting, anxiety
- Phase II: perceptual disturbances (usually visual or auditory)
- Phase III: 10–15% untreated alcohol withdrawal patients reach this phase; seizures (usually tonic-clonic) last 0.5–4 min and can progress to status epilepticus
- Phase IV: Delirium tremens (DTs) usually occurs after 72 h; includes autonomic hyperactivity and severe hyperthermia; mortality rate of patients who reach phase IV is 20%
- Wernicke's encephalopathy can occur in patients with thiamine deficiency

TREATMENT

- In acute intoxication minimize stimulation; effects will diminish as blood alcohol level declines (rate of 4–7 mmol/L per hour)
- Withdrawal reactions following chronic alcohol use may require
  - a) vitamin supplementation (thiamine 50 mg orally or IM)
  - b) benzodiazepine for symptomatic relief and to prevent seizures (chlordiazepoxide, lorazepam, or oxazepam); caution in transferring dependence from alcohol to benzodiazepine

Alcohol (cont.)

c) hydration and electrolyte correction
d) high potency neuroleptic (e.g., haloperidol, zuclopenthixol) to treat behavior disturbances and hallucinations
e) paraldehyde, or haloperidol and lorazepam, to prevent or treat delirium tremens

- SSRIs (e.g., fluoxetine) and buspirone have shown some efficacy in decreasing alcohol consumption by 9–17%, as well as decreasing interest in and craving for alcohol
- Naltrexone reported to be an effective adjunct to treatment for relapse prevention following alcohol detoxification, see pp. 201–202
- See pp. 198–200 for use of anti-alcohol drug in treatment

USE IN PREGNANCY

- Infants born with fetal alcohol syndrome with mental deficiency, irritability, and facial abnormalities
- Withdrawal reactions reported

Breast milk

- Milk levels attain 90–95% of blood levels; prolonged intake can be detrimental

DRUG INTERACTIONS

- Only clinically significant interactions are listed below

Drug of Abuse	Interacting Drugs	Reaction
Alcohol	Acetaminophen	Chronic excessive alcohol use increases susceptibility to acetaminophen-induced hepatotoxicity
	Antibiotics: – cephalosporins	Disulfiram-like reaction with nausea, hypotension, flushing, headache, tachycardia
	– doxycycline	Chronic alcohol use induces metabolism and decreases plasma level of doxycycline
	Anticonvulsants: – barbiturates, phenytoin	Additive CNS effects Decreased plasma level of ethanol Acute intoxication inhibits phenobarbital metabolism; chronic intoxication enhances metabolism
	– valproic acid, divalproex	Displaces alcohol from protein binding and potentiates intoxicating effect
	Antidepressants: – tricyclic	Additive CNS effects Short-term or acute use reduces first-pass metabolism of the antidepressant and increases its plasma level Imipramine and desipramine clearance is increased in chronic alcoholics and during the first month after detoxification; delay in ethanol absorption with antidepressant use
	– SSRI	Rate of fluvoxamine absorption increased by ethanol
	– NaSSA	Additive CNS effects
	Antifungal: metronidazole, ketoconazole, furazolidone	Disulfiram-like reaction
	Antipsychotics	Additive CNS effects Extrapyramidal side effects may be worsened by alcohol
	Ascorbic acid	Increased ethanol clearance

Drug of Abuse	Interacting Drugs	Reaction
	Benzodiazepines	Potentiation of CNS effects Alprazolam reported to increase aggression in moderate alcohol drinkers Brain concentrations of various benzodiazepines altered by ethanol: triazolam and estazolam concentrations decreased, diazepam concentration increased, no change with chlordiazepoxide
	Chloral hydrate	Additive CNS effects Increased plasma level of metabolite of chloral hydrate (trichloroethanol), and of blood ethanol
	Chlorpropamide, tolbutamide	Flushing, sweating, palpitations, headache due to formation of acetaldehyde
	Cocaine	Ethanol promotes the formation of a highly addicting metabolite, cocoethylene Reports of enhanced hepatotoxicity Increased heart rate; variable effect on blood pressure Increased risk of sudden death with combined use (18-fold) Combined use reported to result in more impulsive decision making and poorer performance on tests of learning and memory
	Disulfiram	Flushing, sweating, palpitations, headache due to formation of acetaldehyde (see p. 198)
	H_2 blockers: cimetidine, ranitidine	Peak blood alcohol level increased by 92% with cimetidine and 34% with ranitidine – data contradictory (no effect with famotidine)
	Isoniazid	Increased risk of hepatotoxicity Tyramine-containing alcoholic beverages may cause a hypertensive reaction (MAOI)
	Milk	Decreased ethanol absorption by delaying gastric emptying
	Salicylates	Increased gastric bleeding with ASA; reduced peak plasma concentration of ASA reported ASA may increase blood alcohol concentration by reducing ethanol oxidation by gastric alcohol dehydrogenase
	Tianeptine	Rate of tianeptine absorption decreased; plasma level decreased by 30%
	Verapamil	Increased concentration of ethanol due to inhibited metabolism
	Warfarin	Chronic alcohol use induces warfarin metabolism and decreases hypoprothrombinemic effect. Acute alcohol use can impair warfarin metabolism

Hallucinogens

PHARMACOLOGICAL/ PSYCHIATRIC EFFECTS

Differ somewhat depending on type of drug taken and route of administration (see specific agents below)
- Effects occur rapidly and last from 30 min (e.g., DMT) to several days (e.g., PCP)

Physical
- Increased BP, tachycardia, dilated pupils, nausea, sweating, flushing, chills, hyperventilation, incoordination, muscle weakness, trembling, numbness

Mental
- Alteration of perception and body awareness, impaired attention and short-term memory, disturbed sense of time, depersonalization, euphoria, mystical or religious experiences, grandiosity, anxiety, panic, visual distortions, hallucinations (primarily visual), erratic behavior, aggression

High Doses
- Confusion, restlessness, excitement, anxiety, emotional lability, panic, mania, paranoia, "bad trip"
- Cardiac depression and respiratory depression (mescaline), hypotension, convulsions and coma (PCP)

Chronic Use
- Anxiety, depression, personality changes
- Tolerance (tachyphylaxis) can occur with regular use (except with DMT); reverse tolerance (supersensitivity) has been described
- "Woolly" thinking, delusions and hallucinations reported; may persist for months after drug discontinuation
- Flashbacks – recurrent psychotic symptoms, may occur years after discontinuation
- Regular (weekly) marihuana use has been associated with increased risk of tardive dyskinesia in schizophrenic patients on neuroleptics

TREATMENT
- Provide reassurance and reduction of threatening external stimuli
- In severe cases, the "trip" should be aborted chemically as rapidly as possible. This reduces the likelihood of flashbacks or recurrences in the future; in mild cases "talking down" may be more appropriate
- Avoid low-potency neuroleptics with anticholinergic and α-adrenergic properties (e.g., chlorpromazine) to minimize hypotension, tachycardia, disorientation, and seizures
- Use high-potency neuroleptic (e.g., haloperidol) for psychotic symptoms
- Use benzodiazepine (diazepam, lorazepam) to control agitation and to sedate, if needed
- Propranolol and ascorbic acid may minimize effects of PCP and aid in its excretion

DRUG INTERACTIONS

Drug of Abuse	Interacting Drugs	Reaction
Hallucinogens	Antidepressant:	
Cannabis/Marihuana	Tricyclic, e.g., desipramine	Case reports of tachycardia, light-headedness, mood lability and delirium with combination Cardiac complications reported in children and adolescents
	MAOI: tranylcypromine	Caution: Cannabis increases serotonin levels and may result in a serotonin syndrome
	Antipsychotics, e.g., chlorpromazine, thioridazine	Drugs with anticholinergic and α-adrenergic properties can cause marked hypotension and increased disorientation
	Barbiturates	Additive effect causing anxiety and hallucinations
	Cocaine	Increased heart rate; blood pressure increased with high doses of both drugs; increased plasma level of cocaine and euphoria
	Disulfiram	Synergistic CNS stimulation reported, hypomania
	Lithium	Clearance of lithium may be decreased
	Morphine	THC blocks excitation produced by morphine
LSD	SSRI antidepressant, e.g., fluoxetine	Grand mal seizures reported Recurrence or worsening of flashbacks reported with fluoxetine, sertraline, paroxetine
PCP	Acidifying agents: cranberry juice, ammonium chloride	Increased excretion of PCP

DRUG	COMMENTS
CANNABIS **Marihuana** – crushed leaves, stems, and flowers of female hemp plant, *Cannabis sativa* Smoked (cigarettes or water pipe) Slang: grass, pot, joint, hemp, weed, reefer, smoke, Mary Jane, Indian hay, ace, ganja, gold, J, locoweed, shit, herb, Mexican, ragweed, bhang, sticks, Hydro (hydroponic marihuana) **Hashish** – resin from flowers and leaves; more potent than marihuana Smoked or cooked Slang: hash, hash oil, weed oil, weed juice, honey oil, hash brownies, tea, black, solids, grease, smoke	– Tetrahydrocannabinol (THC) is the active ingredient; 5–11% in marihuana and up to 28% in hashish effects occur rapidly and last up to several hours; accumulates in fat tissue and effects may persist – Tolerance and psychic dependence may occur; reverse tolerance (supersensitivity) described – Combined with other drugs including PCP ("killer weed"), opium ("o.j."), heroin ("A-bomb") or flunitrazepam to enhance effect – Most users experience euphoria with feelings of self-confidence and relaxation; some become dysphoric, anxious, agitated and suspicious. Can cause psychotic symptoms with confusion, hallucinations, emotional lability (very prolonged or heavy use can cause serious and potentially irreversible psychosis) – Increased craving for sweets – Chronic use: bronchitis, weight gain, bloodshot eyes, loss of energy, apathy, "fuzzy" thinking, impaired judgement, decreased testosterone in males – Cannabis cigarettes have a higher tar content than ordinary cigarettes and are potentially carcinogenic – Pregnancy: can retard fetal growth, and cause withdrawal reactions in the infant – Breast-feeding: can reach high levels in milk, especially with heavy use
DIMETHYLTRYPTAMINE (DMT) Synthetic chemical similar to psilocybin Soaked in parsley, dried and snorted or smoked, used as liquid (tea), injected Slang: lunch-hour drug, businessman's lunch	– Appears in nature in several plants in South America; easily synthesized – A monoamine oxidase inhibitor; interacts with a variety of drugs and foods – Effects occur almost immediately and last 30–60 min – Readily destroyed by stomach acids – Often mixed with marihuana – Produces intense visual hallucinations, loss of awareness of surroundings – Anxiety and panic frequent due to quick onset of effects
KETAMINE (Ketalar) General anesthetic in day surgery Taken orally as capsules, tablets, powder, crystals, and solution, injected, snorted Slang: K, special K, vitamin K, ket, green, jet, kit-kat, cat valiums	– NMDA receptor antagonist – Related to PCP – Doses of 60–100 mg injected; consciousness maintained at this dose, but get disorientation – Physical effects: increased tone, nystagmus, stereotypic movements – CNS effects: hallucinations, amnesia – Highly addictive – Toxic effects: respiratory depression, loss of consciousness, catatonia
LYSERGIC ACID DIETHYLAMIDE (LSD) Semi-synthetic drug derived from ergot (grain fungus) White powder: used as tablet, capsule, liquid, snorted, smoked, inhaled, injected Slang: acid, cubes, purple haze, Raggedy Ann, sunshine, LBJ, peace pill, big D, blotters, domes, hits, tabs, doses, window-pane	– $5HT_2$ receptor agonist – Effects occur in less than 1 h and last 2–18 h – Physical effects: mydriasis, nausea, muscle tension – Can cause agitation, visual hallucinations, suicidal, homicidal, and irrational behavior and dysphoria; panic, psychotic reactions can last several days – Flashbacks occur without drug being taken – Tolerance develops rapidly; psychological dependence occurs – Combined with cocaine, mescaline, or amphetamine to prolong effects – Pregnancy: increased risk of spontaneous abortions; congenital abnormalities have been reported

Hallucinogens (cont.)

DRUG	COMMENTS
MESCALINE From peyote cactus buttons; pure product rarely available Cactus buttons are dried, then sliced, chopped, or ground; used as powder, capsule, tablet, inhaled or injected Slang: mesc, peyote, buttons, cactus	– Effects occur slowly and last 10–18 h – Less potent than LSD, but cross-tolerance reported – High doses: anxiety, disorientation, impaired reality testing, headache, dry skin, hypotension, cardiac and respiratory depression – Dependence not reported but tolerance to effects occurs quickly
MORNING GLORY SEEDS Active ingredient is lysergic acid amide; 1/10th as potent as LSD Seeds eaten whole, or ground, mushed, soaked, and solution injected Slang: flying saucers, licorice drops, heavenly blue, pearly gates	– Effects occur after 30–90 min when seeds ingested and immediately when solution injected – Commercial seeds are treated with insecticides, fungicides, and other chemicals and can be poisonous
PEYOTE From cactus *Lophaphora williamsii* Dried, chewed, and swallowed, used as capsules, solution	– Used for centuries by native people of North and South America – Effects occur 1–2 h after ingestion – Geometric brilliant colors, weightlessness, time distortion, anxiety, panic, dizziness, severe nausea
PHENCYCLIDINE General anesthetic used in veterinary medicine; often misrepresented as other drugs Powder, chunks, crystals; used as tablets, capsules, liquid, inhaled, snorted, injected (IM or IV) Slang: PCP, angel dust, hog, horse tranquilizer, animal tranquilizer, peace pill, killer, weed, supergrass, crystal, "CJ," dust, rocket fuel	– Glutamate agonist at NMDA receptor – Effects occur in a few minutes and can last several days to weeks (half-life 18 h) – Frequently sold on street as other drugs (easily synthesized); mis-synthesis yields a product that can cause abdominal cramps, vomiting, coma, and death – Intermittent vomiting, drooling, diaphoresis, miosis, nystagmus, hypertension and ataxia can occur – Can cause apathy, estrangement, feelings of isolation, indifference to pain, delirium, disorientation with amnesia, schizophrenia-like psychosis, and violence (often self-directed); can feel intermittently anxious, fearful, to euphoric – Toxic effects: hypoglycemia, rhabdomyolysis, coma; deaths have occurred secondary to uncontrollable seizures, or to hypertension resulting in intracranial hemorrhage – Flashbacks occur – Psychological dependence occurs – Pregnancy: signs of toxicity have been reported in newborns – Breast-feeding: drug concentrates in milk and detectable for weeks after heavy use

DRUG	COMMENTS
PSILOCYBIN From *Psilocybe mexicana* mushroom Used as dried mushroom, white crystal, powder, capsule, injection; eaten raw, cooked or steeped as tea Slang: magic mushrooms, sacred mushrooms, mushroom, shroom	– Effects occur within 30 min and last several hours – Pure drug rarely available; injection dangerous as foreign particles present – Chemically related to LSD and DMT – Tolerance develops rapidly; cross-tolerance occurs with LSD – Physical or psychological dependence not reported – Mistaken identity with "death-cap" (Amanita) mushroom can result in accidental poisoning
Drugs with Hallucinogenic and Stimulant Properties	
NUTMEG Active ingredient related to trimethoxyamphetamine and to mescaline Seeds eaten whole, ground, powdered; sniffed	– Effects occur slowly and last several hours (duration of hallucinogenic effects is dose related) – Hallucinations are usually preceded by nausea, vomiting, diarrhea, and headache – Lightheadedness, drowsiness, thirst, and hangover can occur
3,4-methylene-dioxymethamphetamine (MDMA) Slang: ecstasy; MDMA, "Adam," XTC, X, E, love drug, business man's special Powder, usually in tablets or capsules	– Causes a calcium-dependent increase in serotonin release into the synaptic cleft and inhibits serotonin reuptake – Many MDMA products are contaminated with other compounds including dextromethorphan, ephedra and PMA – Onset of effects 30–60 min; duration of action 4–6 h – Creates feelings of euphoria and well-being together with derealization, depersonalization, cognitive disturbances and heightened sensations (action believed to be mediated through release of serotonin) – Common effects include salivation, mydriasis, bruxism, trismus – Severe physical reactions including hypotension, tachycardia, dysrhythmia, hyperthermia, seizures, coma; death can occur from excessive physical activity ("raves") that may result in disseminated intravascular coagulation, rhabdomyolysis, hyponatremia and acute renal and hepatic failure – Can precipitate panic disorder, paranoid psychosis, flashbacks, and depression; anxiety can last up to 2 days – After-effects include: drowsiness, muscle aches, generalized fatigue and depression (lasts 1–2 days) – Tolerance to euphoric effects with chronic use – Chronic regular use may result in mood swings, depression, memory loss and parkinsonism
3,4-methylene-dioxyamphetamine (MDA) Chemically related to both mescaline and amphetamine Used orally, liquid, powder, tablet, injection Slang: love drug	– Typical doses: 60–120 mg – Effects occur after 30–60 min (orally), or sooner if injected, and last about 8 h – Hallucinations and perceptual distortions rare; feeling of peace and tranquility occurs – High doses: hyperreactivity to stimuli, agitation, hallucinations, violent and irrational behavior, delirium, convulsions and coma
N-ethyl-3,4-methylene-dioxyamphetamine (MDE) Chemically related to MDMA Slang: Eve	– Effects as for MDMA (above) – Onset of effects within 30 min; duration of action 3–4 h
Paramethoxyamphetamine (PMA) Synthetic drug Used as powder, capsules	– Often sold as MDMA but has more pronounced hallucinogenic and stimulant effects – Causes major increase in BP and pulse, hyperthermia, increased and labored breathing – Highly toxic; convulsions, coma, and death reported

Hallucinogens (cont.)

DRUG	COMMENTS
2,5-dimethoxy-4-methylamphetamine (STP/DOM) Chemically related to both mescaline and amphetamine Used orally Slang: serenity, tranquility, peace	– Effects last 16–24 h – More potent than mescaline, but less potent than LSD – "Bad trips" occur frequently; prolonged psychotic reactions reported in people with psychiatric history – Tolerance reported; no evidence of dependence – Anticholinergic effects, exhaustion, convulsions, excitement, and delirium reported
Trimethoxyamphetamine (TMA) Synthetic drug related to mescaline Used orally, as powder, injection	– Effects occur after 2 h – Often misrepresented as MDA – More potent than mescaline – More toxic if injected or higher doses used – Can cause unprovoked anger and aggression

Stimulants

PHARMACOLOGICAL/ PSYCHIATRIC EFFECTS

- Differ somewhat depending on type of drug taken, dose, and route of administration
- Effects occur rapidly, especially when drug used parenterally
- Acute toxicity reported with doses ranging from 5 to 630 mg of amphetamine; chronic users can ingest up to 1000 mg/day
- Following acute toxicity, psychiatric state usually clears within one week of amphetamine discontinuation

Physical

- Elevated BP, tachycardia, increased respiration and temperature, sweating, pallor, tremors, decreased appetite, dilated pupils, reduced fatigue, insomnia, increased sensory awareness, increased sexual arousal/libido combined with a delay in ejaculation

Mental

- Euphoria, exhilaration, alertness, improved task performance, exacerbation of obsessive-compulsive symptoms
- Methamphetamine reported to induce paranoia and hallucinations in non-schizophrenic subjects; flashbacks reported

High Doses

- Anxiety, excitation, panic attacks, grandiosity, delusions, visual, auditory and tactile hallucinations, paranoia, mania, delirium, increased sense of power, violence
- Fever, sweating, headache, flushing, pallor, hyperactivity, stereotypic behavior, cardiac arrhythmias, respiratory failure, loss of coordination, collapse, cerebral hemorrhage, convulsions, and death

Chronic Use

- Decreased appetite and weight, abdominal pain, vomiting, difficulty urinating, skin rash, increased risk for stroke, high blood pressure, irregular heart rate, impotence, headache, anxiety, delusions of persecution, violence
- Tolerance to physical effects occurs but vulnerability to psychosis remains
- Chronic high-dose use causes physical dependence; psychological dependence frequently results even with regular low-dose use
- Recovery occurs rapidly after amphetamine withdrawal, but psychosis can sometimes become chronic

WITHDRAWAL

- Anxiety, distorted sleep, chronic fatigue, irritability, difficulty concentrating, craving, depression, suicidal or homicidal ideation, and paranoid psychosis
- Nausea, diarrhea, anorexia, hunger, myalgia, diaphoresis, convulsions

COMPLICATIONS

- Exacerbation of hypertension or arrhythmias
- Strokes and retinal damage due to intense vasospasm, especially with "crack"

TREATMENT

- Use calming techniques, reassurance, and supportive measures
- For severe agitation and to prevent seizures, sedate with benzodiazepine (e.g., diazepam)
- For psychosis, use a high-potency neuroleptic (haloperidol); avoid low-potency neuroleptics
- Antidepressants (e.g., desipramine) can be used to treat depression following withdrawal, and to decrease craving. Preliminary data suggests flupenthixol depot injection may be useful in withdrawal; positive results also reported with buspirone, bromocriptine and amantadine

Stimulants (cont.)

DRUG INTERACTIONS

- Only clinically significant interactions are listed below:

Drug of Abuse	Interacting Drugs	Reaction
STIMULANTS (general)	Antipsychotics	Diminished pharmacological effects of stimulants
	Irreversible MAOIs, e.g., phenelzine	Severe palpitations, tachycardia, hypertension, headache, cerebral hemorrhage, agitation, seizures; **AVOID**
Amphetamines	Antidepressants	Enhanced antidepressant effect
	Tricyclics	Increased plasma level of amphetamine due to inhibited metabolism
	Guanethidine	Reversal of hypotensive effects
	Phenothiazines, e.g., chlorpromazine	Increased plasma level of amphetamine due to inhibited metabolism Phenothiazines can decrease CNS excitation from amphetamines
	Urinary acidifiers, e.g., ammonium chloride	Increased elimination of amphetamine due to decreased renal tubular reabsorption and increased elimination
	Urinary alkalizers, e.g., potassium citrate, sodium bicarbonate	Prolonged pharmacological effects of amphetamine due to decreased urinary elimination of unchanged drug
Cocaine	Alcohol	Ethanol promotes the formation of a highly addicting metabolite, cocoethylene Reports of enhanced hepatotoxicity Increased heart rate; variable effect on blood pressure Increased risk of sudden death with combined use (18-fold) Combined use reported to result in more impulsive decision making and poorer performance on tests of learning and memory
	Antidepressants (Cyclic, SSRI)	Decreased craving
	Tricyclics: e.g., desipramine	Decreased seizure threshhold Elevated heart rate and diastolic pressure by 20–30%; increased risk of arrhythmia
	Barbiturates	Reports of enhanced hepatotoxicity
	β-blockers	May increase the magnitude of cocaine-induced myocardial ischemia
	Carbamazepine	Augmentation of cocaine-induced increase in heart rate and diastolic BP
	Catecholamines, e.g., norepinephrine	Potentiation of vasoconstriction and cardiac stimulation
	Disulfiram	Increased plasma level (3-fold) and half-life (60%) of cocaine with possible increased risk of cardiovascular effects
	Flupenthixol	Decreased craving
	Marihuana (cannabis)	Increased heart rate; blood pressure increased only with high doses of both drugs Increased plasma level of cocaine and increased subjective reports of euphoria
	Mazindol	May decrease craving for cocaine Increased lethality and convulsant activity reported
	Narcotics, e.g., heroin, morphine	May potentiate cocaine euphoria
	Yohimbine	Enhanced effect of cocaine on blood pressure

DRUG	COMMENTS
AMPHETAMINE, DEXTROAMPHETAMINE (Dexedrine, Dexampex, Biphetamine) Taken orally as tablet, capsule, sniffed, injected Slang: bennies, hearts, pep-pills, dex, beans, benn, truck-drivers, ice, jolly beans, black beauties, crank, pink football, dexies	– Cause the release of amines (NE, 5-HT, DA) from central and peripheral neurons and inhibit their breakdown – Onset of action: 30 min after oral ingestion – Active drug use usually terminated by a psychotic reaction, or by exhaustion with excessive sleeping – Psychosis can last up to 10 days – Tolerance and psychic dependence occurs with chronic use – Excessive doses can lead to coma, convulsions, and death – Pregnancy: increase in premature births; withdrawal symptoms and behavioral effects (hyperexcitability) noted in offspring
METHAMPHETAMINE (Desoxyephedrine) (Desoxyn, Methampex) Powder: taken as tablets, capsules, liquid, injected, snorted, inhaled Slang: speed, crystal, meth, uppers, shit, moth, crank, crosses, ice, methlies quick, jib	– Enhances release and blocks uptake of catecholamines – Synthetic drug related chemically to amphetamine and ephedrine – Very rapid onset of action; can last 10–12 h – Powerful effects produced are referred to as a "rush" – A "run" refers to the use of the drug several times a day over a period of several days – Physical effects: tachycardia, tachypnea, diaphoresis, hyperthermia, mydriasis, hypertension – Can cause psychosis, paranoia, violence – Chronic use has been associated with neuronal damage – Toxic effects: dysrhythmias, hypertension, hyperthermia, seizures, encephalopathy – After abrupt discontinuation withdrawal effects peak in 2–3 days and include GI distress, headache
COCAINE Extract from leaves of coca plant Leaves chewed, applied to mucous membranes, powder Taken orally, snorted, smoked, injected can last for weeks or months Slang: coke, snow, flake, lady, toot, blow, big C, candy, crack, joy dust, stardust, rock, nose, boulders **"Crack"** Free base cocaine; more potent Volatilized and inhaled	– Inhibits dopamine and serotonin reuptake – stimulates brain's reward pathway – Onset of action and plasma half-life varies depending on route of use (e.g., IV: peaks in 30 s, half-life 54 min; snorting: peaks in 15–30 min, half-life 75 min) – Often adulterated with amphetamine, ephedrine, procaine, xylocaine, or lidocaine – Used with heroin ("dynamite," "speedballs") or morphine ("whizbang") for increased intensity – Used with flunitrazepam to moderate stimulatory effect – CNS effects: rapid euphoria, agitation, delusion, hallucinations – Physical effects: tachycardia, hypertension, pyrexia, diaphoresis, mydriasis, ataxia; tactile hallucinations ("coke bugs") occur – Tolerance develops to some effects (appetite), but increased sensitivity (reverse tolerance) develops to others (convulsions, psychosis) – Powerful psychological dependence occurs; physical dependence seen in crack users; withdrawal symptoms can last for weeks or months – Depression commonly occurs after drug use; dysphoria promotes repetitive use – Chronic users can develop panic disorder, paranoia; with repetitive administration or use of high doses, euphoria may be replaced by dysphoria, irritability, assaultive behavior, paranoia and delirium – Snorting can cause stuffy, runny nose, eczema around nostrils, atrophy of nasal mucosa, bleeding and perforated septum – Smokers are susceptible to respiratory symptoms and pulmonary complications – Sexual dysfunction is common – Chronic users of "crack" can develop microvascular changes in the eyes, lungs and brain; respiratory symptoms include asthma and pulmonary hemorrhage and edema – Dehydration can occur due to effect on temperature regulation, with possible hyperpyrexia – Toxic effects: hyperthermia, seizures, death; fatalities more common with IV use, or when cocaine-filled condoms are swallowed (by smugglers) then burst – Pregnancy: associated with spontaneous labor and abortion; increase in premature births; infants have lower weight, length, and head circumference, jitteriness, irritability, poor feeding, EEG abnormalities, seizures, and genitourinary tract abnormalities

Stimulants (cont.)

DRUG	COMMENTS
KHAT *(Catha edulis)* Leaves chewed	– Grows as a bush in Africa and the Middle East; used by certain communities to attain religious euphoria – Cathinone is principal psychoactive agent – Symptoms occur within 3 h and last about 90 min – Acute symptoms include: euphoria, excitation, grandiosity, increased blood pressure, flushing – Chronic use can cause: anxiety, agitation, confusion, dysphoria, aggression, visual hallucinations, paranoia, emaciation and dehydration
METHYLPHENIDATE Slang: Vitamin R, R-ball, skippy, the smart drug Tablets crushed and snorted	See p. 158 – Large doses can cause seizures, psychosis and stroke
SYMPATHOMIMETICS Ephedrine, phenylpropanolamine, caffeine; taken as capsules, tablets; Slang: look alikes	– Misrepresented as amphetamines and sold in capsules or tablets that resemble amphetamines – After massive doses, death due to stroke can occur

Opiates/Narcotics

GENERAL COMMENTS

- High rate of psychopathology, specifically depression, alcoholism, and antisocial personality disorder, have been demonstrated in opiate abusers (often not clear if these are cause or effect)
- Polydrug use and co-dependence on benzodiazepines appears particularly common among individuals injecting opioids

PHARMACOLOGICAL/ PSYCHIATRIC EFFECTS

- Differ somewhat depending on type of drug taken, the dose, the route of administration, and whether combined with other drugs
- Elderly more sensitive to effects and side effects of opiates

Physical

- Analgesia, "rush" sensation followed by relaxation, decreased tension, slow pulse and respiration, increased body temperature, dry mouth, constricted pupils, decreased GI motility

Mental

- Euphoria, state of gratification, sedation

High Doses

- Respiratory depression, cardiovascular complications, coma and death

Chronic Use

- General loss of energy, ambition, and drive, motor retardation, attention impairment, sedation, slurred speech
- Tolerance and physical dependence; withdrawal
- Cross-tolerance occurs with other narcotics

WITHDRAWAL

- Symptoms include: yawning, runny nose, sneezing, lacrimation, dilated pupils, vasodilation, tachycardia, elevated BP, vomiting and diarrhea, restlessness, tremor, chills, piloerection, bone pain, abdominal pain and cramps, anorexia, anxiety, irritability, insomnia
- Drugs are prescribed for the following reasons:
  a) to reverse effects of toxicity using narcotic antagonists (e.g., naloxone, naltrexone – can precipitate withdrawal)
  b) to treat the immediate withdrawal reaction (e.g., clonidine, methadone)
  c) to aid in detoxification
- Acute symptoms can last 10–14 days (longer with methadone)

TREATMENT

- Opiod withdrawal states are generally not life-threatening; "cold turkey" is acceptable to some addicts
- Non-narcotic alternatives (e.g., benzodiazepines, neuroleptics) usually do not work

- Drugs are prescribed for the following reasons:
  a) to reverse effects of toxicity using narcotic antagonists (e.g., naloxone, naltrexone – can precipitate withdrawal)
  b) to treat the immediate withdrawal reaction (e.g., clonidine, methadone)
  c) to aid in detoxification, or for maintenance therapy in a supervised treatment program (e.g., methadone, buprenorphine)

DRUG INTERACTIONS

- Only clinically significant interactions are listed below:

Drug of Abuse	Interacting Drugs	Reaction
Opiates (general)	CNS drugs, e.g., alcohol, benzodiazepines Cocaine Narcotic antagonist, e.g., naloxone	Additive CNS effects; can lead to respiratory depression May potentiate cocaine euphoria Will precipitate withdrawal reaction
Codeine, oxycodone, hydrocodone	SSRI antidepressants, e.g., fluoxetine, paroxetine Ritonavir	Loss of analgesic efficacy; inhibited biotransformation of narcotic to active moiety via CYP2D6 (e.g., conversion of codeine to morphine, etc.) Moderate decrease in clearance of hydrocodone and oxycodone
Fentanyl, alfentanyl	Erythromycin Ritonavir	Prolonged analgesia Large decrease in clearance of fentanyl and alfentanyl
Heroin	Doxepin	Case reports of delirium when used for heroin withdrawal
Meperidine	Cimetidine MAOIs – irreversible, RIMA Phenothiazines, e.g., chlorpromazine Phenytoin Ritonavir	22% decrease in clearance of meperidine Increased excitation, sweating and hypotension reported; may lead to development of encephalopathy, convulsions, coma, respiratory depression and "serotonin syndrome" Additive analgesic, CNS and cardiovascular effects Decreased plasma level of meperidine due to increased metabolism Large increase in plasma level of meperidine due to inhibited metabolism
Methadone		See p. 205
Opium	Cimetidine Antihistamines: tripelennamine, cyclizine	Enhanced effect of narcotic and increased adverse effects due to decreased metabolism "Opiate high" reported with combination, euphoria
Pentazocine	SSRIs, e.g., fluoxetine	Excitatory toxicity reported (serotonergic)
Propoxyphene	Ritonavir	Large decrease in clearance of propoxyphene

Opiates/Narcotics (cont.)

DRUG	COMMENTS
HEROIN Diacetylmorphine – synthetic derivative of morphine Injected (IV – "mainlining", or SC – "skin popping"), smoked, inhaled, taken orally Slang: "H", horse, junk, snow, stuff, lady, shill, poppy, smack, scag, black tar, Lady Jane, white stuff	– Effects almost immediate following IV injection and last several hours; effects occur in 15–60 min after oral dosing – Risk of accidental overdose as street preparations contain various concentrations of heroin – Physical dependence and tolerance occur within 2 weeks; withdrawal occurs within 8–12 h after last dose and peaks in 48–72 h – Combined with flunitrazepam to enhance effects and to ameliorate heroin withdrawal – Pregnancy: high rate of spontaneous abortions, premature labor and stillbirths – babies are often small and have an increased mortality risk; withdrawal symptoms in newborn reported
MORPHINE Principal active component of opium poppy Taken as powder, capsule, tablet, liquid, injected Slang: "M", dreamer, sweet Jesus, junk, morph, Miss Emma	– Effects as for heroin, but slower onset and longer-acting – Effects occur in 15–60 min after oral dosing and last 1–8 h – Dependence liability high (second to heroin) due to powerful euphoric and analgesic effects
METHADONE (Dolophine) Used as tablets, liquid, injected Slang: the kick pill, dolly, meth	– Drug used in withdrawal and detoxification from opiates, but subject to abuse – Effects occur 30–60 min after oral dosing, and last 7–48 h – Chronic use causes constipation, blurred vision, sweating, decreased libido, menstrual irregularities, joint and bone pain, sleep disturbances – Tolerance unlikely – Pregnancy: dosing needs should be reassessed (decreased between weeks 14 and 32 and increased prior to term); withdrawal effects reported in neonates – Breastfeeding: small amounts of methadone enter milk; nurse prior to taking dose or 2–6 h after
OPIUM Resinous preparation from unripe seed pods of opium poppy; available as dark brown chunks or as powder Soaked, taken as solution, smoked	– Contains a number of alkaloids including morphine (6–12 %) and codeine (0.5–1.5 %) – Nausea common
OTHER FREQUENTLY ABUSED PRESCRIPTION NARCOTICS AND RELATED DRUGS	
CODEINE **Methylmorphine** Used orally, liquid, injected Slang: schoolboy, 3s, 4s	– Naturally occuring alkaloid from opium poppy – Common ingredient of both prescription and over-the-counter analgesics and antitussives (e.g., Fiorinal-C, Tylenol #1, etc.) – Mixed with glutethimide (called loads, pacs) – Tolerance develops gradually; physical dependence is infrequent; withdrawal will occur with chronic high-dose use

DRUG	COMMENTS
FENTANYL (Duragesic, Sublimaze) Slang: tango	– Effects almost immediate following IV injection and last 30–60 min; with IM use, onset slower and duration of action is up to 120 min – Euphoria occurs quickly – Side effects: primarily sedation, confusion, dizziness, dry mouth and GI distress – High doses can produce muscle rigidity (including respiratory muscles) as well as respiratory depression
HYDROCODONE (e.g., Novahistex DH)	– Related to codeine, but more potent – An ingredient in prescription antitussive preparations; sought by abuser due to easy availability and purity of product – Tolerance develops rapidly – Lethal dose: 0.5–1.0 g
HYDROMORPHONE (Dilaudid) Used orally Slang: juice, dillies	– Semisynthetic narcotic – At low doses side effects less common than with other narcotics; high doses more toxic due to strong respiratory depressant effect
LEVORPHANOL (Levo Dromoran)	– Synthetic narcotic analgesic with effects similar to morphine – High doses can produce cardiac arrhythmias, hypotension, respiratory depression, and coma
MEPERIDINE/PETHIDINE (Demerol) Synthetic opioid derivative Used orally, injected	– Metabolite (normeperidine) is highly toxic; may accumulate with chronic use and cause convulsions – High doses produce disorientation, hallucinations, respiratory depression, stupor, and coma
OXYCODONE (Percodan, Percocet) Semisynthetic derivative Used orally; tablets chewed, crushed and snorted, powder boiled for injection Slang: percs, OC, OXY, oxycotton, killers	– An ingredient in combination analgesic products – Very high abuse potential
PENTAZOCINE (Talwin) Used orally, injected Slang: T's, big T, Tee, Tea	– Has both agonist and antagonist properties – Repeated injections can result in tissue damage at injection site – Mixed with tripelennamine (called T's and blues)
PROPOXYPHENE (Darvon) Used orally, injected Slang: yellow football	– Synthetic narcotic analgesic – Abuse results in a state of euphoria – Repeated injections can cause damage to veins and local tissue – Tolerance to analgesic and euphoric effects develops gradually; chronic use results in physical dependence

Inhalants/Aerosols

SUBSTANCES ABUSED

- Volatile gases and solvents: airplane glue, gasoline, toluene, printing fluid, cleaning solvents, benzene, acetone, amyl nitrite ("poppers") etc.
- Aerosols: deodorants, hair spray, freon
- Anesthetic gases: nitrous oxide (laughing gas), chloroform, ether

SLANG

- Glue, gassing, sniffing, chemo

GENERAL COMMENTS

- High rate of psychopathology, specifically alcoholism, depression, and antisocial personality disorder, have been demonstrated in individuals with a history of solvent use
- Considered "poor man's" drug of abuse; used by children, and in third world countries to lessen hunger pain
- Fourth most commonly abused substance among teens in Canada; high use in Aboriginal populations
- Amyl nitrite used to promote sexual excitement and orgasm

METHODS OF USE

- "Bagging" – pouring liquid or discharging gas into plastic bag or balloon
- "Sniffing" – holding mouth over container as gas is discharged
- "Huffing" – holding a soaked rag over mouth or nose
- "Torching" – inhaling fumes discharged from a cigarette lighter, then igniting the exhaled air

PHARMACOLOGICAL/ PSYCHIATRIC EFFECTS

- Differ somewhat depending on type of drug taken
- Fumes sniffed, inhaled; use of plastic bag can lead to suffocation
- Rapid CNS penetration – effects occur quickly and last a short time

Physical

- Drowsiness, dizziness, slurred speech, impaired motor function, light sensitivity, nausea, salivation, sneezing, coughing, decreased breathing and heart rate, hypotension
- Fatalities can arise from cardiac arrest or inhalation of vomit while unconscious

Mental

- Changing levels of awareness, impaired judgement and memory, hallucinations, euphoria, excitation, vivid fantasies, feeling of invincibility, delirium

High Doses

- Loss of consciousness, convulsions, cardiac arrhythmia, seizures, death

Chronic Use

- Fatigue, encephalopathy, hearing loss, visual impairment, sinusitis, rhinitis, laryngitis, kidney and liver damage, bone marrow damage, cardiac arrhythmias, chronic lung disease
- Inability to think clearly, memory disturbances, depression, irritability, hostility, paranoia
- Tolerance develops to desired effect; psychological dependence is frequent

TREATMENT

- Use calming techiques, reassurance
- Effects are usually short-lasting

TOXICITY

- CNS: acute and chronic effects reported, e.g., ataxia, peripheral neuropathy
- Cardiac: an MI can occur, primarily with use of halogenated solvents
- Renal: acidosis, hypokalemia
- Hepatic: hepatitis, hepatic necrosis
- Hematologic: bone marrow suppression primarily with benzene and nitrous oxide use

DRUG INTERACTIONS • Only clinically significant interactions are listed below

Drug of Abuse	Interacting Drug	Reaction
Inhalants	CNS depressants	Increased impairment of judgement, distortion of reality

Gamma Hydroxy Butyrate (GHB)

SLANG

- Liquid ecstasy, liquid X, liquid F, goop, GBH = Grievous Bodily Harm, Easy lay, Ghost Breath, G, Somatomax, Gamma-G, Growth Hormone Booster, Georgia home boy

PHARMACOLOGY

- Produced naturally in the body and is structurally similar to gamma aminobutyric acid (GABA)
- Shown to increase dopamine levels in the CNS
- Used for its hallucinogenic and euphoric effects at raves (or dance parties)
- Has been used in Europe to treat alcohol dependency – reported to reduce alcohol cravings

GENERAL COMMENTS

- Originally researched as an anesthetic; shown to have limited analgesic effects and increased seizure risk
- Promoted illegally as a health food product, an aphrodisiac and for muscle building
- Has been used in "date rapes" because it acts rapidly, produces disinhibition and relaxation of voluntary muscles and causes anterograde amnesia for events that occur under the influence of the drug
- Chronic use may result in psychological dependence
- Products converted to GHB in the body include: gammabutyrolactone (GBL – also called Blue Nitro Vitality, GH Revitalizer, GHR, Remforce, Renewtrient and Gamma G – is sold in health food stores) and the industrial solvent butanediol (BD – also called tetramethyline glycol or Sucol B, and sold as Zen, NRG-3, Soma Solutions, Enliven and Serenity)

METHODS OF USE

- Powder mixed in a liquid; usually sold in vials and taken orally

PHARMACOKINETICS

- Quickly absorbed orally; peak plasma concentration reached in 20–60 min
- Elimination half-life approx. 20 min

PHARMACOLOGICAL/ PSYCHIATRIC EFFECTS

- Deep sleep reported with doses of 2.0 g
- At 10 mg/kg produces anxiolytic effect, muscle relaxation and amnesia
- At 20–30 mg/kg increases REM and slow-wave sleep
- At doses > 60 mg/kg can result in coma

ADVERSE REACTIONS

Physical

- High frequency of drop attacks – "victim" suddenly loses all muscular control and drops to the floor, unable to resist the "attacker"
- Dizziness, nausea, vomiting, hypotension, bradycardia, ataxia, nystagmus, hypotonia, muscle spasms, seizures, decreased respiration; may lead to unconsciousness and coma (particularly dangerous in combination with alcohol). Symptoms usually resolve within 7 h, but dizziness can persist up to 2 weeks

Mental

- Sedation, amnesia, euphoria and hallucinations

Gamma Hydroxy Butyrate (GHB) (cont.)

TOXICITY

- Low therapeutic index; dangerous in combination with alcohol
- Overdoses can occur due to unknown purity and concentration of ingested product
- Symptoms: bradycardia, seizures, apnea, sudden (reversible) coma with abrupt awakening and violence
- Coma reported in doses > 60 mg/kg (4 g)
- Several deaths reported secondary to respiratory failure

Management

- No known antidote

WITHDRAWAL

- Symptoms occur 1–6 h after abrupt cessation and can last for 5–15 days after chronic use
- Initial symptoms include insomnia, anxiety and/or tremor; after chronic use, symptoms can include mild tachycardia, hypertension and can progress to delirium with auditory and visual hallucinations

DRUG INTERACTIONS

- Only clinically significant interactions are listed below

Drug	Example	Effect
CNS Depressant	Alcohol, benzodiazepines	Decreased pharmacological effects and toxicity
Cannabis		Increased pharmacological effects
Stimulant	Amphetamines	Increased pharmacological effects

Flunitrazepam (Rohypnol)

SLANG

- Roofies, R-2s, Roches Dos

PHARMACOLOGY

- Fast-acting benzodiazepine
- See p. 111

GENERAL COMMENTS

- Used as a sedative/tranquilizer in some European countries
- Commonly used as a date-rape drug because it acts rapidly, produces disinhibition and relaxation of voluntary muscles and causes anterograde amnesia for events that occur under the influence of the drug
- Alcohol potentiates the drug's effects

METHOD OF USE

- Purchased in doses of 1 and 2 mg (legal manufacturers have added blue dye to formulation to color beverages and make them murky); illegal manufacturing is common
- Added to alcoholic beverages of unsuspecting victim

ADVERSE REACTIONS

- These reactions are reported following restoration of consciousness

Physical

- Dizziness, impaired motor skills, "rubbery legs,"weakness, unsteadiness
- Decreased blood pressure and pulse

Mental

- Rapid loss of consciousness and amnesia; residual symptoms include drowsiness, confusion, impaired memory and judgment, reduced inhibition
- If some memory of the event remains, the "victim" may describe a disassociation of body and mind – a sensation of being paralyzed, powerless, unable to resist

TOXICITY

- See Benzodiazepines p. 113

DRUG INTERACTIONS

- See Benzodiazepines pp. 114–116

Treatment of Substance Use Disorders

GENERAL COMMENTS

- Drugs available for treatment of substance use disorders may be classified as follows:

Primary Indication	Generic Name	Page
Alcohol dependence	Disulfiram	See p. 198
Alcohol/opiate dependence	Naltrexone	See p. 201
Opiate dependence	Methadone	See p. 203
Nicotine dependence	Bupropion (Zyban)	See p. 14

Disulfiram

PRODUCT AVAILABILITY

Chemical Class	Generic Name	Trade Name[(A)]	Dosage Forms and Strengths
	Disulfiram	Antabuse	Tablets: 250 mg, 500 mg

[(A)] Generic preparations may be available

INDICATIONS*

▲ • Deterrent to alcohol use/abuse
- Double-blind and open studies suggest benefit in decreasing cocaine use and increasing abstinence in patients with comorbid drug abuse (caution – see Interactions, p. 199)

PHARMACOLOGY

- Inhibit alcohol metabolism at the acetaldehyde level; the accumulating acetaldehyde produces an unpleasant reaction consisting of flushing, choking, nausea, vomiting, tachycardia, and hypotension; response is proportional to the dose and amount of alcohol ingested; can occur 10–20 min after alcohol ingestion and may last up to 2 h

DOSING

- 125–500 mg daily (h.s.)

PHARMACOKINETICS

- Onset of action: 3–12 h
- Duration of action: up to 14 days

ADVERSE EFFECTS

- Drowsiness and lethargy frequent, depression, disorientation, headache, restlessness, excitation, optic neuritis and peripheral neuropathy, skin eruptions (up to 5% risk), impotence, garlic-like taste, blood dyscrasias, psychosis
- Transient elevated liver function tests reported in up to 30% of individuals; hepatitis is rare

CONTRAINDICATIONS

- Cardiac and pulmonary disorders, liver disease, renal disorders, epilepsy, diabetes mellitus; psychotic conditions including depression
- Use of alcohol-containing products

* ▲ Approved indications

PRECAUTIONS

- Do not give to intoxicated individuals or within 36 h of alcohol consumption
- Do not administer without patient's knowledge
- If alcohol reaction occurs, general supportive measures should be used; in severe hypotension, vasopressor agents may be required

TOXICITY

- Alcohol reaction is proportional to dose of drug and alcohol ingested; severe reactions may result in respiratory depression, cardiovascular collapse, arrhythmias, convulsions, and death; supportive measures may involve oxygen, vitamin C, antihistamines or ephedrine

PEDIATRIC CONSIDERATIONS

- Anti-alcohol drugs are not recommended in children or adolescents; behavioral approaches to treatment should be used

GERIATRIC CONSIDERATIONS

- Cardiovascular tolerance decreases with age, thus increasing the severity of the alcohol reactions

USE IN PREGNANCY

- Possible teratogenicity: report of limb reduction anomalies

Breast milk

- Unknown

NURSING IMPLICATIONS

- Patient should be made aware of purpose of medication and educated about the consequences of drinking; informed consent to treatment is recommended
- Reactions can occur up to 6 days after a dose
- Daily uninterrupted therapy must be continued until the patient has established a basis for self-control
- Drug should not be used alone, without proper motivation and supportive therapy; will not cure alcoholics, but acts as a motivational aid

PATIENT INSTRUCTIONS

For detailed patient instructions on disulfiram, see the Patient Information Sheet on p. 274.

- Avoid all products (food and drugs) containing alcohol, including tonics, cough syrups, mouth washes, and alcohol-based sauces. A delay in the reaction may be as long as 24 h
- Exposure to alcohol-containing rubs or organic solvents may trigger a reaction
- Carry an identification card stating the name of the drug you are taking
- Take disulfiram once daily in the evening

DRUG INTERACTIONS

- Only clinically significant interactions are listed below

Class of Drug	Example	Interactions
Anticoagulant	Warfarin, coumarins	Increased PT ratio or INR response due to reduced metabolism
Anticonvulsant	Phenytoin	Increased anticonvulsant blood levels and toxicity due to reduced metabolism
Antidepressant		
Cyclic	Amitriptyline, desipramine	Increased plasma level of antidepressant due to reduced metabolism; neurotoxicity reported with combination
Irreversible MAOIs	Tranylcypromine	Report of delirium, psychosis with combination
Antipsychotic	Clozapine	Inhibited metabolism and increased plasma level of clozapine

Disulfiram (cont.)

Class of Drug	Example	Interactions
Benzodiazepine	Diazepam, alprazolam chlordiazepoxide, triazolam	Increased activity of benzodiazepine due to decreased clearance (oxazepam, temazepam, and lorazepam not affected)
Caffeine		Reduced clearance of caffeine by 24–30%
Cocaine		Increased plasma level (3- to 6-fold) and half-life (by 60%) of cocaine; increased risk of cardiovascular effects
Isoniazid		Unsteady gait, incoordination, behavioral changes reported due to reduced metabolism of isoniazid
Methadone		Decreased clearance of methadone
Metronidazole		Acute psychosis, ataxia, and confusional states reported
Paraldehyde		Alcohol-like reaction can occur as paraldehyde is metabolized to acetaldehyde
Protease inhibitor	Ritonavir	Alcohol-like reaction reported (as formulation contains alcohol)
St. John's Wort		Alcohol-like reactions reported
Theophylline	Oxtriphylline, theophylline	Increased plasma level of theophyllines due to reduced metabolism

Naltrexone

PRODUCT AVAILABILITY

Chemical Class	Generic Name	Trade Name[(A)]	Dosage Forms and Strengths
	Naltrexone	Revia, Trexan	Tablets: 50 mg

[(A)] Generic preparations may be available

INDICATIONS*

- ▲ Adjunct in the treatment of alcohol dependence
- ▲ Adjunct in the treatment of opiate addiction
- Early studies suggest efficacy in PTSD
- Early data suggest a role in impulse-control disorders and obsessive-compulsive disorders, e.g., binge-eating behavior in females with bulimia, trichotillomania, pathological gambling, and in the treatment of autism and repetitive self-injurious behavior (data contradictory)
- Case reports of efficacy in decreasing positive symptoms of schizophrenia, and in mitigating hallucinogen-related flashbacks
- Early reports suggest a possible role in augmentation of SSRI effects in depression and mitigation of SSRI tachyphylaxis ("poop-out")
- Preliminary data suggest it may reduce craving in "high-craving" smokers

GENERAL COMMENTS

- Blocks the "craving" mechanism in the brain producing less of a high from alcohol; stops the reinforcing effect of alcohol – promotes abstinence and reduces risk for relapse. Recommended to be used together with psychosocial interventions
- Does not attenuate craving for opioids or suppress withdrawal symptoms; patients must undergo detoxification before starting the drug
- Does not produce euphoria

PHARMACOLOGY

- Synthetic long-acting antagonist at various opiate receptor sites in the CNS; highest affinity for the σ (sigma) receptor

DOSING

- Alcohol dependence: begin at 25 mg/day and increase to 50 mg/day over several days to minimize side effects
- Opioid dependence: initiate dose at 12.5 to 25 mg/day and monitor for withdrawal signs; increase dose gradually based on response. Maintenance dose can be given every 2 to 3 days to a total of 350 mg weekly
- Dosage requirements in impulse-control disorders may be higher (up to 200 mg/day)

PHARMACOKINETICS

- Rapidly and completely absorbed from the GI tract
- Undergoes extensive first-pass metabolism; only about 20% of drug reaches the systemic circulation
- Widely distributed; 21–28% is protein bound
- Onset of effect occurs in 15–30 minutes in chronic morphine users
- Duration of effect is dose-dependent; blockade of opioid receptors lasts 24–72 h
- Metabolized in liver; major metabolite, 6-β-naltrexone is active as an opiate antagonist
- Elimination half-life is 96 h; excreted primarily by the kidneys

ADVERSE EFFECTS

- GI effects – abdominal pain, cramps, nausea and vomiting (approx 10%) and weight loss; women are more sensitive to GI side effects
- Headache (6.6%), insomnia, lassitude, anxiety, dysphoria, depression, confusion, nervousness
- Joint and muscle pain

* ▲ Approved indications

- Dose-related elevated enzymes and hepatocellular injury reported; liver function tests recommended at start of treatment and monthly for the first 6 months
- Case reports of naltrexone-induced panic attacks

WITHDRAWAL

- No data available

PRECAUTIONS

- Since naltrexone is an opiate antagonist, do not give to patients who have used narcotics in the previous 10 days – may result in symptoms of opiate withdrawal
- Do not use in patients with liver disorders; baseline liver function tests recommended; repeat monthly for 6 months. Liver toxicity has been reported in very obese individuals on high doses
- Attempts to overcome blockade of naltrexone with high doses of opioid agonists (e.g., morphine) may lead to respiratory depression and death

CONTRAINDICATIONS

- Patients receiving opioids, or those in acute opioid withdrawal
- Acute hepatitis or liver failure

TOXICITY

- No experience in humans; 800 mg dose for 1 week showed no evidence of toxicity

PEDIATRIC CONSIDERATIONS

- Has been studied in children for aggression, self-injurious behavior, autism and mental retardation (dose: 0.5–2 mg/kg/day)
- Effects noted within first hour of administration

GERIATRIC CONSIDERATIONS

- No data

USE IN PREGNANCY

- No adequate well-controlled studies done

Breast milk

- Unknown whether naltrexone is excreted into breast milk

NURSING IMPLICATIONS

- Naltrexone should be used in conjunction with established psychotherapy or self-help programs
- As naltrexone does not attenuate craving for opioids or suppress withdrawal symptoms, compliance problems may occur; individuals must undergo detoxification prior to starting drug

PATIENT INSTRUCTIONS

For detailed patient instructions on naltrexone, see the Patient Information Sheet on p. 275.

- Notify your physician, dentist and pharmacist that you are on naltrexone

DRUG INTERACTIONS

Class	Example	Interaction Effects
Antipsychotic	Chlorpromazine	Lethargy, somnolence with combination
Opiate-containing agent	Codeine, morphine	Decreased efficacy

Methadone

PRODUCT AVAILABILITY

Chemical Class	Generic Name	Trade Name(A)	Dosage Forms and Strengths
	Methadone	Roxane(B), Metadol(C) Dolophine(B)	Bulk powder Oral liquid: 5 mg/5 ml(B), 10 mg/5 ml(B), 10 mg/ml Tablets(B): 5 mg, 10 mg, 40 mg (dispersable) Injection(B): 10 mg/ml

(A) Generic preparations may be available, (B) Not marketed in Canada, (C) Not marketed in USA

INDICATIONS*

- ▲ A substitute drug in narcotic analgesic dependence therapy
- Long-acting analgesic for moderately severe to severe pain

GENERAL COMMENTS

- Useful drug in opiate-dependent patients who desire maintenance opiate therapy and who relapse with alternative interventions, because:
  - effective orally and can be administered once daily, due to its long half-life
  - suppresses withdrawal symptoms of other narcotic analgesics
  - suppresses chronic craving for narcotics without developing tolerance
  - does not produce euphoria in users already tolerant to euphoric effects of narcotic analgesics
- Patients receiving methadone remain in treatment longer, demonstrate a decreased use of illicit opiates, show decreased antisocial behavior and maintain social stability
- Methadone is a narcotic and its prescribing, dispensing and usage is governed by Federal regulations (regulations vary in different countries). It is prepared as a liquid, mixed with orange juice. Most patients receive their methadone, on a daily basis, from the pharmacy and are required to drink the contents of the bottle in the presence of the pharmacist. Some patients (who are stable on their medication) are permitted to carry several days' supply of methadone

PHARMACOLOGY

- A synthetic opiate acting on the μ-opiate receptor; blocks reinforcing euphorigenic effects of other administered opiates
- Analgesic and sedative properties – similar in degree to morphine, but with a longer duration of action

DOSING

- Initially 30–40 mg/day, given once daily; increase by 10 mg every 2–3 days to a stable maintenance dose (up to 200 mg/day)
- Oral methadone doses are approximately twice the intravenous dose (due to decreased bioavailability)
- Patients vary in dosage requirements; dosage is adjusted to control abstinence symptoms without causing marked sedation or respiratory depression
- Doses below 60 mg/day are considered to be inadequate in preventing relapse
- In rare cases patients who are rapid metabolizers of methadone may require a divided (split) dose rather than one single daily dose; the situation should be carefully evaluated by the physician

PHARMACOKINETICS

- Bioavailabilty: 70–80%
- Half-life: 13–55 h (average: 25 h); half-life increases with repeated dosing
- Peak plasma level: 2–3 h
- 70–85% protein bound
- Metabolized primarily by the liver
- Plasma level measurements are not considered useful, except in specific circumstances where stabilization has posed difficulties (threshold range suggested to be 150–220 ng/ml)
- Urine testing may be done to detect illicit drug use and/or compliance with methadone

* ▲ Approved indications

Methadone (cont.)

ONSET AND DURATION OF ACTION

- Onset of effect: 30–60 minutes
- Duration of action increases with chronic use

ADVERSE EFFECTS

1. CNS Effects

- Drowsiness, insomnia, euphoria, dysphoria, confusion, cognitive impairment, depression and weakness; tolerance develops to sedating and analgesic effects
- With chronic use: sleep disturbances
- Headache

2. Anticholinergic Effects

- Sweating, flushing
- Chronic constipation

3. Cardiovascular

- Dizziness, lightheadedness

4. GI Effects

- Nausea, vomiting, decreased appetite
- Weight changes

5. Sexual Side Effects

- Impotence, ejaculatory problems

6. Other Side Effects

- Rarely, pulmonary edema and respiratory depression
- With chronic use: menstrual irregularities, pain in joints and bones

WITHDRAWAL

- Rapid withdrawal can result in opiate withdrawal syndrome, which includes CNS effects: restlessness, agitation, insomnia, headache; Autonomic effects: increased blood pressure, heart rate, body temperature and respiration, lacrimation, perspiration, congestion, itching, "gooseflesh"; Neurological effects: muscle twitching, cramps, tremors, seizures; GI effects: nausea, vomiting, diarrhea, anorexia
- Symptoms may begin 24–48 h after the last dose, peak in 72 h, and may last for 6–7 weeks

Management

- Reinstitute dose to previous level; restabilize patient and monitor while tapering dose at a slower rate
- Clonidine may ameliorate withdrawal symptoms

PRECAUTIONS

- Methadone has a high physical and psychological dependence liability, therefore withdrawal symptoms will occur on abrupt discontinuation – decrease the dose slowly

TOXICITY

- With excessive doses can get marked shallow breathing, pinpoint pupils, flaccidity of skeletal muscles, low blood pressure, slowed heart rate, cold and clammy skin; can progress to cyanosis, coma, severe respiratory depression, circulatory collapse and cardiac arrest

PEDIATRIC CONSIDERATIONS

- Has been used for postoperative pain in children at doses of 0.2 mg/kg; longer duration of action than with morphine. Drug must be tapered (by 5–10% every 1–2 days) if used for longer than 5–7 days; the patient must be continually assessed for withdrawal symptoms

GERIATRIC CONSIDERATIONS

- No data

USE IN PREGNANCY

- Dosing needs should be assessed during pregnancy: decreased between weeks 14 and 32 and increased prior to term
- Withdrawal effects reported in infants

Breast milk

- A small amount of methadone enters breast milk; nurse prior to a dose of methadone, or 2–6 h after dose

NURSING IMPLICATIONS

- Methadone must be prescribed in sufficient doses, on a maintenance basis, to prevent relapse; long-term treatment may be required. Premature withdrawal may lead to relapse

- Methadone is a narcotic and must be prescribed according to Federal regulations. It is prepared as a liquid mixed in orange juice. Many patients pick up their methadone, from the pharmacy, on a daily basis, and drink the medication in the presence of the pharmacist. Some patients (who are stable on their medication) are permitted to carry several days' supply of methadone
- Each time the patient is to be medicated, he/she should be assessed for impairment (i.e., drowsiness, slurred speech, forgetfulness, lack of concentration, disorientation and ataxia); patients should not be medicated if they appear impaired or smell of alcohol the physician should be contacted as to management of the patient

PATIENT INSTRUCTIONS

For detailed patient instructions on methadone, see the Patient Information Sheet on p. 276.
- Take your methadone once daily, as prescribed
- Carry a card in your wallet stating that your are taking methadone
- Do not share this medication with anyone. If you receive "carries" of methadone, store them out of the reach of children; methadone can be poisonous to individuals who do not take opiates

DRUG INTERACTIONS

Only clinically significant interactions are listed below:

Class of Drug	Example	Interaction Effects
Alcohol		Acute alcohol use can decrease methadone metabolism and increase the plasma level Chronic alcohol use can induce methadone metabolism and decrease the plasma level
Antacid	Al/Mg antacids	Decreased absorption of methadone
Anticonvulsant	Phenytoin, carbamazepine, barbiturates	Decreased plasma level of methadone due to enhanced metabolism (by 50% with phenytoin)
Antidepressant		Increased plasma level of desipramine (by about 108%)
Cyclic	Desipramine, amitriptyline	Increased giddiness, euphoria; suspected potentiation of methadone's "euphoric" effects – abuse with amitriptyline reported
SSRI	Fluvoxamine	Increased plasma level for methadone by 20–100% with fluvoxamine, due to decreased clearance
Antifungal	Fluconazole	Increase in methadone peak and trough plasma levels by 27% and 48% respectively; clearance decreased by 24%
Antipsychotic	Risperidone	Case reports of precipitation of narcotic withdrawal symptoms (mechanism unclear)
Antitubercular drug	Isoniazid Rifampin	Decreased clearance and increased plasma level of methadone Decreased plasma level of methadone due to enhanced metabolism
Antiviral	Nelfinavir, efavirenz, nevirapine	Increased clearance of methadone and decreased total concentration (AUC) (by up to 60% with efavirenz and nevirapine)
	Didanosine, stavudine	Decreased bioavailability of antiretrovirals due to increased degradation in GI tract by methadone (C_{max} and AUC decreased by 66% and 63%, respectively, for didanosine, and by 44% and 25% for stavudine)
	Zidovudine (AZT)	Inhibited metabolism of AZT by methadone (AUC increased by 43%)
Benzodiazepine	Diazepam, clonazepam Diazepam	Enhanced risk of respiratory depression "Opiate high" reported with combined use
Cimetidine		Decreased clearance of methadone
Disulfiram		Decreased clearance of methadone

Methadone (cont.)

Class of Drug	Example	Interaction Effects
Narcotics	Pentazocine, nalbuphine, butorphanol	Occurrence of withdrawal symptoms due to partial antagonist effects of these narcotics
Protease inhibitor	Ritonavir	Large decrease in clearance of methadone
Urine acidifier	Ascorbic acid	Increased elimination of methadone
Urine alkalizer	Sodium bicarbonate	Decreased elimination of methadone

New Unapproved Treatments of Psychiatric Disorders

PRODUCT AVAILABILITY Biochemical theories on the etiology of specific psychiatric disorders have initiated investigations of various drugs/chemicals that may influence brain neurotransmitters and thereby play a role in the treatment of psychiatric disorders. Several drugs traditionally used to treat medical conditions have been found to be of benefit in ameliorating or preventing symptoms of certain psychiatric disorders. This section presents a summary of some of these drugs and their uses. **As a rule, unapproved treatments should be reserved for patients highly resistant to conventional therapies. Clinicians should always be cognisant of medicolegal issues when prescribing drugs for non-approved indications.**

	Anxiety Disorders	Depression	Bipolar Disorder (cycling)	Mania	Schizo-phrenia	SDAT	Antisocial Behavior/ Aggression	ADHD	Drug Dependence Treatment
Aminoglutethimide (p. 215)		PR							
Anticonvulsants (pp. 213–214), e.g.,									
Oxycarbazine				PR					
Phenytoin							C/P		
Tiagabine	PR								
Topiramate	PR		PR	PR	S				
Vigabatrin	PR								
Azathioprine (p. 215)					PR				
β-Blockers, e.g., propranolol, atenolol, pindolol (p. 210)	+	+/S			C/S		+		
Bromocriptine (pp. 212–213)		+			C/S				
Buprenorphine (p. 216)									+ (opioids)
Calcium-channel blockers (pp. 211–212),									
nifedipine					PR				
nimodipine			+/S			PR			
verapamil			+/S						

	Anxiety Disorders	Depression	Bipolar Disorder (cycling)	Mania	Schizo-phrenia	SDAT	Antisocial Behavior/ Aggression	ADHD	Drug Dependence Treatment
Clonidine (p. 209)	P				+		P(PR)/S	+/S	+
Cyproheptadine (p. 214–215)					C				
Dexamethasone (pp. 216)		PR							
Estrogen/progesterone (p. 216)		+/S				PR	+		
Famotidine (p. 216–217)					PR				
Guanfacine (p. 210)								PR	
Ketoconazole (p. 215)		PR							
Lecithin (p. 212)						P			
Modafinil (p. 213)		PR/S						PR	
NSAIDS (p. 217)						+			
Ondansetron (p. 215)					PR				PR/S (alcohol)
Pergolide (p. 213)		PR/S							
Prazosin (p. 211)	PR								
Selegiline (p. 217)					C/PR	PR		+	
Testosterone (p. 217)		PR/S							
Thyroid hormones (p. 211)		S	C						
Vitamins (p. 217)					C/S	PR			

C = contradictory results, P = partial improvement, + = positive, S = synergistic effect, PR = preliminary data

Adrenergic Agents

Central stimulating or blocking agents of noradrenergic receptors

CLONIDINE

A central and peripheral α-adrenergic agonist; acts on presynaptic neurons and inhibits noradrenergic transmission at the synapse

Antisocial Behavior/ Aggression

- Dose: 0.4–0.6 mg/day as tablets or transdermal patch; in children, doses of 0.15 to 0.4 mg/day
- Improvement in behavior or impulsivity noted when used alone or in combination with methylphenidate (use with caution); may reduce hyperarousal behaviors in pervasive developmental disorder and ADHD
- May have synergistic effect with anticonvulsant regimens in controlling aggression and impulsivity

(Weller, E.B. et al., J. Clin. Psychiatry 60 (suppl. 15), 5–11, 1999; Connor, D.F. et al., J. Pediatr. (Phila) 39(1), 15–25, 2000)

Anxiety Disorders

- Postulated that abnormally high reactivity of brain noradrenergic systems is related to some clinical forms of anxiety
- Dose: 0.15–0.5 mg/day
- Of some benefit in generalized anxiety disorder, panic attacks, phobic disorders, and obsessive-compulsive disorders; may be effective in PTSD alone and in combination with cyclic antidepressants
- May augment effects of SSRIs in social phobia
- Psychological symptoms respond better than somatic symptoms
- Anxiolytic effects may be short-lived

(Ahmed, I. et al., CNS Drugs 6(1), 53–70, 1996; Van Ameringen, M. et al., J. Affect. Dis. 39, 115–121, 1996)

ADHD

- Dose: 5–8 µg/kg body weight per day (0.05–0.3 mg/day)
- Children metabolize clonidine faster than adults and may require more frequent dosing (4–6 times a day)
- Meta-analysis of studies demonstrate a moderate benefit in children and adolescents
- Promising on ADHD target symptoms; reduces hyperarousal, agitation and aggression; useful in patients with tic disorders or oppositional/conduct disorders
- Some benefit in combining with methylphenidate or dextroamphetamine in resistant patients; may be useful in ameliorating sleep disturbance caused by psychostimulants – use caution with combination – case reports of sudden death
- Sedation common on initiation; less common: anxiety, irritability, decreased memory, headache, dry mouth, hypotension
- Taper on drug discontinution to prevent tic rebound in Tourette's patients

(Swanson, J.M. et al., J. Child Adol. Psychopharmacology 5(4), 301–304, 1995; Connor, D.F. et al., J. Am. Acad. Child Adolesc. Psychiatry 38(12), 1551–1559, 1999)

Schizophrenia

- Dose: 0.25–0.9 mg/day
- Shown to decrease psychotic symptoms; may be particularly helpful in decreasing paranoid ideation
- Response in both positive and negative symptoms seen
- Improvement in hallucinogen-related flashbacks reported
- Reported efficacy for clozapine-induced sialorrhea
- Rebound psychotic symptoms reported on withdrawal
- May relieve neuroleptic-induced akathisia; gradual improvement in tardive dyskinesia reported
- May increase agitation and produce depressive symptoms

(Maas, J.W. et al., J. Clin. Psychopharmacology, 15(5), 361–364, 1995; Lerner, A.G. et al., Am. J. Psychiatry 155(10), 1460, 1998)

Drug Dependence

- Dose: 0.1–0.3 mg tid
- Used in heroin and nicotine withdrawal to reduce autonomic hyperactivity and increase patient comfort. Opioid antagonists (e.g., naltrexone) often given concomitantly
- Adverse effects include dizziness, hypotension, dry mouth and lack of energy

(Gowing, L. et al., Cochrane Database Syst. Rev. (2): CD002021, 2000 and (1) CD002024, 2001)

Adrenergic Agents (cont.)

β-BLOCKERS e. g., propranolol

Have membrane-stabilizing effect and GABA-mimetic activity; 5-HT antagonist properties

Antisocial Behavior/ Aggression

- Propranolol dose: 80–960 mg/day
- Response may take up to 8 weeks
- Useful in controlling rage, violence, irritability, and aggression due to a number of causes (e.g., SDAT, autism)
- May be effective in controlling aggressive behavior in children and adolescents with organic brain dysfunction
- Positive response reported also with nadolol (40–160 mg/day), pindolol (10–60 mg/day), and metoprolol (100–200 mg/day)
- Rebound rage reactions on drug withdrawal reported; taper dose gradually

(Bailly, D., CNS Drugs 5(2), 115–136, 1996; Simeon, J.G., Child Adol. Psychopharmacology News 2(3), 11–12, 1997; Silver, J.M. et al., J. Neuropsychiatry Clin. Neuroscience 1(3), 328–335, 1999)

Anxiety Disorders

- Propranolol dose: up to 320 mg/day
- Beneficial for somatic or autonomically mediated symptoms of anxiety (e.g., tremor, palpitations) as seen in social phobia and acute panic
- Efficacy reported in adults and children with posttraumatic stress disorder
- Positive response also reported with oxprenolol (40–240 mg/day), metoprolol (100 mg/day), and atenolol (50 mg/day)
- Pindolol 2.5–7.5 mg/day may augment response to SSRIs in OCD

(Bailly, D., CNS Drugs 5(2), 115–136, 1996; Koran, L.M. et al., J. Clin. Psychopharmacology 16(3), 253–254, 1996; Le Melledo, J.M. et al, Biol. Psychiatry 1:44(5), 364–366, 1998)

Depression

- Pindolol dose: 2.5 mg bid to 5 mg tid (5-HT_{1A} receptor blocker)
- 4 placebo-controlled and 4 open-label studies show positive results in combination with some antidepressants (e.g., SSRIs, tranylcypromine); used as augmentation therapy (and to speed up the onset of response); data contradictory as 4 studies report lack of efficacy
- Preliminary data suggest usefulness in treating seasonal affective disorder
- β-blockers are used to treat akathisia caused by SSRI antidepressants

(Moreno, F.A. et al., J. Clin. Psychiatry 58(10), 437–439, 1997; Blier, P. et al., J. Clin. Psychiatry 59 (suppl 5), 16–23, 1998; Bordet, R. et al., Am. J. Psychiatry 155(10), 1346–1351, 1998)

Schizophrenia

- Propranolol dose: up to 5800 mg/day (more commonly: 120–640 mg/day); pindolol 5 mg tid
- Contradictory results seen
- May be beneficial in acute schizophrenia; may increase plasma level of antipsychotic
- Some response seen on negative symptoms
- Efficacy may be related to treatment of neuroleptic-induced akathisia; improvement reported in tardive akathisia
- May be useful in controlling aggressive behavior in schizophrenic patients; nadolol reported to decrease overall psychotic symptoms and extrapyramidal side effects in aggressive schizophrenic patients; pindolol decreased the number and severity of aggressive acts
- Case reports of encephalopathy with doses over 1000 mg of propranolol

(Bailly, D., CNS Drugs 5(2), 115–136, 1996; Allan, E.R. et al., J. Clin. Psychiatry 57(10), 455–459, 1996; Caspi, N. et al., Int. Clin. Psychopharmacology 16(2), 111–115, 2001)

GUANFACINE

Antihypertensive; α_{2A} agonist

ADHD

- Dose: 0.5–3 mg/day given bid
- Children metabolize guanfacine faster than adults and may require more frequent dosing (2–3 times a day)
- Uncontrolled studies suggest efficacy in treatment-refractory patients nonresponsive to other medication or in patients with comorbid Tourette's syndrome

- Case reports of induced mania
- May cause withdrawal effects if stopped abruptly

(Hunt, R.D. et al., Am. Acad. Child Adolesc. Psychiatry 34(1), 50–54, 1995; Horrigan, J.P. et al., J Child Adolesc. Psychopharmacol. 8(2), 149–150, 1998)

THYROID HORMONES

Modulate adrenergic receptor function and permit a given concentration of catecholamines to be more effective; metabolic enhancers

Depression

- Dose: liothyronine (T_3): 0.005–0.05 mg/day, L-thyroxine 0.15–0.5 mg/day
- In refractory depression, may potentiate effects of antidepressants; positive effects seen in up to 60% of refractory patients within 2 weeks – may be more beneficial in women than in men
- Suggested T_3 may actually be treating subclinical hypothyroidism
- May exacerbate mania

(Joffe, R.T., J. Clin. Psychiatry 59 (suppl 5), 26–29, 1998; Bauer, M. et al. Neuropsychopharmacology 18, 444–455, 1998)

Bipolar Disorder

- Dose: L-thyroxine: 0.3–0.5 mg/day
- Controversial results seen
- May be treating unidentified hypothydroidism
- Reported to alleviate symptoms and increase cycle length in rapid-cycling female patients; adjunctive to other therapies of bipolar disorder

(Dubovsky, S.L. et al., J. Clin. Psychiatry 58(5), 224–242, 1997)

PRAZOSIN

α_1-adrenergic antagonist

Anxiety Disorders

- Dose: 2–5 mg/day
- Preliminary data suggest benefit in ameliorating nightmares in individuals with PTSD

(Raskind, M.A. et al., J. Clin. Psychiatry, 61, 129–133, 2000)

Block the influx of calcium into brain tissue, which may decrease the release of a number of neurotransmitters

Calcium Channel Blockers

NIFEDIPINE

Schizophrenia

- Dose: up to 60 mg/day
- Possible effects on negative symptoms when used with a neuroleptic; nifedipine may alter the plasma level of the neuroleptic
- Potential benefit in treating tardive dyskinesia; may also enhance learning and memory in these patients

(Cates, M. et al., Ann. Pharmacotherapy 27(2), 191–196, 1993; Schwartz, B.L. et al., Clin. Neuropharmacology 20(4), 364–370, 1997)

NIMODIPINE

Bipolar Disorder

- Dose: up to 510 mg/day (as tid or qid dosing)
- Response seen in 33% of patients with treatment-refractory affective disorder
- May augment effects of carbamazepine and lithium
- Reports of efficacy in stabilizing patients with rapid-cycling and ultrarapid-cycling bipolar disorder used alone or in combination with other mood stabilizers
- Improvements in mania scales and BPRS noted

(Pazzaglia, P.S. et al., J Clin. Psychopharmacology 18(5), 404–413, 1998; Davanzo, P.A. et al., J. Child Adolescent Psychopharmacology 9, 51–61, 1999; Dubovsky, S.L. et al, J. Clin. Psychiatry 58:5, 224–242, 1997)

Calcium Channel Blockers (cont.)

SDAT

- Dose: 90 mg/day
- Improvement reported in cognitive function, in several studies of patients with multi-infarct dementia and Alzheimer's disease; progression of disease less than with placebo
- Early data suggest efficacy in management of coexisting depression in dementia

(DeVry, J. et al., Clin. Neuropharmcology 20(1), 22–35, 1997; Pautoni, L. et al., Clin. Neuropharmacology 19(6), 497–506, 1996; Flynn, B. et al., Annals of Pharmacotherapy 33, 188–197, 1999)

VERAPAMIL

Bipolar Disorder

- Dose: 160–480 mg/day
- Useful adjunctive drug in combination with lithium or a neuroleptic; may be alternative to other mood stabilizers during pregnancy
- Some studies report efficacy in acute treatment of rapid-cycling BAD and in prophylaxis – may be more effective in lithium-responsive than in lithium-resistant patients
- May prevent antidepressant-induced switches into mania

(Walton, S.A. et al., J. Clin. Psychiatry 57(11), 543–546, 1996; Dubovsky, S.L. et al., J. Clin. Psychiatry 58(5), 224–242, 1997; Hollister, L.E. et al., Can. J. Psychiatry 44, 658–664, 1999)

Cholinergic Agents

LECITHIN

Increases the activity of acetylcholine (acetylcholine precursor)

SDAT

- Dose: up to 24 g/day
- Meta-analysis of studies suggests little improvement in functioning or cognition
- Contradictory data as to efficacy when combined with tacrine (THA)

(Higgins, J.P. et al., Cochrane Database Syst. Rev. (4) CD001015, 2000)

Dopaminergic Agents

BROMOCRIPTINE

Biphasic effect hypothesized: Acts on presynaptic autoreceptors to inhibit dopaminergic transmission at lower doses, while acting as a dopamine postsynaptic receptor agonist at high doses

Depression

- Dose: 2.5–60 mg/day (doses up to 220 mg/day have been used)
- Response seen after 4–14 days therapy
- Several double-blind studies show beneficial effect; may alleviate depressive recurrence in patients who initially responded to SSRIs; up to 57% of treatment-refractory patients responded in open trials
- Case reports of efficacy as augmentation therapy with cyclic antidepressants; may alleviate SSRI-induced apathy syndrome
- Hypomania has been reported

(Inoue, T. et al. Biol. Psychiatry 40, 151–153, 1996; Nierenberg, A.A. et al., J. Clin. Psychiatry 59 (suppl. 5), 60–63, 1998; Wada, T. et al., Prog. Neuropsychopharmacol. Biol. Psychiatry 25(2), 457–462, 2001)

Schizophrenia

- Dose: 0.25–2.5 mg/day
- Controlled studies show worsening, no change, or improvement in psychotic symptoms
- Selected patients have responded to bromocriptine alone or combined with a neuroleptic; reported to augment effect of clozapine on negative symptoms in refractory patients

- Symptoms most responsive include suspiciousness, hostility, thought disorder, hallucinations, somatic concerns, and sexual preoccupation
- Useful in alleviating side effects due to neuroleptic-induced high prolactin level (e.g., amenorrhea, sexual dysfunction)
- Reported to alleviate symptoms of neuroleptic malignant syndrome (NMS) if started very early; dose: 2.5–60 mg/day
- Some efficacy reported in treatment of neuroleptic-induced extrapyramidal symptoms
- Low doses may decrease symptoms of tardive dyskinesia (0.75–7.5 mg/day)
- High doses may increase psychotic symptoms

(Biol. Therapies in Psychiatry 16(1), 1–2, 1993; Al-Semaan, Y. Can. J. Psychiatry 41(7), 484–485, 1996)

MODAFINIL

Psychostimulant which exhibits weak affinity for dopamine uptake carrier sites; may work by reducing GABA release and increasing the release of glutamate

Depression

- Dose: 100–400 mg/day
- Shown to augment effects of antidepressants, within 1–2 weeks in treatment-refractory patients, particularly those with residual tiredness or fatigue
- Has a low abuse potential
- Induces CYP1A2, 2B6 and 3A4; may decrease levels of drugs metabolized by these enzymes

(Menza, M.A. et al., J. Clin. Psychiatry, 61(5), 378–381, 2000)

ADHD

- Dose: 100–300 mg/day in divided doses
- Beneficial results reported in open trial of children, aged 5–15, for average treatment of 4 weeks
- Good response reported in double-blind placebo-controlled study of modafinil (mean dose 206.8 mg/day) with dextroamphetamine, in adults

(Rugino, T.A. et al., J. Am. Acad. Child Adolesc. Psychiatry 40(2), 230–235, 2001; Taylor, F.B. et al., J. Child. Adolesc. Psychopharmacol. 10(4), 311–320, 2000)

PERGOLIDE

Dopamine agonist at D1 and D2 receptors

Depression

- Preliminary data suggest may augment antidepressant response in treatment-refractory patients

(Nierenberg, A.A. et al., J. Clin. Psychiatry 59 (suppl. 5), 60–63, 1998)

GABA-Agents / Anticonvulsants

OXYCARBAZINE

Anticonvulsant; inhibits voltage-dependent sodium channels and possibly potassium channels
A 10-keto analog of carbamazepine

Mania

- Dose: 600–1200 mg/day in divided doses
- Reported to reduce manic symptoms
- Considered to be better tolerated than carbamazepine, with a lesser degree of drug interactions due to enzyme induction
- Side effects include: sedation, dizziness, hypotension, sialorrhea, hyponatremia (2.5% – monitor sodium levels), rash

(Ghaemi, S.N., Int. Drug Therapy Newsletter 36(3), 20–22, 2001)

PHENYTOIN

Anticonvulsant; stabilizes membranes, has 5-HT potentiating and GABA-agonist properties

Antisocial Behavior/ Aggression

- Dose: 100–600 mg/day
- Contradictory results seen in ability to alter emotional lability, impulsivity, irritability, and aggression when used alone or with neuroleptics (high doses may produce deterioration in behavior); greater benefit in reducing impulsive aggressive acts
- Reports of behavior improvement in adults and children with EEG abnormalities

(Barratt, E.S. et al., J. Clin. Psychopharmacology 17(5), 341–349, 1997; Stanford, M.S. et al., Psychiatry Res. 103(2–3), 193–203, 2001)

GABA-Agents / Anticonvulsants (cont.)

TIAGABINE

Anticonvulsant; increases GABA

Anxiety Disorders

- Dose: 15 mg/day
- Case reports of improvement in panic attacks and agoraphobia

(Zwanzger, P. et al., J. Clin. Psychiatry 62(8), 656–657, 2001)

TOPIRAMATE

Anticonvulsant; GABA agonist; blocks glutamate/kainate/AMPA receptors and modulates neuronal conductance channels

Bipolar Disorder

- Dose: 50–1300 mg/day; some suggest a response at lower doses (e.g., 25 mg bid)
- Double-blind study suggests benefit in Bipolar I disorder
- Open label studies suggest efficacy in acute mania, in Bipolar II disorder, in rapid-cycling BAD and when used adjunctively with other mood stabilizers
- Onset of side effects may be delayed by 1–2 weeks; suggested to increase dose slowly
- Reported to cause weight loss
- Cognitive side effects (especially confusion and difficulty with verbal processing), sedation, fatigue, headache, dizziness, paresthesias
- Renally excreted; maintain adequate hydration; has been associated with kidney stones in 1.5% of patients; reduce dose in patients with creatinine clearance < 70 ml/min
- Cases of severy myopia and secondary angle-closure glaucoma
- Interaction: can reduce efficacy of oral contraceptives; reported to increase carbamazepine level by 20%

(Currents in Affective Illness 18(4), 5–13, 1999; Psychopharmacology Update 9(7), 9, 1998; Ghaemi, SN et al., Int. Drug Therapy Newsletter 34(5), 33–37, 1999; Calabrese, J.R., Presentation APA Chicago, May 2000; Gelenberg, A.J., Biolog. Therapies in Psychiatry, 23(8), 30–31, 2000, and 24(8), 30, 2001; Marcotte, D., J. Affective Disorders 50, 245–251, 1998)

Anxiety Disorders

- Open-label study suggests benefit in treatment-refractory PTSD – reported to decrease nightmares and flashbacks; no tolerance to effects reported

(Biolog. Therapies in Psychiatry 22(12), 50, 1999)

Schizophrenia

- Dose: up to 125 mg/day
- Used in combination with clozapine to decrease myoclonic jerks; reported to minimize weight gain

(Dursun, S.M. et al., Can. J. Psychiatry, 45, 198, 2000)

VIGABATRIN

Irreversible GABA transaminase inhibitor

Anxiety Disorders

- Dose: 250–500 mg/day
- Preliminary data suggest efficacy in decreasing startle response and improving sleep in patients with PTSD

(MacLeod, A. J. Clin. Psychopharmacology 16(2), 190–191, 1996)

Serotonin Antagonists

CYPROHEPTADINE

5-HT$_{2A}$ and 5-HT$_{2C}$ antagonist

Schizophrenia

- Dose: 12–24 mg/day
- Contradictory data suggest beneficial effects on negative symptoms of schizophrenia when added to a typical antipsychotic
- Improvement of clozapine-withdrawal syndrome noted; may be related somewhat to stabilizing sleep architecture

- Early studies report efficacy in neuroleptic-induced EPS

(Meltzer, H.Y. et al., Psychopharmacology 104, 176–181, 1996; Akhohdzadeh, S. et al., J. Clin. Pharm. Ther. 24(1), 49–52, 1999; Chaudhry, I.B. et al., Schizophr. Res. 53(1–2), 17–24, 2002)

ONDANSETRON

5-HT_3 receptor antagonist

Schizophrenia

- Dose: 4–12 mg/day (high doses found less effective)
- Efficacy in acute schizophrenia reported
- Improvement seen in symptoms of tardive dyskinesia
- Report of moderate to marked improvement in hallucinations, paranoid delusions, confusion and functional impairment in 15 of 16 patients with Parkinson's disease; doses of 12–24 mg/day used

(Zoldan, J., Neurology 45, 1305–1308, 1995; Sirota, P. et al., Am. J. Psychiat. 157(2), 287–289, 2000)

Alcohol Dependence

- Dose: 4 μg/kg/day
- Randomized controlled trial suggests that patients under age 25 with early-onset alcoholism (but not those with late-onset alcoholism) show a significant reduction in the number of drinks per day and have improved abstinence
- Reported to reduce craving in predisposed alcoholics in combination with naltrexone 25 mg bid

(Johnson, B.A. et al., JAMA 284, 963–971, 2000; Ait-Daoud, N. et al, Psychopharmacol. 154(1), 23–27, 2001)

Steroid Biosynthesis Inhibitors

AMINOGLUTETHIMIDE

Glucocorticoid antagonist

Depression

- Preliminary data suggests efficacy in treatment-refractory depression, alone or in combination with cortisol and metyrapone or ketoconazole

(Murphy, B.E., Psychoneuroendocinology 22(suppl. 1), S125–S132, 1997; Murphy, B.E. et al., Can. J. Psychiat 43(3), 279–286, 1998)

KETOCONAZOLE

Glucocorticoid antagonist (cortisol synthesis inhibitor)

Depression

- Dose 200–1000 mg/day
- Meta-analysis of reports suggest efficacy in select patients with treatment-refractory depression, alone or in combination with metyrapone and cortisol; may have efficacy in atypical depression
- Side effects include nausea, pruritis and increase in liver function enzymes; hepatotoxicity occurs occasionally
- Cortisol (20 mg/day) supplementation used

(Price, L.H. et al., CNS Drugs 5(5), 311–320, 1996; Wolkowitz, O.M. et al., Psychosomatic Med. 61(5), 698–711, 1999; Murphy, B.E. et al., Can. J. Psychiat. 43(3), 279–286, 1998)

Miscellaneous

AZATHIOPRINE

Immunosuppressant

Schizophrenia

- Dose: 150 mg/day
- Case report and an open study suggest improvement in psychosis in some patients. Platelet associated antibodies (which block dopamine uptake) were related to response
- Monitor for leucopenia

(Levine, J. et al., Lancet 344, 59–60, 1994; Levine, J. et al., Neuropsychobiology 36(4), 172–176, 1997)

Miscellaneous (cont.)

BUPRENOPHRINE

Opioid Dependence

- Dose: up to 12 mg/day (sublingual)
- Analysis of controlled studies suggests buphrenorphine may be an effective aid in heroin withdrawal; causes minimal withdrawal symptoms due to partial agonist activity
- Double blind studies suggest utility of buprenorphine as a maintenance therapy for the treatment of opioid dependence, improvement noted in psychosocial adjustment and global functioning
- Side effects most commonly seen in first 2–3 days of treatment include: headache, sedation, nausea, constipation, dizziness and anxiety

(Pani, P.P. et al., Drug Alcohol Depend. 60(1), 39–50, 2000; Eder, H. et al., Eur. Addict. Res. 4(Suppl. 1), 3–7, 1998; Gowing, L. et al., Cochrane Database Syst. Rev. (3) CD0020, 25, 2000; Barnett, P.G. et al., Addiction 96, 683–690, 2001)

DEXAMETHASONE

Glucocorticoid involved in hypothalamic-pituitary-adrenal (HPA) axis; increases rate of tyrosine hydroxylase mRNA synthesis; modulates stress-induced changes in serotonin metabolism

Depression

- Dose: 4–8 mg/day
- Two studies describe response in some patients with unipolar depression and bipolar depression

(Arana, G.W. et al., J. Clin. Psychiatry 52, 304–306, 1991; Arana, G.W. et al., Am. J. Psychiatry 152, 265–267, 1995)

ESTROGENS & PROGESTERONE

***Estrogens* increase central bioavailability of norepinephrine, serotonin and acetylcholine; may increase binding sites on platelets for antidepressants; decrease dopaminergic concentrations in limbic structures. Chronic use causes increase in dopaminergic receptor density resulting in dopamine supersensitivity. May have dopamine agonist properties.**
***Progesterone* enhances serotonergic activity (chronic estrogen use augments activity of progesterone in CNS)**

Antisocial Behavior/ Aggression

- Dose: conjugated estrogens 0.625–3.75 mg/day; diethylstilboestrol 1–2 mg/day
- Used in elderly males with dementia exhibiting aggressive behavior
- Feminizing effects and risk of thrombosis minimal with low doses; peripheral edema has been reported

(Shelton, P.S. et al., Annals of Pharmacotherapy 33(7/8), 808–812, 1999)

Depression

- Dose: conjugated estrogens 4.375–25 mg/day for 21 days followed by progesterone 5 mg/day for 5 days
- Found useful in combination with antidepressant in some refractory female patients (post-menopausal women more likely to respond)
- Maximum clinical effect may take up to 4 weeks to occur
- Estradiol patches and sublingual 17β-estradiol reported effective in treating severe postpartum depression

(Epperson, C.N. et al., Psychosomatic Med. 61(5), 676–697, 1999; Burt, V.K. et al., Harv. Rev. Psychiatry 6(3), 121–132, 1998; Ahokas, A. et al., J. Clin. Psychiatry 65, 332–336, 2001)

SDAT

- Studies suggest a protective effect of estrogen therapy on age of onset of Alzheimer's disease; women with a history of long-term use had the lowest risk – data contradictory
- Improvement noted in memory and attention
- May enhance response to tacrine

(Flynn, B.L., Annals of Pharmacotherapy 33, 178–181, 1999; Mulnard, R.A. et al., JAMA 283, 1007–1015, 2000; Asthana, S. et al., Neurology 57, 605–612, 2001)

FAMOTIDINE

H_2 receptor inhibitor

Schizophrenia

- Dose 40–100 mg/day

- Improvement in positive and negative symptoms noted in treatment-resistant patients when prescribed alone or in combination with neuroleptics

(Deutsch, S.I. et al., CNS Drugs 8(4), 276–284, 1997; Martinez, M.C., Annals of Pharmacotherapy 33, 742–744, 1999)

NSAIDS

SDAT

Nonsteroidal antiinflammatory drug

- Inhibit CNS inflammatory response
- Data suggest that NSAIDS confer protection against Alzheimer's disease by stabilizing cognitive function, but do not protect against vascular dementia

(Stewart, W.F. et al., Neurology 48, 626–632, 1997; Flynn, B.L. et al., Annals of Pharmacotherapy 33(7/8), 840–849, 1999; Bas A. in't Veld, et al., NEJM 345, 1515–1521, 2001)

SELEGILINE

Inhibitor of MAO-B, possibly nonselective at higher doses; stimulates nitric oxide production

ADHD

- Positive effects on ADHD and tic symptoms reported in double-blind placebo controlled crossover studies and in open trials

(Popper, C.W., J. Clin. Psychiatry 58 (suppl 14), 14–29, 1997)

Schizophrenia

- Dose: 5 mg bid
- Contradictory data as to efficacy in treating depressive symptoms and negative symptoms of schizophrenia
- Benefit in the treatment of extrapyramidal symptoms reported

(Gupta, S. et al., Compr. Psychiat. 40(2), 148–150, 1999; Jungerman, T. et al., J. Clin. Psychopharmacol. 19(6), 522–525, 1999; Rapoport, A. et al., J. Neural Trans. 106(9–10), 911–918, 1999)

SDAT

- Dose: 5 mg bid
- Preliminary data suggest improvement in cognitive function, behavior and activities of daily living in patients with Alzheimer's disease; combination with Vitamin E 2000 IU/day may improve response
- Meta-analysis of studies suggests improvement in memory, mood and behavior
- May slow down the progression of Alzheimer's disease of moderate severity; suggested to reduce the concentration of free radicals and other neurotoxins

(Sano, M. et al., New Engl. J. Med. 336(17), 1216–1222, 1997; Birks, J. et al., Cochrane Database Syst. Rev. (2) CD00442, 2000; Thomas, T., Neurobiol. Aging 21(2), 343–348, 2000)

TESTOSTERONE

Depression

- Dose: 400 mg im every 2 wks
- Early data suggests benefit as augmentation strategy in men, with low-normal serum testosterone, refractory to SSRIs

Seidman, S.N. et al., J. Affective Disorders 48, 157–161, 1998)

VITAMINS

Schizophrenia

- Reports that *ascorbic acid* in doses up to 8g/day may antagonize dopamine neurotransmission and potentiate activity of the neuroleptic (may antagonize the metabolism of the neuroleptic)
- Doses of *vitamin E* of 600 IU/day reported to reduce severity of acute EPS in patients treated with antipsychotics; doses of up to 1600 IU daily reported useful in decreasing symptoms of tardive dyskinesia (anti-oxidant)

(Adler, L.A. et al., Biol. Psychiatry 43, 868–872, 1998; Int. Drug Ther. Newsletter 34(1), 3, 1999; Dorfman-Etrog, P. et al., Eur. Neuropsychopharmacol. 9(6), 475–477, 1999)

SDAT

- Vitamin E at 2000 IU/day reported to slow down the progression of Alzheimer's disease of moderate severity due to anti-oxidant effect; no improvement in cognitive function occurred

(Sano, M. et al., New Engl. J. Med. 336(17), 1216–1222, 1997)

Herbal and "Natural" Products

PRODUCT AVAILABILITY

Herbal (natural) products have been traditionally used by many cultures to treat a variety of psychiatric conditions. Very few of these products, however, have been subjected to scientific scrutiny through standardized research methods. Clinicians should always be cognisant of medicolegal issues when recommending herbal products for non-approved indications.

CAUTION: Quality control of herbal/natural products is variable, depending on the preparation used. As these products are not standardized in North America, the amount of active constituents can vary between preparations, and some products may be adulterated with other herbs, chemicals and drugs.

Drug	Anxiety	Depression	Bipolar Disorder	Sleep Disorders	Schizophrenia	SDAT	Drug Dependence Treatment
Ginkgo Biloba (p. 218)		PR				C	
Inositol (p. 219)	PR	PR					
Kava Kava (p. 219)	+						
Kudzu (p. 219)							PR (alcohol)
Melatonin (pp. 219–220)		PR		C			
Omega 3 Fatty Acids (p. 220)			PR		PR	PR	
S-Adenosyl-methionine (p. 220)		+				C	
St. John's Wort (p. 221)	PR	+*					
Valerian (p. 221)				+			

C = contradictory results, P = partial improvement, + = positive, PR = preliminary data. *Mild to moderate depression only

GINKGO BILOBA

Active ginkgolides obtained from the nuts and leaves of the oldest deciduous tree in the world (ginkgo – also called Maidenhair tree or kew tree)

Standardized products contain flavone glycosides (24%) and terpenoids (6%)

SDAT

- Dose: 120–240 mg/day in divided doses; 1–3 months treatment, at full dose, required for full therapeutic effect
- Increases vasodilation and peripheral blood flow in capillary vessels and end arteries; may have antioxidant action (free radical scavenger); may increase cholinergic transmission by inhibiting acetylcholinesterase
- A number of controlled studies suggest that ginkgo extracts can improve vascular perfusion and decrease thrombosis; used in dementia, chronic cerebrovascular insufficiency and cerebral trauma. Improvement noted in memory, concentration, fatigue, anxiety and depressed mood; data contradictory
- Side effects are rare, and include: headache, dizziness, palpitations, GI upset and contact dermatitis; spontaneous bruising and bleeding have been reported. Very large doses may cause restlessness, diarrhea, nausea and vomiting
- Caution in patients on anticoagulants or ASA, due to possible enhanced effect and risk of bleeding

(Wong, A.H. et al., Arch. Gen. Psychiat. 55(11), 1033–1044, 1998; Curtis-Prior, P. et al., J. Pharm. Pharmacol. 51(5), 531–541, 1999; Muller, J.L. et al., Drug Benefit Trends 10(5), 43–50, 1998; Martien, C. et al, J. Am. Geriatric Society 48, 1183–1194, 2000)

Depression

- May have MAOI properties; some evidence suggests it may inhibit reuptake of serotonin and dopamine – use caution with co-prescribed drugs

- Early data suggest that ginkgo may augment antidepressants in treatment refractory depression
- Suggested that doses of 240–900 mg/day may be effective in treating SSRI-induced sexual dysfunction

(Wong, A.H. et al., Arch. Gen. Psychiat. 55(11), 1033–1044, 1998; Carpenter, V.G., APA Conference June 4/98, Toronto)

INOSITOL

Simple isomer of glucose and a precursor of a "second messenger" system (the phosphotidyl-inositol cycle) used by various receptors including α_1 and 5-HT_2

Anxiety Disorders

- 12–18 g/day
- Preliminary data suggest efficacy in treating panic, phobic disorders, obsessive-compulsive disorder and trichotillomania
- May aggravate symptoms of ADHD in children

(Fux, M. et al., Am. J. Psychiatry 153(9), 1219–1221, 1997; Levine, J., Eur. Neuropsychoharmacol. 7, 147–155, 1997; Seedat, S. et al. J. Clin. Psychiatry 62:1, 60–61, 2001)

Depression

- Dose: up to 27 g/day
- One study suggests response in 6 out of 13 patients with depression
- Reported not to augment antidepressant effect in SSRI refractory patients
- Mild psychotic symptoms and mania reported

(Levine, J. et al., Am. J. Psychiatry 152(5), 192–194, 1995; Nemets, B. et al., J. Neurol. Transm. 106(7–8), 795–798, 1999

KAVA KAVA

Made from the roots of *Piper methysticum*; active ingredients felt to be kava lactones.
May have activity at GABA receptor, antagonize dopamine, and block voltage dependent sodium ion channels
Slang name: AWA.

Anxiety Disorders

- Dose: 60–240 mg kavalactones daily
- Used throughout the Pacific Islands as a ceremonial drink to induce relaxation and sleep and to decrease anxiety; may have anticonvulsant and muscle relaxant activity
- Meta-analysis of placebo-controlled studies suggests benefit in the treatment of anxiety, tension and agitation
- Does not adversely affect cognition, mental acuity or coordination
- Adverse effects are rare at lower doses, and include: yellow skin discoloration with chronic use; at doses above 400 mg/day: dry flaking skin, red eyes, facial puffiness, muscle weakness, dystonic reactions, dyskinesias, and choreoathetosis
- Liver dysfunction has been reported; use with caution in patients with a history of liver disease – periodic liver function tests recommended
- May potentiate other CNS depressants (including alcohol and benzodiazepines), causing increased side effects and toxicity

(Volz, H.P. et al., Pharmacopsychiatry 30(1), 1–5, 1997; Wong, A.H. et al., Arch. Gen. Psychiatry 55(11), 1033–1044, 1998; Pittler, M.H. et al., J. Clin. Psychopharm. 20(1), 84–89, 2000)

KUDZU

Alcohol Treatment

From the tropical vine *Radix puerariae*; active ingredients include daidzin, daidzein and puerarin (a β-blocker)

- Animal studies suggest suppression of alcohol intake in rodents; used in humans to treat alcohol intoxication and to decrease alcohol intake (controlled studies not available)

(Keung, W.M. et al. Phytochemistry 47(4), 499–506, 1998)

MELATONIN

Hormone produced by the pineal gland involved in regulation of circadian rhythms

- Dietary supplement in the USA, not regulated by FDA with regard to purity, efficacy or safety; not permitted to be sold in Canada

Sleep Disorders

- Dose: 0.3–10 mg/day (0.3 mg = physiological dose – considered most effective)
- Promotes sleep onset without producing drowsiness; not associated with rebound insomnia or withdrawal effects
- Useful in circadian-based sleep disorders (e.g., jet lag) – can shift circadian rhythms at a rate of 1–2 h/day with taken when physiological plasma levels of melatonin are low (i.e., noon to bedtime)
- Hypnotic effect not fully established, as studies show inconsistent results (due to different populations and variable doses used in trials); shown to decrease sleep latency and increase total sleep time in some studies; may be more effective given 2 h before bedtime, or may exert hypnotic effect only when endogenous concentrations of melatonin are low

Herbal and Natural Products (cont.)

- May be useful in elderly, who have decreased nocturnal secretion of melatonin
- May facilitate withdrawal from benzodiazepines (which can decrease nocturnal melatonin production)
- May be helpful for medically ill patients with insomnia for whom conventional hypnotics may be problematic
- Reported to improve sleep quality in patients with diabetes with high HbA1C concentrations
- Early data suggest it may be beneficial in multidisabled children (with neurological or behavioral disorders) with severe insomnia in doses of 2–10 mg
- Shown to improve sleep efficiency in patients with schizophrenia, in double-blind study
- Adverse effects are rare: abdominal cramps with high doses, fatigue, headache, dizziness and increased irritability; very high doses can exacerbate depression

(Wagner, J. et al., Annals of Pharmacotherapy 32(6), 680–691, 1998; Brown, G.M., CNS Drugs 3(3), 209–226, 1995; Hung, J.C. et al., J. Pediatr. Pharm. Pract. 3, 250–256, 1998; Shamir, E. et al., J. Clin. Psychiatry 61, 373–377, 2000; Chittaranjan Andrade et al. J. Clin. Psychiatry 62:41–45, 2001; Garfinkel, D. 17th Congress of the Intl. Assoc. of Gerontology, July 6, 2001, Vancouver, BC)

Depression

- Used in combination with light therapy in the treatment of seasonal affective disorder

(Lam, R., Psychopharmacology Update 5(9), 2, 1995)

OMEGA 3 POLYUNSATURATED FATTY ACIDS

Contained in fish oil (e.g., mackerel, halibut, salmon), green leafy vegetables, nuts, flaxseed oil and canola oil; may affect cell membrane composition at neuron synapses and interfere with signal transduction; may also affect monoamine oxidase

Bipolar Disorder

- Preliminary double-blind study suggests that bipolar patients who took supplements of fish oil, in addition to their usual medication, had longer remission than those on placebo
- Epidemiological data suggest a relationship between depression and low consumption of fish
- Case reports of induced hypomania, mania or mixed states with supplements of omega 3 fatty acids

(Stoll, A.L. et al., Arch. Gen. Psychiatry 56, 407–412, 1999; Int. Drug. Therapy Newsletter 35(10), 73, 2000; Hibbeln, J.R. Lancet 351, 1213, 1998; Pomerantz, J.M., Drug Benefit Trends 13:6, 2–3, 2001)

Schizophrenia

- Preliminary data suggest a relationship between high consumption of omega 3 fatty acids and less severe symptoms of schizophrenia and decreased symptoms of tardive dyskinesia

(Pomerantz, J.M., Drug Benefit Trends 13(6), 2–3, 2001; Freeman, M.P., Ann. Clin. Psychiatry 12, 159–165, 2000)

SDAT

- Early data suggest a possible relationship between first consumption and decreased dementia risk

(Pomerantz, J.M., Drug Benefit Trends 13(6), 2–3, 2001; Kalmijn, S. et al., Ann. Neurol. 42, 776–782, 1997)

S-ADENOSYL-METHIONINE

Naturally occurring brain methyl group donor in the methylation process, increasing membrane fluidity and influencing both monoamine and phospholipid metabolism; may increase the turnover of serotonin, norepinephrine, and dopamine

Depression

- Dose: 150–2400 mg/day
- Meta-analysis of all studies suggests comparable efficacy to tricyclic antidepressants
- Rapid onset reported; response may depend on folate and vitamin B_{12} levels
- May augment effects of other antidepressants – caution as to increased serotonergic effects; DO NOT COMBINE with MAOIs
- Few adverse effects: nausea with higher doses; may induce mania in bipolar patients

(Fava, M. et al., Psychiatry Research 56, 295–297, 1995; Spillman, M. et al., CNS Drugs 6(6), 416–425, 1996; Pies, R., J. Clin. Psychiatry 61(11), 815–820, 2000)

SDAT

- Contradictory data; improvement in cognition and vigilance reported in some studies

(Spillman, M. et al., CNS Drugs 6(6), 416–425, 1996)

ST. JOHN'S WORT

Active ingredients thought to be the naphthodianthrone, hypericum, hyperforin, and other flavonoids; standardized products contain 0.3% hypericin (approximately equivalent to 2–4 g of dried herb); mechanism of action still unclear, but affects number of systems, including NE, 5-HT$_{1A}$, DA, GABA, and MAO enzymes; suggested to inhibit 5-HT reuptake

Depression

- Dose: 300–1500 mg/day in divided doses
- Meta-analysis of clinical trials suggests efficacy in patients with mild to moderate depression; lack of data regarding long-term use
- Double-blind study suggests lack of efficacy in major depression
- Double-blind study of 250 mg hypericum extract showed equal efficacy to 150 mg imipramine, with fewer adverse effects, in mild to moderate depression
- Adverse effects are rare: GI problems, dry mouth, sedation, fatigue, headache, restlessness, constipation, hair loss, photosensitivity and hypersensitivity reactions; cases of mania and hypomania in bipolar patients, including irritability, disinhibition, agitation, anger, decreased concentration, and disrupted sleep
- Contraindicated in pregnancy, lactation, cardiovascular disease and pheochromocytoma
- Due to possible MAOI activity, use caution with foods containing tyramine and with sympathomimetic or serotonergic drugs
- Interactions
  - Potent inducer of CYP3A4; IA2 and/or the p-glycoprotein transporter; reported to decrease plasma level of cyclosporin, resulting in rejection of transplanted organ; also reported to decrease plasma level of indinavir (57% decrease in AUC), digoxin (25% decrease in AUC), theophylline and warfarin; breakthrough bleeding reported in patients on oral contraceptives; may interact with other drugs metabolized by these enzymes
  - May increase levels of serotonin in the CNS; several cases of serotonin syndrome reported in combination with serotonergic drugs

(Bennett Jr., D.A. et al., Annals of Pharmacotherapy 32(11), 1291–1208, 1998; Wong, A.H. et al., Arch. Gen. Psychiatry 55(11), 1033–1044, 1998; Linde, K. et al., Brit. Med. J. 313, 253–258, 1996; Singer A. et al., J. Pharmacol. Exp. Ther. 290(3), 1363–1368, 1999; Gelenberg, A.J. (ed.), Biolog. Therapies in Psychiatry, 23(6), 22–24, 2000; Woelk, H., Br. Med.J. 321, 536–539, 2000; Shelton, R.C. et al. JAMA 285: 1978–1986, 2001)

Anxiety Disorders

- Efficacy reported in seasonal affective disorder and compulsive anxiety
- Open trial suggests efficacy in obsessive compulsive disorder

(Interview with N.E. Rosenthal, Currents in Affective Illness 17(11), 5–10, 1998; Taylor, L.v.H. et al., J. Clin. Psychiatry, 61(8), 575–578, 2000)

VALERIAN

From the plant *Valeriana officinalis*; active ingredients associated with sedative properties thought to be valepotriates, mono- and sesquiterpenes (e.g., valerenic acid) and pyridine alkaloids; the composition and relative proportions of these compounds vary between species. Interacts with central GABA$_A$ receptors; causes CNS depression and muscle relaxation

Sleep Disorders

- Dose: 200–1200 mg/day
- Two placebo-controlled crossover studies showed improvement in sleep quality, decrease in sleep latency and a decrease in the number of awakenings; response better in females and individuals less than 40 years of age; one study did not show benefit
- Adverse effects rare: include nausea, excitability, blurred vision, headache and morning hangover with higher doses
- Liver dysfunction reported; use with caution in patients with a history of liver disease – periodic liver function tests recommended
- Four cases of hepatotoxicity reported when valerian combined with herbal product, skullcap
- Withdrawal symptoms, including delirium, reported after abrupt discontinuation of chronic use

(Wagner, J. et al., Annals of Pharmacotherapy 32(6), 680–691, 1998)

GLOSSARY

ADHD Attention deficit hyperactivity disorder

Agranulocytosis Reduction of neutrophil white blood cells to very low levels

Akathisia Inability to relax, compulsion to change position, motor restlessness

Akinesia Absence of voluntary muscle movement

Alopecia Hair loss

Amenorrhea Absence of menstruation

Anorexia Lack of appetite for food

Anterocollis Forward spasm of the neck

Anticholinergic Block effects of acetylcholine

Antiemetic Helps prevent nausea and vomiting

Arrhythmia Any variation of the normal rhythm (usually of the heart beat)

Arteriosclerosis Hardening and degeneration of the arteries due to fibrous tissue formation

Arthralgia Pain in the joints

Asterixis Spots before the eyes

Asthenia Weakness, fatigue

Ataxia Incoordination, especially the inability to coordinate voluntary muscular action

Atherosclerosis Degeneration of the walls of the arteries due to fatty deposits

AUC Area under the concentration vs time curve (on graph depicting drug in the plasma after a single dose) – represents the extent of systemic exposure of the body to the drug

Autonomic The part of the nervous system that is functionally independent of thought control (involuntary)

BAD Bipolar affective disorder (manic-depressive illness)

Ballismus Jerking, twisting

Bipolar I Disorder Cyclical mood disorder with depression alternating with mania or mixed mania

Bipolar II Disorder Cyclical mood disorder with depression alternating with hypomania

Blepharospasm Forceful sustained eye closure

BMI (body mass index) Weight (in kg) divided by height (in m^2)

Bradycardia Abnormally slow heart beat

Bruxism Teech clenching, grinding

Cataplexy Loss of muscle tone and collapse

Choreiform Purposeless, uncontrolled sinuous movements,

Choreoathetosis Slow, repeated, involuntary sinuous movements or twitching of muscles

Chronic brain syndrome Irreversible damage to brain cells = dementia

CNS Central nervous system

CNS depression Drowsiness, ataxia, incoordination, slowing of respiration which in severe cases may lead to coma and death

Cortex The external layer (superficial gray matter) of the brain

Coryza "Head cold," acute catarrhal inflammation of nasal mucosa

Cycloplegia Paralysis of accommodation of the eye

CYP Cytochrome P-450 enzymes, involved in drug metabolism

DDAVP Desmopressin acetate

Dermatitis Inflammation of the skin

Diaphoresis Perspiration

Diplopia Double vision

Dysarthria Impaired, difficult speech

Dysgeusia Unpleasant taste

Dyspepsia Pain or discomfort in upper abdomen or chest (gas, feeling of fullness, or burning pain)

Dysphagia Difficulty in swallowing

Dyskinesia Abnormal movements, i.e., twitching, grimacing, spasm

Dystonia Disordered muscle tone leading to spasms or postural change

ECG Electrocardiogram (tracing of electrical activity of the heart muscle)

ECT Electroconvulsive therapy, "shock therapy"

EEG Electroencephalogram (tracing of electrical activity of the brain)

Edema Swelling of body tissues due to accumulation of fluid

Emesis Vomiting

Endocrine A gland that secretes internally, a ductless gland

Endogenous depression Depression from within; in DSM-IV, called major depression

Enzyme Organic compound that acts upon specific fluids, tissues, or chemicals in the body to facilitate chemical action

Enuresis Involuntary discharge of urine

Eosinophilia myalgia syndrome (EMS) Connective tissue disease with eosinophilia and myalgia (Eosinophils are blood cells that are usually in low quantities)

Epigastric Referring to the upper middle region of the abdomen

Epistaxis Nose bleed

Exacerbation Increase in severity of symptoms or disease

Extrapyramidal Refers to certain nuclei of the brain close to the pyramidal tract

Extrapyramidal syndrome	Parkinsonian-like effects of drugs
Fasciculation	Twitching of muscles
Fibrosis	Formation of fibrous or scar tissue
FSH	Follicle stimulating hormone
GABA	Gamma-amino butyric acid; an inhibitory neuro-transmitter
Galactorrhea	Excretion of milk from breasts
GI	Gastrointestinal
Glaucoma	Increased pressure within the eye
Glomerular	Pertaining to small blood vessels of the kidney that serve as filtering structures in the excretion of urine
Gynecomastia	Increase in breast size in males
Histological	Pertaining to microscopic tissue anatomy
Hypercalcemia	An excessive amount of calcium in the blood
Hyperkinetic	Abnormal increase in activity
Hyperpara-thyroidism	Increased secretion of the parathyroid
Hyperreflexia	Increased action of the reflexes
Hypertension	High blood pressure
Hyperthyroid	Excessive activity of the thyroid gland
Hypertrophy	Enlargement
Hypnotic	Inducing sleep
Hypotension	Low blood pressure
Hypothyroid	Insufficiency of thyroid secretion
Induration	Area of hardened tissue
INR	International Normalization Ratio; measures coagulation of blood
Jaundice	Yellow skin caused by excess of bile pigment
Kindling	Epileptogenesis caused by adaptive changes in neurons due to repeated electrical discharges
LDH	Lactic dehydrogenase (an enzyme)
LH	Luteinizing hormone
Libido	Drive or energy usually associated with sexual interest
Limbic system	A system of brain structures common to the brains of all mammals (deals with emotions)
Leukocytosis	Increase in the white blood cells in the blood
Leukopenia	Decrease in the white blood cells in the blood
Locomotor activity	Movement using muscles
MAOI	Monoamine oxidase (an enzyme) inhibitor
Manic depressive psychosis	Conspicuous mood swings ranging from normal to elation or depression, or alternating of the two; in DSM-IV, called bipolar affective disorder
MDD	Major depressive disorder
Micrographia	Decrease in size of handwriting; may be a form of akinesia
Miosis	Constricted pupils

Myalgia	Tenderness or pain in muscles
Mydriasis	Dilated pupils
Narcolepsy	Condition marked by an uncontrollable desire to sleep
Nephritis	Inflammation of the kidneys
Nystagmus	Involuntary movement of the eyeball or abnormal movement on testing
OCD	Obsessive compulsive disorder
Oculogyric crisis	Rolling up of the eyes and the inability to focus
Occipital	In the back part of the head
Ophthalmoplegia	Paralysis of the extraocular eye muscles
Opisthotonus	Arching (spasm) of the body due to contraction of back muscles
Orthostatic hypotension	Faintness caused by suddenly standing erect (leading to a drop in blood pressure)
Palinopsia	Visual perseveration, "tracking" or shimmering
Papilledema	Edema of the optic disc
Paresthesia	Feeling of "pins and needles," tingling or stiffness in distal extremities
Parkinsonism	A condition marked by mask-like facial appearance, tremor, change in gait and posture (resembles Parkinson's disease)
Perioral	Around the mouth
Peripheral neuropathy	Pathological changes in the peripheral nervous system
Petechiae	Small purplish hemorrhagic spots on skin
Photophobia	Sensitivity of the eyes to light
Photosensitivity	Easily sunburned
Piloerection	"Goose-bumps" or hair standing up
Pisa syndrome	A condition where an individual leans to one side
PMS	Premenstrual syndrome
Polydipsia	Excessive thirst
Polyuria	Excessive urination
Postural hypotension	Lowered blood pressure caused by a change in position
Priapism	Abnormal, continued erection of the penis
Prostatic hypertrophy	Enlargement of the prostate gland
Pruritis	Itching
Psychosis	A major mental disorder of organic or emotional origin in which there is a departure from normal patterns of thinking, feeling and acting; commonly characterized by loss of contact with reality
Psychomotor excitement	Physical and emotional overactivity
Psychomotor retardation	Slowing of physical and psychological reactions
Pyloric	Referring to the lower opening of the stomach

Glossary (cont.)

Rabbit syndrome Perioral tremor, particularly of the lower lip

Retardation Slowing

Retrocollis Spasm of neck muscles causing the head to twist up and back

Schizophrenia A severe disorder of psychotic depth characterized by a retreat from reality with delusions and hallucinations

SDAT Senile dementia Alzheimer's type

Sedative Producing calming of activity or excitement

Serotonin syndrome Hypermetabolic syndrome resulting from serotonergic excess. Symptoms include: disorientation, confusion, agitation, tremor, myoclonus, hyperreflexia, twitching, shivering, ataxia, hyperactivity

SIADH Syndrome of inappropriate secretion of antidiuretic hormone

Sialorrhea Excessive flow of saliva

Somnambulism Sleep-walking

Stereotypic Rhythmic and repetitive

Syncope A sudden loss of strength or fainting

Tachycardia Abnormally rapid heart rate

Tachyphylaxis Tolerance to effects

Tardive dyskinesia Persistent dyskinetic movements that appear late in neuroleptic therapy

Tardive dystonia Persistent abnormal muscle tone that appears late in neuroleptic therapy

Therapeutic index Ratio of median lethal dose of a drug to its median effective dose: i.e.,

$$\text{therapeutic index} = \frac{\text{median lethal dose}}{\text{median effective dose}}$$

Tinnitus A noise in the ears (ringing, buzzing, or roaring)

Torticollis Spasm on one side of the neck causing the head to twist

Tortipelvis Twisting of pelvis due to muscle spasm

Tracking A reaction in which the medication leaves the original injection site and moves to another

TRH Thyrotropin-releasing hormone, releases TSH and prolactin

Trismus Severe spasm of the muscles of the jaw resembling tetanus (lock jaw)

TSH Thyroid-stimulating hormone

UGT Uridine diphosphate glucuronosyltransferase enzyme, involved in drug metabolism

Ulceration An open lesion on the skin or mucous membrane

Vasoconstrictor Causes narrowing of the blood vessels

Wernicke-Korsakoff syndrome Syndrome characterized by confusion, ataxia, ophthalmoplegia, recent memory impairment and confabulation

Suggested Readings

ANTIDEPRESSANTS

- Burry, L., Kennie, N. (2000). Withdrawal reactions. *Pharmacy Practice 16(4)*, 46–54.
- Caccia, S. (1998). Metabolism of the newer antidepressants; an overview of the pharmacological and pharmacokinetic implications. *Clin. Pharmacokinetics 34(4)*, 281–302.
- Fava, M. (2001). Augmentation and combination strategies in treatment-resistant depression. *J. Clin. Psychiatry 62 (Suppl. 18)*, 4–11.
- Findling, R.L.(2001). Antidepressant pharmacology of children and adolescents with ADHD. *Int. Drug. Therapy Newsletter 36(12)*, 89–93.
- Gerber, P.E., Lynd, L.D. (1998). Selective serotonin-reuptake inhibitor-induced movement disorders. *Annals of Pharmacotherapy 32(6)*, 692–698.
- Greenblatt, D.J., von Moltke, L.L, Harmatz, J.S. et al. (1998). Drug interactions with newer antidepressants: Role of human cytochromes P450. *J. Clin. Psychiatry 58 (Suppl. 15)*, 19–27.
- Kornstein, S.G., McEnany, G. (2000). Enhancing pharmacologic effects in the treatment of depression in women. *J. Clin. Psychiatry 61 (suppl. 11)*, 18–27.
- Montejo, A.L., Llorca, G., Izquierdo, J.A. et al. (2001). Incidence of sexual dysfunction associated with antidepressant agents: A prospective multicenter study of 1022 outpatients. *J. Clin. Psychiatry 62 (suppl. 3)*, 10–21.
- Nelson, J.C. (1997). Safety and tolerability of new antidepressants. *J. Clin. Psychiatry 58 (Suppl. 6)*, 26–31.
- Nelson, J.C. (2000). Augmentation strategies in depression 2000. *J. Clin. Psychiatry 61 (Suppl. 2)*, 13–19.
- Richelson, E. (1996). Synaptic effects of antidepressants. *J. Clin. Psychopharmacology 16(3) (Suppl. 2)*, 1–9.
- Rosen, R.C., Lane, R.M., Menza, M. (1999). Effects of SSRIs on sexual function: A critical review. *J. Clin. Psychopharm. 19(1)*, 67–85.
- Shulman, R.W. (1995). The serotonin syndrome: A tabular guide. *Can. J. Clin. Pharmacology 2(3)*, 139–144.
- Stahl, S.M. (1998). Basic psychopharmacology of antidepressants. Part 1: Antidepressants have seven distinct mechanisms of action. *J. Clin. Psychiatry 59 (Suppl. 4)*, 5–14.
- Sweet, R.A., Brown, E.J., Heimberg, R.G. et al. (1995). Monoamine oxidase inhibitor dietary restrictions: What are we asking patients to give up? *J. Clin. Psychiatry 56(5)*, 196–201.

ELECTROCONVULSIVE THERAPY

- American Psychiatric Association Task Force on Electroconvulsive Therapy (1990). *The practice of electroconvulsive therapy: Recommendations for treatment, training, and privileging*. Washington D.C.: APA.
- Fink, M. (1994). Combining electroconvulsive therapy and drugs: A review of safety and efficacy. *CNS Drugs 1(5), 370–376.*
- Lalla, F.R. & Milroy, T. (1996). The current status of seizure duration in the practice of electroconvulsive therapy. *Can. J. Psychiatry 41(5)*, 299–304.

ANTIPSYCHOTICS

- American Psychiatric Association (1997). Practice guidelines for the treatment of patients with schizophrenia. *Am. J. Psychiatry 154(4) (Apr. Suppl.)*, 1–63.
- Blin, O., Micallef, J. (2001). Antipsychotic-associated weight gain and clinical outcome parameters. *J. Clin. Psychiatry 62 (Suppl. 7)*, 11–21.
- Czekalla, J., Kollack-Walker, S., Beasley, C.M. (2001). Cardiac safety parameters of olanzapine: Comparison with other atypical and typical antipsychotics. *J. Clin. Psychiat. 62 (Suppl. 2)*, 35–40.
- Hoehns, J.D., Stanford, R.H., Geraets, D.R. et al. (2001). Torsades des pointes associated with chlorpromazine: Case report and review of associated ventricular arrhythmias. *Pharmacotherapy 21(7)*, 871–883.
- Hummer, M. & Fleischhacker, W.W. (1996). Compliance and outcome in patients treated with antipsychotics. The impact of extrapyramidal syndromes. *CNS Drugs 5 (Suppl. 1)*, 13–20.

Suggested Readings (cont.)

- Jalenques, I. (1996). Drug-resistant schizophrenia: Treatment options. *CNS Drugs 5(1),* 8–23.
- Javitt, D.C. (2001). Management of negative symptoms of schizophrenia. *Curr. Psychiatry Rep. 3(5),* 413–417.
- Kinon, B.J., Basson, B.R., Gilmore, J.A. et al. (2000). Strategies for switching from conventional antipsychotic drugs or risperidone to olanzapine. *J. Clin. Psychiatry 61,* 833–840.
- Potenza, M.N., McDougle, C.J. (1998). Potential of atypical antipsychotics in the treatment of nonpsychotic disorders. *CNS Drugs 9(3),* 213–232.
- Remington, G.J., Adams, M.E. (1995). Depot neuroleptic therapy: Clinical considerations. *Can. J. Psychiatry 40(3) (Suppl. 1),* 5–11.
- Remschmidt, H., Schulz, E. & Herpertz-Dahlmann, B. (1996). Schizophrenic psychosis in childhood and adolescents: A guide to diagnosis and drug choice. *CNS Drugs 6(2),* 100–112.
- Richelson, E. (1999). Receptor pharmacology of neuroleptics: Relation to clinical effects. *J. Clin. Psychiatry 60 (Suppl. 10),* 5–14.
- Seeman, P., Corbett, R., Van Tol, H.H.M. (1997). Atypical neuroleptics have low affinity for dopamine D_2 receptors or are selective for D_4 receptors. *Neuropsychopharmacology 16(2),* 93–135.
- Simpson, G.M. (2000). The treatment of tardive dyskinesia and tardive dystonia. *J. Clin. Psychiatry 61 (Suppl. 4),* 39–44.
- Stahl, S. (2001). "Hit-and-run" action's at dopamine receptors, Part 1 and Part 2. *J. Clin. Psychiat. 62(9),* 670–671 and *62(10),* 747–748.
- Treatment of schizophrenia: The expert consensus guideline series (1996). *J. Clin. Psychiatry 15 (Suppl. 12B),* 1–58.
- Weiden, P.J., Aquila, R., Emanuel, M. et al. (1998). Long-term considerations after switching antipsychotics. *J. Clin. Psychiatry 59 (Suppl. 19),* 36–49.

ANTIPARKINSONIAN AGENTS

- Barnes, T.R.E. & McPhillips, M.A. (1996). Antipsychotic-induced extrapyramidal symptoms: Role of anticholinergic drugs in treatment. *CNS Drugs 6(4),* 315–330.
- Casey, D.E. (1996). Extrapyramidal syndromes: Epidemiology, pathophysiology and the diagnostic dilemma. *CNS Drugs 5 (Suppl. 1),* 1–12.

ANXIOLYTICS

- Apter, J.T., Allen, LA. (1999). Buspirone: Future directions. *J. Clin. Psychopharmacology 19(1),* 86–93.
- Fulton, B., Brogden, R.N. (1997). Buspirone: An updated review of its clinical pharmacology and therapeutic applications. *CNS Drugs 7(1),* 68–88.
- Labellarte, M.J., Ginsburg, G.S., Walkup, J.T. et al. (1999). The treatment of anxiety disorders in children and adolescents. *Biol. Psychiatry 46(11),* 1567–1578.
- Nelson, J., Chouinard, G. (1999). Guidelines for the clinical use of benzodiazepines: Pharmacokinetics, dependency, rebound and withdrawal. *Can. J. Clinical Pharmacology 6(2),* 69–83.

HYPNOTICS/SEDATIVES

- Lader, M. (1998). Withdrawal reactions after stopping hypnotics in patients with insomnia. *CNS Drugs 10(6),* 425–440.
- Wagner, J., Wagner, M.L., Hening, W.A. (1998). Beyond benzodiazepines: Alternative pharmacological agents for the treatment of insomnia. *The Annals of Pharmacotherapy 32(6),* 680–691.

MOOD STABILIZERS

- Davis, L.L., Ryan, W., Adinoff, B. et al. (2000). Comprehensive review of the psychiatric users of valproate. *J. Clin. Psychopharmacology 20(1) (Suppl. 1),* 1S–17S.
- Dunner, D.L. (2000). Optimizing lithium treatment. *J. Clin. Psychiatry 61 (Suppl. 9),* 76–81.
- Goldberg, J.F. (2000). Treatment guidelines: Current and future management of bipolar disorder. *J. Clin. Psychiatry 61 (Suppl. 13),* 12–18.
- Hebert, A.A., Ralston, J.P. (2001). Cutaneous reactions to anticonvulsant medications. *J. Clin. Psychiatry 62 (Suppl. 14),* 22–26.
- Knowles, S.R. (1999). Adverse effects of antiepileptics. *Canadian J. Clinical Pharmacology 6(3),* 137–148.
- McDonald, W.M. (2000). Epidemiology, etiology and treatment of geriatric mania. *J. Clin. Psychiatry 61 (Suppl. 13),* 3–11.

- Swann, A.C. (2001). Major system toxicities and side effects of anticonvulsants. *J. Clin. Psychiatry 62 (Suppl. 14)*, 16–21.
- Yonkers, K.A., Little, B.B., March, D. (1998). Lithium during pregnancy; drug effects and their therapeutic implications. *CNS Drugs 9(4)*, 261–269.

PSYCHOSTIMULANTS

- Biederman, J. (1998). Attention-Deficit/Hyperactivity Disorder: A life-span perspective. *J. Clin. Psychiatry 59 (Suppl. 7)*, 4–16.
- Wender, P.H., Wolf, L.E., Wasserstein, J. (2001). Adults with ADHD. An overview. *Ann. N.Y. Acad. Sci. 931*, 1–16.

COGNITION ENHANCERS

- Bryson, H.M., Benfield, P. (1997). Donepezil. *Drugs & Aging 10(3)*, 234–239.
- Flynn, B.L. (1999). Pharmacologic management of Alzheimer Disease, Part I: Hormonal and emerging investigational drug therapies. *The Annals of Pharmacotherapy 33*, 178–187.
- Flynn, B.L., Ranno, A.E. (1999). Pharmacologic management of Alzheimer Disease, Part II: Antioxidants, antihypertensives and ergoloid derivatives. *The Annals of Pharmacotherapy 33*, 188–197.
- McGuffey, E.C. (1997). Alzheimer's disease: An overview for the pharmacist. *J. Am. Pharmaceutical Assoc. NS37(3)*, 347–352.
- Naranjo, C.A., Best, T.S. (1998). Advances in the pharmacotherapy of cognitive deficits in dementia. *Can. J. Clin. Pharmacology 5(2)*, 98–109.
- Schneider, L.S. (1998). New therapeutic approaches to cognitive impairment. *J. Clin. Psychiatry 59 (Suppl. 11)*, 8–13.

SEX-DRIVE DEPRESSANTS

- Bradford, J.M. (2001). The neurobiology, neuropharmacology and pharmacological treatment of the paraphilias and compulsive sexual behaviour. *Can. J. Psychiatry 46(1)*, 26–34.

DRUGS OF ABUSE

- Anton, R.F. (2001). Pharmacologic approaches to the management of alcoholism. *J. Clin. Psychiatry 62 (Suppl. 20)*, 11–17.
- Buck, M.L. (2000). Managing iatrogenic opioid dependence with methadone. *Pediatric Pharmacotherapy 6(7)*, 1–7.
- Naranjo, C.A., Bremner, K.E. (1994). Pharmacotherapy of substance use disorders. *Can. J. Clin. Pharmacology 1(2)*, 55–71.
- Schwartz, R.H., Milteer, R. (2000). Drug-facilitated sexual assault ("date rape"). *South Medical J. 93(6)*, 558–561.
- Soyka, M. (1996). Dual diagnosis in patients with schizophrenia: Issues in pharmacological treatment. *CNS Drugs 5(6)*, 414–425.
- Swift, R.M. (2001). Can medication successfully treat substance addiction? *Psychopharmacology Update 12(1)*, 4–5.

NEW TREATMENTS OF PSYCHIATRIC DISORDERS

- Reneric, J.-P., Bouvard, M.P. (1998). Opioid receptor antagonists in psychiatry: Beyond drug addiction. *CNS Drugs 10(5)*, 365–382.

MISCELLANEOUS

- Ackerman, S., Nolan, L.S. (1998). Body weight gain induced by psychotropic drugs: Incidence, mechanisms, and management. *CNS Drugs 9(2)*, 135–151.
- Cohen, L.S., Rosenbaum, J.F. (1998). Psychotropic drug use during pregnancy: Weighing the risks. *J. Clin. Psychiatry 59 (Suppl. 2)*, 18–28.
- Lin, K.-M. (2001). Biological differences in depression and anxiety across races and ethnic groups. *J. Clin. Psychiatry 62 (Suppl. 13)*, 13–19.
- Herrmann, N., Lanctôt, K.L. & Naranjo, C.A. (1996). Behavioural disorders in demented elderly patients. *Current Issues in Pharmacotherapy 6(4)*, 280–300.
- Llewellyn, A., Stowe, Z.N. (1998). Psychotropic medication in lactation. *J. Clin. Psychiatry 59 (Suppl. 2)*, 41–52.
- Rasmussen, S.A., Eisen, J.L. (1997). Treatment strategies for chronic and refractory obsessive-compulsive disorder. *J. Clin. Psychiatry 58 (Suppl. 13)*, 9–13.
- Spiqset, O., Hagg, S. (1998). Excretion of psychotropic drugs into breast-milk: Pharmacokinetic overview and therapeutic implications. *CNS Drugs 9(2)*, 111–134.
- Szabodi, E. ,Tavernor, S. (1999). Hypo- and hypersalivation induced by psychoactive drugs. *CNS Drugs 11(6)*, 449–466.

Suggested Readings (cont.)

HERBAL AND NATURAL PRODUCTS

- Facts and Comparisons. The Review of Natural Products (updated loose-leaf binder). Facts and Comparisons Publ., St. Louis, MO.
- Wong, A.H., Smith, M., Boon, M.S. (1998). Herbal remedies in psychiatric practice. *Arch. Gen. Psychiatry 55(11),* 1033–1044.
- Pies, R. (2000). Adverse neuropsychiatric reactions to herbal and over-the-counter "antidepressants." *J. Clin. Psychiatry 61(11),* 815–820.

Index of Drugs*

*Page numbers in **bold type** indicate main entries.

Index of Drugs (cont.)

Index of Drugs (cont.)

Index of Drugs (cont.)

Patient Information Sheets

This section in the *Clinical Handbook of Psychotropic Drugs* contains information that may be passed on to patients about some of the most frequently used psychotropic medications. The sheets reproduced on the following pages, designed to be easily understood by patients, give details on such matters as the uses of the drug, how quickly it starts working, how long it should be taken, side effects and what to do if they occur, what to do if a dose is forgotten, drug interactions, and precautions. Information sheets such as these of course cannot replace a proper consultation with and advice from the physician or other medical professional, but can serve as a useful tool to enhance compliance, improve efficacy, and enhance safety. The authors and the publisher would welcome feedback and suggestions from readers (for contact addresses, see the front of the book). Information sheets are included here on the drugs and classes of drug shown at the right.

Registered users can download the patient information sheets (as Adobe Acrobat® PDF files) in a form suitable for printing and handing out directly to patients from our Web site, at the address www.hhpub.com/psychotropic-drugs. There is a one-time registration fee of US $50.00, which entitles the user to unlimited access until a new edition is released. To obtain your user name and password, simply fill in the form below.

Contents

PATIENT INFORMATION on SELECTIVE SEROTONIN REUPTAKE INHIBITOR (SSRI) ANTIDEPRESSANTS

The name of your medication is ______________________________.

Use

SSRI antidepressants are used in the treatment of a number of disorders including:

- Major depressive disorder, depression associated with Manic Depressive Illness (Bipolar Disorder)
- Obsessive compulsive disorder
- Panic disorder
- Bulimia
- Social phobia

These drugs have also been found effective in several other disorders, including dysthymia, premenstrual dysphoria or depression, post-traumatic stress disorder and impulsive behavior, though they are currently not approved for these indications.

How quickly will the drug start working?

Antidepressants begin to improve sleep and appetite and to increase energy within about one week; however, feelings of depression may take from 4 to 6 weeks to improve. Because antidepressants take time to work, **do not decrease or increase the dose or stop the medication** without discussing this with your doctor.

Improvement in symptoms of obsessive compulsive disorder, panic disorder and bulimia also occur gradually.

How long should you take this medication?

Following the first episode of depression it is recommended that antidepressants be continued for a minimum of one year; this decreases the chance of being ill again. The doctor may then decrease the drug slowly and monitor for any symptoms of depression; if none occur, the drug can gradually be stopped.

For individuals who have had several episodes of depression, antidepressant medication should be continued indefinitely.

DO NOT STOP taking your medication if you are feeling better, without first discussing this with your doctor.

Long-term treatment is generally recommended for obsessive compulsive disorder, panic disorder and bulimia.

Side effects

Side effects occur, to some degree, with all medication. They are usually not serious and do not occur in all individuals. They may sometimes occur before beneficial effects of the medication are noticed. If a side effect continues, speak to your doctor about appropriate treatment.

Common side effects that should be reported to your doctor at the next appointment include:

- Drowsiness and lethargy – This problem goes away with time. Use of other drugs that make you drowsy will worsen the problem. Avoid driving a car or operating machinery if drowsiness persists.
- Energizing/agitated feeling – Some individuals may feel nervous or have difficulty sleeping for a few days after starting this medication. Report this to your doctor; he/she may advise you to take the medication in the morning.
- Headache – This tends to be temporary and can be managed by taking analgesics (aspirin, acetaminophen) when required.
- Nausea or heartburn – If this happens, take the medication with food.
- Muscle tremor, twitching – Speak to your doctor as this may require an adjustment in your dosage.
- Changes in sex drive or sexual performance – Discuss this with your doctor.
- Blurred vision – This usually occurs at start of treatment and tends to be temporary. Reading under a bright light or at a distance may help; a magnifying glass can be of temporary use. If the problem continues, advise your doctor.
- Dry mouth – Sour candy and sugarless gum help increase saliva in your mouth; try to avoid sweet, calorie-laden beverages. Drink water and brush your teeth regularly.
- Constipation – Increase bulk foods in your diet (e.g., salads, bran) and drink plenty of fluids. Some individuals find a bulk laxative (e.g., Metamucil, Fibyrax) or a stool softener (Colace, Surfak) helps regulate their bowels. If these remedies are not effective, consult your doctor or pharmacist.
- Nightmares – Can be managed by changing the dosing schedule.
- Loss of appetite.

Rare side effects you should report to your doctor **IMMEDIATELY** include:

- Soreness of the mouth, gums, or throat
- Skin rash or itching, swelling of the face
- Any unusual bruising or bleeding
- Nausea, vomiting, loss of appetite, lethargy, weakness, fever, or flu-like symptoms

- Yellow tinge in the eyes or to the skin; dark-colored urine
- Inability to pass urine (more than 24 hours)
- Tingling in the hands and feet, severe muscle twitching
- Severe agitation or restlessness
- Switch in mood to an unusual state of happiness, excitement, irritability, or a marked disturbance in sleep

Let your doctor know **as soon as possible** if you miss your period or suspect you may be **pregnant**.

What should you do if you forget to take a dose of your medication?

If you take your total dose of antidepressant in the morning and you forget to take it for more than 6 hours, skip the missed dose and continue with your schedule the next day. **DO NOT DOUBLE THE DOSE**. If you take the drug several times a day, take the missed dose when you remember, then continue with your regular schedule.

Interactions with other medication

Because SSRI antidepressant drugs can change the effect of other medication, or may be affected by other medication, always check with your doctor or pharmacist before taking other drugs, including over-the-counter medication such as cold remedies. Always inform any doctor or dentist that you see that you are taking an antidepressant drug.

Precautions

1. Do not increase or decrease your dose without consulting your doctor.
2. Take your drug with meals or with water, milk, orange or apple juice; avoid grapefruit juice as it may interfere with the effect of the drug.
3. This drug may impair the mental and physical abilities required for driving a car or operating machinery. Avoid these activities if you feel drowsy or slowed down.
4. This drug may increase the effects of alcohol, making you more sleepy, dizzy and lightheaded.
5. Do not stop your drug suddenly as this may result in withdrawal symptoms such as muscle aches, chills, tingling in your hands or feet, nausea, vomiting, and dizziness.
6. Report any changes in mood or behavior to your physician.
7. This drug may interact with medication prescribed by your dentist, so let him/her know the name of the drug you are taking.
8. Store your medication in a clean, dry area at room temperature. Keep all medication out of the reach of children.

If you have any questions regarding this medication, do not hesitate to contact your doctor, pharmacist, or nurse.

PATIENT INFORMATION on the ANTIDEPRESSANT BUPROPION

Bupropion belongs to a class of antidepressants called Selective Norepinephrine Dopamine Reuptake Inhibitors (NDRI).

Use

Bupropion is primarily used in the treatment of Major Depressive Disorders and depression associated with Manic Depressive Illness (Bipolar Disorder). It has also been approved in the management of smoking cessation.

Though not approved for these indications, bupropion has also been found useful in children and adults with Attention Deficit Hyperactivity Disorder, and has been used as an add-on treatment to increase the effects of other classes of antidepressants.

How quickly will the drug start working?

Bupropion is usually prescribed twice a day, morning and evening. It begins to improve sleep and appetite and to increase energy within about one week; however, feelings of depression may take from 4–6 weeks to improve. Because antidepressants take time to work, **do not decrease or increase the dose or stop the medication** without discussing this with your doctor. Improvement in smoking cessation/withdrawal also occurs over a period of 6 weeks.

How long should you take this medication?

Following the first episode of depression it is recommended that antidepressants be continued for a minimum of one year; this decreases the chance of being ill again. The doctor may then decrease the drug slowly and monitor for any symptoms of depression; if none occur, the drug can gradually be stopped.

For individuals who have had several episodes of depression, antidepressant medication should be continued indefinitely.

DO NOT STOP taking your medication if you are feeling better, without first discussing this with your doctor.

Use of bupropion for smoking cessation is recommended as a one-time treatment for a period of 6 weeks.

Side effects

Side effects occur, to some degree, with all medication. They are usually not serious and do not occur in all individuals. They may sometimes occur before beneficial effects of the medication are noticed. If a side effect continues, speak to your doctor about appropriate treatment.

Common side effects that should be reported to your doctor at the next appointment include:

- Energizing/agitated feeling – Some individuals may feel nervous or have difficulty sleeping for a few days after starting this medication. Report this to your doctor; he/she may advise you to take the medication in the morning.
- Vivid dreams or nightmares – This can occur at the start of treatment.
- Headache – This can be managed by taking analgesics (e.g., aspirin, acetaminophen) as required. If the headache persists or is "troubling" contact your doctor.
- Muscle tremor, twitching – Speak to your doctor as this may require an adjustment in your dosage.
- Nausea or heartburn – If this happens, take the medication with food.
- Loss of appetite.
- Dry mouth – Sour candy and sugarless gum help increase saliva in your mouth; try to avoid sweet, calorie-laden beverages. Drink water and brush your teeth regularly.
- Sweating – You may sweat more than usual; frequent showering, use of deodorants and talcum powder may help.
- Blood pressure – A slight increase in blood pressure can occur with this drug. If you are taking medication for high blood pressure, tell your doctor, as this medication may have to be adjusted.

Rare side effects you should report to your doctor **IMMEDIATELY** include:

- Persistent, troubling headache
- Seizures; these usually occur with high doses – should you have a seizure, stop taking your drug and contact your physician
- Chest pain, shortness of breath
- Soreness of the mouth, gums, or throat
- Skin rash or itching, swelling of the face
- Nausea, vomiting, loss of appetite, lethargy, weakness, fever, or flu-like symptoms
- Muscle pain and tenderness or joint pain accompanied by fever and rash
- Yellow tinge in the eyes or to the skin; dark-colored urine
- Tingling in the hands and feet, severe muscle twitching
- Severe agitation or restlessness
- **Switch in mood to an unusual state of happiness, excitement, irritability, or a marked disturbance in sleep**

Let your doctor know **as soon as possible** if you miss your period or suspect you may be **pregnant**.

What should you do if you forget to take a dose of your medication?

If you forget to take the morning dose of antidepressant by more than 4 hours, skip the missed dose and continue with your schedule for the evening dose. **DO NOT DOUBLE THE DOSE** as seizures may occur.

Interactions with other medication

Because antidepressant drugs can change the effect of other medication, or may be affected by other medication, always check with your doctor or pharmacist before taking other drugs, including over-the-counter medication such as cold remedies. Always inform any doctor or dentist that you see that you are taking an antidepressant drug.

Precautions

1. Do not increase or decrease your dose without consulting your doctor.
2. Do not chew or crush the tablet, but swallow it whole.
3. If you have been advised by your doctor to break a bupropion sustained release tablet in half, do so just prior to taking your medication; discard the second half unless you can use it within 24 hours (store the half tablet in a tightly-closed container away from light).
4. Do not stop your drug suddenly as this may result in withdrawal symptoms such as muscle aches, chills, tingling in your hands or feet, nausea, vomiting, and dizziness.
5. Report any changes in mood or behavior to your physician.
6. This drug may interact with medication prescribed by your dentist, so let him/her know the name of the drug you are taking.
7. Store your medication in a clean, dry area at room temperature and away from high humidity. Keep all medication out of the reach of children.

If you have any questions regarding this medication, do not hesitate to contact your doctor, pharmacist, or nurse.

PATIENT INFORMATION on the ANTIDEPRESSANT VENLAFAXINE

Venlafaxine belongs to a class of antidepressants called Selective Serotonin and Norepinephrine Reuptake Inhibitors (SNRI).

Use

Venlafaxine is primarily used in the treatment of Major Depressive Disorders, depression associated with Manic Depressive Illness (Bipolar Disorder) and for Generalized Anxiety Disorder.

Though not approved for these indications, venlafaxine has also been found effective in several other disorders including obsessive compulsive disorder, panic disorder, social phobia, premenstrual dysphoria and in children and adults with Attention Deficit Hyperactivity Disorder.

How quickly will the drug start working?

Venlafaxine begins to improve sleep and appetite and to increase energy within about one week; however, feelings of depression may take from 4 to 6 weeks to improve. Because antidepressants take time to work, **do not decrease or increase the dose or stop the medication** without discussing this with your doctor.

Improvement in symptoms of obsessive compulsive disorder, panic disorder and social phobia also occur gradually over several weeks.

How long should you take this medication?

Following the first episode of depression it is recommended that antidepressants be continued for a minimum of one year; this decreases the chance of being ill again. The doctor may then decrease the drug slowly and monitor for any symptoms of depression; if none occur, the drug can gradually be stopped. For individuals who have had several episodes of depression, antidepressant medication should be continued indefinitely.

DO NOT STOP taking your medication if you are feeling better, without first discussing this with your doctor.

Long-term treatment is generally recommended for obsessive compulsive disorder, panic disorder, and social phobia.

Side effects

Side effects occur, to some degree, with all medication. They are usually not serious and do not occur in all individuals. They may sometimes occur before beneficial effects of the medication are noticed. If a side effect continues, speak to your doctor about appropriate treatment.

Common side effects that should be reported to your doctor at the next appointment include:

- Energizing/agitated feeling – Some individuals may feel nervous or have difficulty sleeping for a few days after starting this medication. Report this to your doctor; he/she may advise you to take the medication in the morning.
- Headache – This can be managed by taking analgesics (e.g., aspirin, acetaminophen) as required. If the headache persists or is "troubling" contact your doctor.
- Nausea or heartburn – If this happens, take the medication with food.
- Dry mouth – Sour candy and sugarless gum help increase saliva in your mouth; try to avoid sweet, calorie-laden beverages. Drink water and brush your teeth regularly.
- Constipation – Increase bulk foods in your diet (e.g., salads, bran) and drink plenty of fluids. Some individuals find a bulk laxative (e.g., Metamucil, Fibyrax) or a stool softener (Colace, Surfak) helps regulate their bowels. If these remedies are not effective, consult your doctor or pharmacist.
- Sweating – You may sweat more than usual; frequent showering, use of deodorants and talcum powder may help.
- Blood pressure – A slight increase in blood pressure can occur with this drug. If you are taking medication for high blood pressure, tell your doctor, as this medication may have to be adjusted.
- Changes in sex drive or sexual performance – Discuss this with your doctor.

Rare side effects you should report to your doctor **IMMEDIATELY** include:

- Persistent, troubling headache
- Soreness of the mouth, gums, or throat
- Skin rash or itching, swelling of the face
- Nausea, vomiting, loss of appetite, lethargy, weakness, fever, or flu-like symptoms
- Yellow tinge in the eyes or to the skin; dark-colored urine
- Tingling in the hands and feet, severe muscle twitching
- Severe agitation or restlessness
- **Switch in mood to an unusual state of happiness, excitement, irritability, or a marked disturbance in sleep**

Let your doctor know **as soon as possible** if you miss your period or suspect you may be **pregnant**.

What should you do if you forget to take a dose of your medication?

If you take your total dose of antidepressant in the morning and you forget to take it for more than 6 hours, skip the missed dose and continue with your schedule the next day. **DO NOT DOUBLE THE DOSE**. If you take the drug several times a day, take the missed dose when you remember, then continue with your regular schedule.

Interactions with other medication

Because antidepressant drugs can change the effect of other medication, or may be affected by other medication, always check with your doctor or pharmacist before taking other drugs, including over-the-counter medication such as cold remedies. Always inform any doctor or dentist that you see that you are taking an antidepressant drug.

Precautions

1. Do not increase or decrease your dose without consulting your doctor.
2. Do not chew or crush the sustained-release tablet (Effexor XR), but swallow it whole.
3. This drug may impair the mental and physical abilities required for driving a car or operating machinery. Avoid these activities if you feel drowsy or slowed down.
4. This drug may increase the effects of alcohol, making you more sleepy, dizzy and lightheaded.
5. Do not stop your drug suddenly as this may result in withdrawal symptoms such as muscle aches, chills, tingling in your hands or feet, nausea, vomiting, and dizziness.
6. Report any changes in mood or behavior to your physician.
7. This drug may interact with medication prescribed by your dentist, so let him/her know the name of the drug you are taking.
8. Store your medication in a clean, dry area at room temperature. Keep all medication out of the reach of children.

If you have any questions regarding this medication, do not hesitate to contact your doctor, pharmacist, or nurse.

PATIENT INFORMATION on SEROTONIN-2 ANTAGONIST/REUPTAKE INHIBITOR (SARI) ANTIDEPRESSANTS

The name of your medication is ____.

Use

SARI antidepressants are used in the treatment of Major Depressive Disorder and depression associated with Manic Depressive Illness (Bipolar Disorder). These drugs have also been found effective in several other disorders including dysthymia, premenstrual dysphoria or depression and impulsive behavior, though they are currently not approved for these indications.

How quickly will the drug start working?

Antidepressants begin to improve sleep and appetite and to increase energy within about one week; however, feelings of depression may take from 4–6 weeks to improve. Because antidepressants take time to work, **do not decrease or increase the dose or stop the medication** without discussing this with your doctor. Improvement in symptoms of premenstrual dysphoria or impulsive behavior also occur gradually.

How long should you take this medication?

Following the first episode of depression it is recommended that antidepressants be continued for a minimum of one year; this decreases the chance of being ill again. The doctor may then decrease the drug slowly and monitor for any symptoms of depression; if none occur, the drug can gradually be stopped. For individuals who have had several episodes of depression, antidepressant medication should be continued indefinitely.

DO NOT STOP taking your medication if you are feeling better, without first discussing this with your doctor.

Side effects

Side effects occur, to some degree, with all medication. They are usually not serious and do not occur in all individuals. They may sometimes occur before beneficial effects of the medication are noticed. If a side effect continues, speak to your doctor about appropriate treatment.

Common side effects that should be reported to your doctor at the next appointment include:

- Drowsiness and lethargy – This problem goes away with time. Use of other drugs that make you drowsy will worsen the problem. Avoid driving a car or operating machinery if drowsiness persists.
- Energizing/agitated feeling – Some individuals may feel nervous or have difficulty sleeping for a few days after starting this medication.
- Headache – This tends to be temporary and can be managed by taking analgesics (aspirin, acetaminophen) when required.
- Nausea or heartburn – If this happens, take the medication with food.
- Muscle tremor, twitching – Speak to your doctor as this may require an adjustment in your dosage.
- Changes in sex drive or sexual performance – Though rare, should this problem occur, discuss it with your doctor.
- Dry mouth – Sour candy and sugarless gum help increase saliva in your mouth; try to avoid sweet, calorie-laden beverages. Drink water and brush your teeth regularly.
- Loss of appetite.

Rare side effects you should report to your doctor **IMMEDIATELY** include:

- Soreness of the mouth, gums, or throat
- Skin rash or itching, swelling of the face
- Any unusual bruising or bleeding
- Nausea, vomiting, loss of appetite, lethargy, weakness, fever, or flu-like symptoms
- Persistent abdominal pain, pale stools
- Yellow tinge in the eyes or to the skin; dark-colored urine
- Tingling in the hands and feet, severe muscle twitching
- Severe agitation or restlessness
- **Switch in mood to an unusual state of happiness, excitement, irritability, or a marked disturbance in sleep**

Let your doctor know **as soon as possible** if you miss your period or suspect you may be **pregnant**.

What should you do if you forget to take a dose of your medication?

If you take your total dose of antidepressant in the morning and you forget to take it for more than 6 hours, skip the missed dose and continue with your schedule the next day. **DO NOT DOUBLE THE DOSE**. If you take the drug several times a day, take the missed dose when you remember, then continue with your regular schedule.

Interactions with other medication

Because SARI antidepressant drugs can change the effect of other medication, or may be affected by other medication, always check with your doctor or pharmacist before taking other drugs, including over-the-counter medication such as cold remedies. Always inform any doctor or dentist that you see that you are taking an antidepressant drug.

Precautions

1. Do not increase or decrease your dose without consulting your doctor.
2. Take your drug with meals or with water, milk, orange or apple juice; avoid grapefruit juice as it may interfere with the effect of the drug.
3. This drug may impair the mental and physical abilities required for driving a car or operating machinery. Avoid these activities if you feel drowsy or slowed down.
4. This drug may increase the effects of alcohol, making you more sleepy, dizzy and lightheaded.
5. Do not stop your drug suddenly as this may result in withdrawal symptoms such as muscle aches, chills, tingling in your hands or feet, nausea, vomiting, and dizziness.
6. Report any changes in mood or behavior to your physician.
7. This drug may interact with medication prescribed by your dentist, so let him/her know the name of the drug you are taking.
8. Store your medication in a clean, dry area at room temperature. Keep all medication out of the reach of children.

If you have any questions regarding this medication, do not hesitate to contact your doctor, pharmacist, or nurse.

PATIENT INFORMATION on the ANTIDEPRESSANT MIRTAZAPINE

Mirtazapine belongs to a class of antidepressants called Noradrenergic/Specific Serotonergic Antidepressants (NaSSA)

Use

Mirtazapine is primarily used in the treatment of Major Depressive Disorders, depression associated with Manic Depressive Illness (Bipolar Disorder).

Though not approved for these indications, mirtazapine has also been found effective in several anxiety disorders including obsessive compulsive disorder, panic disorder, generalized anxiety disorder, posttraumatic stress disorder and premenstrual dysphoria.

How quickly will the drug start working?

Mirtazapine begins to improve sleep and appetite and to increase energy within about one week; however, feelings of depression may take from 4 to 6 weeks to improve. Because antidepressants take time to work, **do not decrease or increase the dose or stop the medication** without discussing this with your doctor.

Improvement in symptoms of anxiety disorder also occur gradually over several weeks.

How long should you take this medication?

Following the first episode of depression it is recommended that antidepressants be continued for a minimum of one year; this decreases the chance of being ill again. The doctor may then decrease the drug slowly and monitor for any symptoms of depression; if none occur, the drug can gradually be stopped. For individuals who have had several episodes of depression, antidepressant medication should be continued indefinitely.

DO NOT STOP taking your medication if you are feeling better, without first discussing this with your doctor.

Long-term treatment is generally recommended for anxiety disorders.

Side effects

Side effects occur, to some degree, with all medication. They are usually not serious and do not occur in all individuals. They may sometimes occur before beneficial effects of the medication are noticed. If a side effect continues, speak to your doctor about appropriate treatment.

Common side effects that should be reported to your doctor at the next appointment include:

- Drowsiness and lethargy – This problem goes away with time. Use of other drugs that make you drowsy will worsen the problem. Avoid driving a car or operating machinery if drowsiness persists.
- Dry mouth – Sour candy and sugarless gum help increase saliva in your mouth; try to avoid sweet, calorie-laden beverages. Drink water and brush your teeth regularly.
- Constipation – Increase bulk foods in your diet (e.g., salads, bran) and drink plenty of fluids. Some individuals find a bulk laxative (e.g., Metamucil, Fibyrax) or a stool softener (Colace, Surfak) helps regulate their bowels. If these remedies are not effective, consult your doctor or pharmacist.
- Increased appetite and weight gain – Monitor your food intake and try to avoid foods with a high fat content (e.g., cakes and pastry).
- Joint pain or worsening of arthritis – Discuss this with your doctor.

Rare side effects you should report to your doctor **IMMEDIATELY** include:

- Soreness of the mouth, gums, or throat
- Skin rash or itching, swelling of the face
- Nausea, vomiting, loss of appetite, lethargy, weakness, fever, or flu-like symptoms
- Yellow tinge in the eyes or to the skin; dark-colored urine
- Severe agitation or restlessness
- **Switch in mood to an unusual state of happiness, excitement, irritability, or a marked disturbance in sleep**

Let your doctor know **as soon as possible** if you miss your period or suspect you may be **pregnant**.

What should you do if you forget to take a dose of your medication?

If you take your total dose of antidepressant at bedtime and you forget to take your medication, skip the missed dose and continue with your schedule the next day. **DO NOT DOUBLE THE DOSE**. If you take the drug several times a day, take the missed dose when you remember, then continue with your regular schedule.

Interactions with other medication

Because antidepressant drugs can change the effect of other medication, or may

be affected by other medication, always check with your doctor or pharmacist before taking other drugs, including over-the-counter medication such as cold remedies. Always inform any doctor or dentist that you see that you are taking an antidepressant drug.

Precautions

1. Do not increase or decrease your dose without consulting your doctor.
2. This drug may impair the mental and physical abilities required for driving a car or operating machinery. Avoid these activities if you feel drowsy or slowed down.
3. This drug may increase the effects of alcohol, making you more sleepy, dizzy and lightheaded.
4. Do not stop your drug suddenly as this may result in withdrawal symptoms such as muscle aches, chills, tingling in your hands or feet, nausea, vomiting, and dizziness.
5. Report any changes in mood or behavior to your physician.
6. This drug may interact with medication prescribed by your dentist, so let him/her know the name of the drug you are taking.
7. Store your medication in a clean, dry area at room temperature. Keep all medication out of the reach of children.

If you have any questions regarding this medication, do not hesitate to contact your doctor, pharmacist, or nurse.

PATIENT INFORMATION on CYCLIC ANTIDEPRESSANTS

The name of your medication is ____.

Use

Cyclic antidepressants are primarily used in the treatment of major depressive disorders and depression associated with Manic Depressive Illness (Bipolar Disorder).

Certain drugs in this class have also been found effective in several other disorders including obsessive compulsive disorder, panic disorder, bulimia, management of chronic pain conditions (e.g., migraines) and bed-wetting in children.

How quickly will the drug start working?

Antidepressants begin to improve sleep and appetite and to increase energy within about one week; however, feelings of depression may take from 4 to 6 weeks to improve. Because antidepressants take time to work, **do not decrease or increase the dose or stop the medication** without discussing this with your doctor.

Improvement in symptoms of obsessive compulsive disorder, panic disorder and bulimia, pain management and enuresis also occur gradually.

How long should you take this medication?

Following the first episode of depression it is recommended that antidepressants be continued for a minimum of one year; this decreases the chance of being ill again. The doctor may then decrease the drug slowly and monitor for any symptoms of depression; if none occur, the drug can gradually be stopped.

For individuals who have had several episodes of depression, antidepressant medication should be continued indefinitely.

DO NOT STOP taking your medication if you are feeling better, without first discussing this with your doctor.

Long-term treatment is generally recommended for obsessive compulsive disorder, panic disorder, bulimia, pain management and enuresis.

Side effects

Side effects occur, to some degree, with all medication. They are usually not serious and do not occur in all individuals. They may sometimes occur before beneficial effects of the medication are noticed. If a side effect continues, speak to your doctor about appropriate treatment.

Common side effects that should be reported to your doctor at the next appointment include:

- Drowsiness and lethargy – This problem goes away with time. Use of other drugs that make you drowsy will worsen the problem. Avoid driving a car or operating machinery if drowsiness persists.
- Energizing/agitated feeling – Some individuals may feel nervous or have difficulty sleeping for a few days after starting this medication. Report this to your doctor; he/she may advise you to take the medication in the morning.
- Blurred vision – This usually occurs at the start of treatment and tends to be temporary. Reading under a bright light or at a distance may help; a magnifying glass can be of temporary use. If the problem continues, advise your doctor.
- Dry mouth – Sour candy and sugarless gum help increase saliva in your mouth; try to avoid sweet, calorie-laden beverages. Drink water and brush your teeth regularly.
- Constipation – Increase bulk foods in your diet (e.g., salads, bran) and drink plenty of fluids. Some individuals find a bulk laxative (e.g., Metamucil, Fibyrax) or a stool softener (Colace, Surfak) helps regulate their bowels. If these remedies are not effective, consult your doctor or pharmacist.
- Headache – This tends to be temporary and can be managed by taking analgesics (aspirin, acetaminophen) when required.
- Nausea or heartburn – If this happens, take the medication with food.
- Dizziness – Get up from a lying or sitting position slowly; dangle your legs over the edge of the bed for a few minutes before getting up. Sit or lie down if dizziness persists or if you feel faint, then contact your doctor.
- Sweating – You may sweat more than usual; frequent showering, use of deodorants and talcum powder may help.
- Muscle tremor, twitching – Speak to your doctor as this may require an adjustment in your dosage.
- Changes in sex drive or sexual performance – Discuss this with your doctor.
- Nightmares – Can be managed by changing the dosing schedule.

Rare side effects you should report to your doctor **IMMEDIATELY** include:

- Soreness of the mouth, gums, or throat
- Skin rash or itching, swelling of the face
- Nausea, vomiting, loss of appetite, lethargy, weakness, fever, or flu-like symptoms
- Yellow tinge in the eyes or to the skin; dark-colored urine
- Inability to pass urine (more than 24 hours)
- Inability to have a bowel movement (more than 2–3 days)

- Tingling in the hands and feet, severe muscle twitching
- Severe agitation or restlessness
- **Switch in mood to an unusual state of happiness, excitement, irritability, or a marked disturbance in sleep**

Let your doctor know **as soon as possible** if you miss your period or suspect you may be **pregnant**.

What should you do if you forget to take a dose of your medication?

If you take your total dose of antidepressant in the morning and you forget to take it for more than 6 hours, skip the missed dose and continue with your schedule the next day. **DO NOT DOUBLE THE DOSE**. If you take the drug several times a day, take the missed dose when you remember, then continue with your regular schedule.

Interactions with other medication

Because antidepressant drugs can change the effect of other medication, or may be affected by other medication, always check with your doctor or pharmacist before taking other drugs, including over-the-counter medication such as cold remedies. Always inform any doctor or dentist that you see that you are taking an antidepressant drug.

Precautions

1. Do not increase or decrease your dose without consulting your doctor.
2. Take your drug with meals or with water, milk, orange or apple juice; avoid grapefruit juice as it may interfere with the effect of the drug.
3. Avoid taking high-fiber foods (e.g., bran) or laxatives (e.g., psyllium) together with your medication, as this may reduce the antidepressant effect.
4. This drug may impair the mental and physical abilities required for driving a car or operating machinery. Avoid these activities if you feel drowsy or slowed down.
5. This drug may increase the effects of alcohol, making you more sleepy, dizzy and lightheaded.
6. Avoid exposure to extreme heat and humidity since this drug may affect your body's ability to regulate temperature.
7. Do not stop your drug suddenly as this may result in withdrawal symptoms such as muscle aches, chills, tingling in your hands or feet, nausea, vomiting, and dizziness.
8. Report any changes in mood or behavior to your physician.
9. This drug may interact with medication prescribed by your dentist, so let him/her know the name of the drug you are taking.
10. Store your medication in a clean, dry area at room temperature. Keep all medication out of the reach of children.

If you have any questions regarding this medication, do not hesitate to contact your doctor, pharmacist, or nurse.

PATIENT INFORMATION on the ANTIDEPRESSANT MOCLOBEMIDE

The name of your medication is moclobemide. It belongs to a class of antidepressants called RIMA (Reversible Inhibitor of Monoamine Oxidase-A).

Use

Moclobemide is primarily used in the treatment of major depressive disorders and depression associated with Manic Depressive Illness (Bipolar Disorder). It has also been approved in the management of chronic dysthymia. Though not approved for these indications, moclobemide has also been found effective in seasonal affective disorder and social phobia.

How quickly will the drug start working?

Moclobemide begins to improve sleep and appetite and to increase energy within about one week; however, feelings of depression may take from 4–6 weeks to improve. Because antidepressants take time to work, **do not decrease or increase the dose or stop the medication** without discussing this with your doctor. Improvement in symptoms of seasonal affective disorder and social phobia also occur gradually.

When should I take this medication?

Moclobemide is usually prescribed to be taken twice daily, morning and evening. Take this drug after meals to minimize side effects. If a meal is missed, the drug should still be taken, but a large meal should not be eaten for at least 1 hour.

How long should you take this medication?

Following the first episode of depression it is recommended that antidepressants be continued for a minimum of 1 year; this decreases the chance of being ill again. The doctor may then decrease the drug slowly and monitor for any symptoms of depression; if none occur, the drug can gradually be stopped. For individuals who have had several episodes of depression, antidepressant medication should be continued indefinitely.

DO NOT STOP taking your medication if you are feeling better, without first discussing this with your doctor.

Long-term treatment is generally recommended for social phobia; while cyclical therapy may be effective for seasonal affective disorder.

Side effects

Side effects occur, to some degree, with all medication. They are usually not serious and do not occur in all individuals. They may sometimes occur before beneficial effects of the medication are noticed. If a side effect continues, speak to your doctor about appropriate treatment.

Common side effects that should be reported to your doctor at the next appointment include:

- Energizing/agitated feeling – Some individuals may feel nervous or have difficulty sleeping for a few days after starting this medication. Report this to your doctor; he/she may advise you to take the medication in the morning and afternoon (rather than the evening).
- Headache – This can be managed by taking analgesics (e.g., aspirin, acetaminophen) as required. If the headache persists or is "troubling" contact your doctor.
- Dizziness – Get up from a lying or sitting position slowly; dangle your legs over the edge of the bed for a few minutes before getting up. Sit or lie down if dizziness persists or if you feel faint, – then call the doctor.
- Nausea or heartburn – If this happens, take the medication with food.
- Sweating – You may sweat more than usual; frequent showering, use of deodorants and talcum powder may help.

Rare side effects you should report to your doctor **IMMEDIATELY** include:

- Persistent, throbbing headache
- Soreness of the mouth, gums, or throat
- Skin rash or itching, swelling of the face
- nausea, vomiting, loss of appetite, lethargy, weakness, fever, or flu-like symptoms
- Yellow tinge in the eyes or to the skin; dark-colored urine
- Severe agitation or restlessness
- **Switch in mood to an unusual state of happiness, excitement, irritability, or a marked disturbance in sleep**

Let your doctor know **as soon as possible** if you miss your period or suspect you may be **pregnant**.

Treatment with moclobemide does NOT require special diet restrictions as with other MAOI's. However, you should avoid eating excessive amounts of aged, overripe cheeses or yeast extracts. If a **hypertensive reaction** should occur, the symptoms usually come on suddenly, so be alert for these signs:

- Severe, throbbing headache which starts at the back of the head and radiates forward. Often the headache is accompanied by nausea and vomiting
- Neck stiffness
- Heart palpitations, fast heart beat, chest pain
- Sweating, cold and clammy skin
- Enlarged (dilated) pupils of the eyes
- Sudden unexplained nose bleeds

If a combination of these symptoms does occur, **contact your doctor IMMEDIATELY**; if you are unable to do so, go to the Emergency Department of your nearest hospital.

Moclobemide should always be taken after meals to avoid any food-related side effects (e.g., headaches).

What should you do if you forget to take a dose of your medication?

If you take your total dose of antidepressant in the morning and you forget to take it for more than 6 hours, skip the missed dose and continue with your schedule the next day. **DO NOT DOUBLE THE DOSE**. If you take the drug several times a day, take the missed dose when you remember, then continue with your regular schedule.

Interactions with other medication

Because antidepressant drugs can change the effect of other medication, or may be affected by other medication, always check with your doctor or pharmacist before taking other drugs, including over-the-counter medication such as cold remedies. Always inform any doctor or dentist that you see that you are taking the antidepressant drug moclobemide.

Precautions

1. Do not increase or decrease your dose without consulting your doctor.
2. Do not stop your drug suddenly as this may result in withdrawal symptoms such as muscle aches, chills, tingling in your hands or feet, nausea, vomiting, and dizziness.
3. Report any changes in mood or behavior to your physician.
4. This drug may interact with medication prescribed by your dentist, so let him/her know the name of the drug you are taking.
5. Take no other medication (including over-the-counter or herbal products) without consulting with your doctor or pharmacist. Avoid all products containing dextromethorphan.
6. Store your medication in a clean, dry area at room temperature. Keep all medication out of the reach of children.

If you have any questions regarding this medication, do not hesitate to contact your doctor, pharmacist, or nurse.

PATIENT INFORMATION
on
MONOAMINE OXIDASE INHIBITOR (MAOI) ANTIDEPRESSANTS

The name of your medication is ______________________________.

Use

This medication is primarily used in the treatment of major depressive disorders and depression associated with Manic Depressive Illness (Bipolar Disorder). It has also been approved in the management of atypical depression, phobic anxiety states or social phobia.

Though not approved for these indications, MAOIs have also been found effective in dysthymia, panic disorder and obsessive-compulsive disorder.

How quickly will the drug start working?

MAOIs begin to improve sleep and appetite and to increase energy within about one week; however, feelings of depression may take from 4 to 6 weeks to improve. Because antidepressants take time to work, **do not decrease or increase the dose or stop the medication** without discussing this with your doctor.

Improvement in symptoms of atypical depression, phobic anxiety or social phobia, dysthymia, panic disorder and obsessive-compulsive disorder also occur gradually.

How long should you take this medication?

Following the first episode of depression it is recommended that antidepressants be continued for a minimum of one year; this decreases the chance of being ill again. The doctor may then decrease the drug slowly and monitor for any symptoms of depression; if none occur, the drug can gradually be stopped. For individuals who have had several episodes of depression, antidepressant medication should be continued indefinitely.

DO NOT STOP taking your medication if you are feeling better, without first discussing this with your doctor.

Long-term treatment is generally recommended for atypical depression, phobic anxiety or social phobia, dysthymia, panic disorder or obsessive-compulsive disorder.

Side effects

Side effects occur, to some degree, with all medication. They are usually not serious and do not occur in all individuals. They may sometimes occur before beneficial effects of the medication are noticed. If a side effect continues, speak to your doctor about appropriate treatment.

Common side effects that should be reported to your doctor at the next appointment include:

- Drowsiness and lethargy – This problem goes away with time. Use of other drugs that make you drowsy will worsen the problem. Avoid driving a car or operating machinery if drowsiness persists.
- Energizing/agitated feeling – Some individuals may feel nervous or have difficulty sleeping for a few days after starting this medication. Report this to your doctor; he/she may advise you to take the medication in the morning and afternoon (rather than the evening).
- Headache – This can be managed by taking analgesics(e.g., aspirin, acetaminophen) as required. If the headache persists or is "troubling" contact your doctor.
- Dizziness – Get up from a lying or sitting position slowly; dangle your legs over the edge of the bed for a few minutes before getting up. Sit or lie down if dizziness persists or if you feel faint – then call the doctor.
- Nausea or heartburn – If this happens, take the medication with food.
- Dry mouth – Sour candy and sugarless gum help increase saliva in your mouth; try to avoid sweet, calorie-laden beverages. Drink water and brush your teeth regularly.
- Blurred vision – This usually occurs at start of treatment and tends to be temporary. Reading under a bright light or at a distance may help; a magnifying glass can be of temporary use. If the problem continues, advise your doctor.
- Constipation – Increase bulk foods in your diet (e.g., salads, bran) and drink plenty of fluids. Some individuals find a bulk laxative (e.g., Metamucil, Fibyrax) or a stool softener (Colace, Surfak) helps regulate their bowels. If these remedies are not effective, consult your doctor or pharmacist.
- Muscle tremor, twitching, jerking – Speak to your doctor as this may require an adjustment in your dosage.
- Sweating – You may sweat more than usual; frequent showering, use of deodorants and talcum powder may help.
- Loss of appetite.

Rare side effects you should report to your doctor **IMMEDIATELY** include:

- Persistent, throbbing headache
- Soreness of the mouth, gums, or throat
- Skin rash or itching, swelling of the face
- Nausea, vomiting, loss of appetite, lethargy, weakness, fever, or flu-like symptoms

- Yellow tinge in the eyes or to the skin; dark-colored urine
- Inability to pass urine (more than 24 hours)
- Severe agitation or restlessness
- **Switch in mood to an unusual state of happiness, excitement, irritability, or a marked disturbance in sleep**

Let your doctor know **as soon as possible** if you miss your period or suspect you may be **pregnant**.

Caution

Certain foods and drugs contain chemicals which are degraded by the enzyme monoamine oxidase. Since this drug inhibits this enzyme, these chemicals increase in the body and may raise the blood pressure and cause a severe reaction called a **hypertensive crisis**.

Listed below are the foods and drugs which should be **avoided** while taking this drug.

Do not consume the following foods:
- All matured or aged cheeses (Cheddar, Brick, Mozzarella, Parmesan, Blue, Gruyere, Stilton, Brie, Camembert, Swiss, Roquefort)
- Broad bean pods (e.g., Fava Beans)
- Meat extract ("Bovril," "Oxo"), concentrated yeast extracts ("Marmite")
- Sausage (if aged, especially salami, mortadella, pepperoni, pastrami)
- Overripe bananas (especially banana peel), e.g., used in baking banana bread
- Dried salted fish
- Sauerkraut
- Soya sauce or soybean condiments, tofu
- Tap (draft) beer, alcohol-free beer

A time interval of 14 days should elapse after stopping a MAOI drug before restarting to eat the above foods.

Hypertensive reactions have been reported, by some individuals, with the following foods; try small portions to determine if these foods will cause a reaction:
- Pickled herring, smoked fish, caviar, snails, tinned fish, shrimp paste
- Sour cream, yogurt
- Meat tenderizers
- Homemade red wine, Chianti, canned/bottled beer, sherry, champagne
- Tea, coffee, cola
- Tinned and packet soup (especially miso)
- Sausage: bologna, summer sausage, or other unrefrigerated fermented meats; game meat that has been hung
- Chocolate
- Overripe fruit, avocados, raspberries
- Oriental foods
- Spinach
- Nuts

It is SAFE to use the following foods, in moderate amounts (only if fresh):
- Cottage cheese, cream cheese, farmer's cheese, processed cheese, Cheez Whiz, ricotta, Havarti, Boursin
- Liver (as long as it is fresh), fresh or processed meats (e.g., hot dogs)
- Spirits (in moderation)
- Soy milk
- Salad dressings
- Worcestershire sauce
- Yeast-leavened bread

Make sure all food is fresh, stored properly, and eaten soon after being purchased. Never touch food that is fermented or possibly "off." Avoid restaurant sauces, gravy and soup.

Do not use the following over-the-counter drugs without prior consultation with your doctor or pharmacist:
- Cold remedies, decongestants (including nasal sprays and drops), some antihistamines and cough medicine
- Narcotic painkillers (e.g., products containing codeine)
- All stimulants including pep-pills (Wake-ups, Nodoz), or appetite suppressants
- Anti-asthma drugs (Primatine P)
- Sleep aids and Sedatives (Sominex, Nytol)
- Yeast, dietary supplements (e.g., Ultrafast, Optifast)

It is SAFE to use:
- Plain ASA (aspirin), acetaminophen (e.g., Tylenol), or ibuprofen (e.g., Motrin, Advil)
- Antacids (e.g., Tums, Maalox)
- Throat lozenges

If a **hypertensive reaction** should occur, the symptoms usually come on suddenly, so be alert for these signs:
- Severe, throbbing headache which starts at the back of the head and radiates forward; often the headache is accompanied by nausea and vomiting
- Neck stiffness
- Heart palpitations, fast heart beat, chest pain
- Sweating, cold and clammy skin
- Enlarged (dilated) pupils of the eyes
- Sudden unexplained nose bleeds

If a combination of these symptoms does occur, **contact your doctor IMMEDIATELY**; if you are unable to do so, go to the Emergency Department of your nearest hospital.

What should you do if you forget to take a dose of your medication?

If you take your total dose of antidepressant in the morning and you forget to take it for more than 6 hours, skip the missed dose and continue with your schedule the next day. **DO NOT DOUBLE THE DOSE**. If you take the drug several times a day, take the missed dose when you remember, then continue with your regular schedule.

Interactions with other medication

Because antidepressant drugs can change the effect of other medication, or may be affected by other medication, always check with your doctor or pharmacist before taking other drugs, including over-the-counter medication such as cold remedies. Always inform any doctor or dentist that you see that you are taking an antidepressant drug.

Precautions

1. Do not increase or decrease your dose without consulting your doctor.
2. Be aware of foods to avoid with this medication.
3. Take no other medication (including over-the-counter or herbal products) without consulting with your doctor or pharmacist. Avoid all products containing dextromethorphan.
4. This drug may interact with medication prescribed by your dentist, so let him/her know the name of the drug you are taking.
5. This drug may impair the mental and physical abilities required for driving a car or operating other machinery. Avoid these activities if you feel drowsy or slowed down.
6. Do not stop your drug suddenly as this may result in withdrawal symptoms such as muscle aches, chills, tingling in your hands or feet, nausea, vomiting, and dizziness.
7. Report any changes in mood or behavior to your physician.
8. Store your medication in a clean, dry area at room temperature. Keep all medication out of the reach of children.

If you have any questions regarding this medication, do not hesitate to contact your doctor, pharmacist, or nurse.

PATIENT INFORMATION
on
ELECTROCONVULSIVE THERAPY (ECT)

Use

ECT is a procedure used primarily to treat patients with severe Depression. It has also been found effective in the manic phase of Manic Depressive Illness (Bipolar Affective Disorder), and in some patients with Schizophrenia.

What is the ECT procedure?

ECT is done after the patient has been given an anesthetic to induce sleep; a muscle relaxant is also given to decrease the effect of the procedure on the muscles, bones and joints.

ECT involves passing a small, controlled electric current between two metal discs (electrodes) which are applied on the surface of the scalp. The two electrodes may be placed on one side of the head for unilateral ECT or on both sides of the forehead for bilateral ECT. The electric current passes between the two electrodes and through part of the brain in order to stimulate the brain; that electrical stimulation induces a convulsion or seizure which usually lasts from 20 to 90 seconds.

The procedure takes approximately 10 minutes from the time the anesthetic is given until its effect wears off. Oxygen is given throughout this time and the patient is monitored continuously by the physician. The treatment is not painful and the electric current and seizure are not felt by the patient.

How does ECT work?

As is the case with many medical treatments, the actual way that ECT relieves symptoms of illness is not totally understood. It is believed that ECT affects some of the chemicals which transfer impulses or messages between nerve cells in the brain, perhaps more strongly and quickly than some medications. The treatment may correct some of the biochemical changes which accompany the illness.

How effective is ECT?

Studies comparing the effectiveness of ECT and drug therapy in depression have consistently shown that ECT is the most effective treatment of depression, especially in patients whose illness does not respond adequately to drug treatment.

The total number of treatments required to get the full benefit from ECT may range from 6 to 20, depending on the patient's diagnosis and response to treatment. In some patients, a response may be evident after 3 treatments, however a full course is generally recommended to obtain a full response. Some patients require periodic treatments to sustain their improvement.

How safe is ECT and what are the potential side effects?

ECT is considered a safe treatment, when given according to modern standards. It has been demonstrated to be safe when given to elderly patients as well as during pregnancy, with proper monitoring. Side effects that can occur include the following:

- Memory – The most common side effect seen following ECT is some degree of memory loss. Recovery from that memory loss begins a few weeks after treatment and is usually complete in most patients after 6 to 9 months. There may be a permanent loss of memory for details of some events, particularly those which occurred some time before and during the weeks the treatment was given. Also, there may be some difficulty learning and remembering new information for a short period after ECT. However, the ability to acquire new memories recovers completely, usually a few months after treatment. A very small number of patients report severe problems with memory that remain for months or years.
- Confusion – Some patients experience a brief period of confusion after waking from the anesthetic.
- Headache – Common, but not usually severe.
- Muscle aches – Usually temporary.
- Increased heart rate and blood pressure – This can occur during treatment and last for several minutes. Monitoring of patients during and following ECT includes temperature, pulse, blood pressure and electrocardiogram (ECG).
- Prolonged seizure – Occurs rarely; seizure activity is monitored during the procedure by an electroencephalogram (EEG). Rarely a patient may have a spontaneous seizure following the ECT.
- Dental injury (e.g., broken teeth) or bone fractures – Occur very rarely.

The risk of death is very rare (2 to 4 per 100,000 treatments) and is similar to that seen with any treatment given under a general anesthetic.

What else do I need to know about the ECT procedure?

1. Ensure that you understand the information that has been provided to you by your doctor or nurse regarding ECT; ask them to explain anything about the treatment which you do not understand.
2. Do not eat or drink anything for approximately 8 hours before each treatment (and nothing after midnight).
3. Any essential medication (e.g., for high blood pressure) which your physician has told you must be taken before ECT, should be swallowed only with a very small sip of water.
4. Any other medication which you usually take in the morning should be withheld until after the ECT procedure.

PATIENT INFORMATION
on
ANTIPSYCHOTIC (NEUROLEPTIC) DRUGS

The name of your medication is ____.

Use

The primary use of this medication is to **treat symptoms of acute or chronic psychosis**, including schizophrenia, mania, psychotic depression, delusional disorders and organic disorders. There are several other uses for these drugs (e.g., Tourette's Syndrome, impulsive/aggressive behavior, etc.)

What symptoms will this drug help control?

Symptoms of psychosis differ between individuals, both as to the type of symptom and severity. Some common symptoms which antipsychotics have been found to help include:

- Hallucinations (e.g., hearing voices, seeing things, smelling odors, feeling unusual body sensations)
- Fixed beliefs, often of a paranoid nature (i.e., someone is persecuting or following you; people are talking about you) or of a gradiose nature (i.e., you are a special or famous person)
- Disorganized thoughts (difficulty in focusing on a thought), or speeded-up thoughts
- Irritability, agitation, hyperexcitement, over-elated mood

Some antipsychotics may also help symptoms of social withdrawal, lack of interest in oneself and in others, and poor motivation.

How quickly will the drug start working?

Antipsychotics begin to relieve agitation and sleep disturbances in about 1 week, help control mood changes in about 2 weeks, and help difficulties in thoughts and awareness in 6–8 weeks; voices (hallucinations) will decrease in intensity and frequency over 2–8 weeks. Feelings of apathy and lack of motivation may decrease gradually over 3–6 months.

Because antipsychotics require time to work, **do not decrease or increase the dose or stop the medication** without discussing this with your doctor.

How long should you take this medication?

Following the first episode of psychosis, it is recommended that antipsychotic medication be continued for at least 1–2 years; this decreases the chance of being ill again.

For individuals that have had a psychotic illness for several years or repeated psychotic episodes, antipsychotic medication should be continued indefinitely. The physician may adjust the dose from time to time.

Preparations of antipsychotics

Antipsychotics are available in different forms:

- Fast-acting injection – To help control symptoms quickly, when the patient is in distress
- Oral liquid – Convenient for individuals who have difficulty swallowing tablets
- Oral tablets – The usual, most common form, e.g., pills, capsules, sublingual tablets
- Long-acting (depot) injection – Convenient for patients who have been stabilized on an oral antipsychotic. An injection is given every 1 to 4 weeks; this eliminates the need for the patient to remember to take his/her medication daily, helps in compliance with treatment and has been shown to lower the risk of relapse.

Side effects

Side effects occur, to some degree, with all medication. They are usually not serious and do not occur in all individuals. Most will decrease or disappear with time. If a side effect continues, speak to your doctor about appropriate treatment.

Common side effects that should be reported to your doctor **IMMEDIATELY** include:

- Muscle spasms, excessive rigidity, shaking, or restlessness. These symptoms can be controlled with antiparkinsonian agents (e.g., Cogentin, Akineton, Kemadrin, etc.)

Common side effects that should be reported to your doctor at the next appointment include:

- Drowsiness and lethargy – This problem usually goes away with time. Use of other drugs that make you drowsy will worsen the problem. Avoid driving a car or operating machinery if drowsiness persists.
- Dizziness – Get up from a lying or sitting position slowly; dangle your legs over the edge of the bed for a few minutes before getting up. Sit or lie down if dizziness persists or if you feel faint, then contact your doctor.
- Dry mouth – Sour candy and sugarless gum help increase saliva in your mouth; try to avoid sweet, calorie-laden beverages. Drink water and brush your teeth regularly.

- Blurred vision – This usually occurs at start of treatment and may last 1–2 weeks. Reading under a bright light or at a distance may help; a magnifying glass can be of temporary assistance. If the problem continues, advise your doctor.
- Constipation – Increase bulk foods in your diet (e.g., salads, bran), drink plenty of fluids, and exercise regularly. Some individuals find a bulk laxative (e.g., Metamucil, Fibyrax) or a stool softener (Colace, Surfak) helps regulate their bowels. If these remedies are not effective, consult your doctor or pharmacist.
- Stuffy nose – Increase humidity. Temporary use of a decongestant nose spray (e.g., Otrivin) may help.
- Weight changes – Monitor your food intake; you may notice a craving for carbohydrates (e.g., sweets, potatoes, rice, pasta), but try to avoid foods with high fat content (e.g., cakes and pastry).
- Nausea or heartburn – If this happens, take the medication with food.
- Breast tenderness, liquid discharge from breasts, or missed periods.
- **Tardive dyskinesia** can occur in some patients who have been treated with neuroleptics, usually for many years. It involves involuntary movements of certain muscles, usually those of the lips and tongue, and sometimes those of the hands, neck, and other parts of the body. Movements initially tend to increase over several years, but then stabilize and in some patients will decrease with time; in a few patients symptoms worsen. Withdrawal of the antipsychotic at the first signs of tardive dyskinesia, or switching to a "second generation" class of drug, improves the chance that this adverse effect with disappear with time. This has to be balanced against the risk of recurrent illness.

Rare side effects you should report to your doctor **IMMEDIATELY** include:
- Skin rash or itching
- Unusual headache, persistent dizziness or fainting
- Nausea, vomiting, loss of appetite, lethargy, weakness, fever, or flu-like symptoms
- Soreness of the mouth, gums, or throat
- Yellow tinge in the eyes or to the skin; dark colored urine
- Inability to pass urine (more than 24 hours)
- Inability to have a bowel movement (more than 2–3 days)
- Fever (high temperature) with muscle stiffness/rigidity
- Increased thirst and/or frequent urinating or loss of bladder control

Let your doctor know **as soon as possible** if you miss your period or suspect you may be **pregnant**.

What should you do if you forget to take a dose of medication?

If you take your total dose of antipsychotic at bedtime and you forget to take it, DO NOT take the dose in the morning, but continue with your schedule the next day. If you take the drug several times a day, take the missed dose when you remember, then continue with your regular schedule.

Interactions with other medication

Because antipsychotic drugs can change the effect of other medication, or may be affected by other medication, always check with your doctor or pharmacist before taking other drugs, including over-the-counter medication such as cold remedies. Always inform any doctor or dentist that you see that you are taking an antipsychotic medication.

Precautions

1. Do not increase or decrease your dose without consulting your doctor.
2. Take your drug with meals or with water, milk or orange juice; avoid apple or grapefruit juice as they may interfere with the effect of the drug.
3. Do not break or crush your medication unless you have been advised to do so by your doctor.
4. This drug may impair the mental and physical abilities required for driving a car or operating machinery. Avoid these activities if you feel drowsy or slowed down.
5. This drug may increase the effects of alcohol, making you more sleepy, dizzy and lightheaded.
6. Avoid exposure to extreme heat and humidity (e.g., saunas) since this drug may affect your body's ability to regulate temperature changes and blood pressure.
7. Antacids (e.g., Gelusil, Maalox, Amphogel, etc.) interfere with absorption of these drugs in your stomach and therefore may decrease their effect. To avoid this, take the antacid at least 2 h before or 1 hour after taking your antipsychotic drug.
8. Some patients may get a serious sunburn with little exposure to sunlight. Avoid direct sun, wear protective clothing and use a sunscreen preparation on exposed areas.
9. Excessive use of caffeinated beverages (coffee, tea, colas, etc.) can cause anxiety, agitation and restlessness and counteract some of the beneficial effects of your medication.
10. Cigarette smoking can change the amount of antipsychotic that remains in your bloodstream; inform your doctor if you make any changes to your current smoking habit.
11. Do not stop your drug suddenly as this may result in withdrawal symptoms such as nausea, dizziness, sweating, headache, sleeping problems, agitation and tremor, and also result in the return of psychotic symptoms.
12. Store your medication in a clean, dry area at room temperature. Keep all medication out of the reach of children.

If you have any questions regarding this medication, do not hesitate to contact your doctor, pharmacist, or nurse.

PATIENT INFORMATION on CLOZAPINE

Clozapine belongs to the class of drugs called **Antipsychotics**.

Use

The primary use of this medication is to **treat symptoms of acute or chronic schizophrenia**; it is used in patients who have not had an adequate response to other antipsychotic drugs. Clozapine has been found effective in other psychotic disorders, including psychosis in Parkinson's Disease, Bipolar Disorder and organic disorders. Though not approved for this indication, it has also been used in the treatment of impulsive/aggressive behavior.

What symptoms will this drug help control?

Symptoms of psychosis differ between individuals, both as to the type of symptom and severity. Some common symptoms which antipsychotics have been found to help include:

- Hallucinations (e.g., hearing voices, seeing things, smelling odors, feeling unusual body sensations)
- Fixed beliefs, often of a paranoid nature (i.e., someone is persecuting or following you; people are talking about you)
- Disorganized thoughts (difficulty in focusing on a thought), or speeded-up thoughts
- Irritability, agitation, hyperexcitement, overelated mood

Clozapine may also help symptoms of social withdrawal, lack of interest in oneself and in others and poor motivation.

How quickly will the drug start working?

Clozapine begins to relieve agitation within a few days, helps control mood changes in about 2 weeks, and help difficulties in thoughts and awareness in 6–8 weeks; voices (hallucinations) will decrease in intensity and frequency over 2–8 weeks. Some patients respond to clozapine gradually over a period of months. Because antipsychotics require time to work, **do not decrease or increase the dose or stop the medication** without discussing this with your doctor.

How long should you take this medication?

For individuals that have had a psychotic illness for several years or repeated psychotic episodes, clozapine should be continued indefinitely. The physician may adjust the dose, from time to time, based on results of blood levels of clozapine and response to treatment.

DO NOT STOP taking your medication if you are feeling better, without first discussing this with your doctor.

Why are blood tests necessary with clozapine, and why is medication given for a week at a time?

A rare side effect (affects less than 1% of people) has been reported with clozapine; it is called **agranulocytosis.** With this side effect, the white cells in the blood decrease in quantity, which makes it difficult for the body to fight off any infections. Because this can result in a serious problem, if identified early, agranulocytosis can be reversed by stopping clozapine. It is therefore necessary to measure the amount of white blood cells in the body on a weekly basis to identify those individuals who may be at risk for agranulocytosis.

After taking clozapine for 6 months, individuals are no longer considered at as great a risk for agranulocytosis and may have their bloodwork done, and be given prescriptions, for 2 weeks at a time.

Side effects

Side effects occur, to some degree, with all medication. They are usually not serious and do not occur in all individuals. Most will decrease or disappear with time. If a side effect continues, speak to your doctor about appropriate treatment.

Common side effects that should be reported to your doctor at the next appointment include:

- Drowsiness and lethargy – This problem usually goes away with time. Use of other drugs that make you drowsy will worsen the problem. Avoid driving a car or operating machinery if drowsiness persists.
- Dizziness – Get up from a lying or sitting position slowly; dangle your legs over the edge of the bed for a few minutes before getting up. Sit or lie down if dizziness persists or if you feel faint, then contact your doctor.
- Dry mouth – Sour candy and sugarless gum help increase saliva in your mouth; try to avoid sweet, calorie-laden beverages. Drink water and brush your teeth regularly.
- Blurred vision – This usually occurs at start of treatment and may last 1–2 weeks. Reading under a bright light or at a distance may help; a magnifying glass can be of temporary use. If the problem continues, advise your doctor.

- Constipation – Increase bulk foods in your diet (e.g., salads, bran), drink plenty of fluids, and exercise regularly. Some individuals find a bulk laxative (e.g., Metamucil, Fibyrax) or a stool softener (Colace, Surfak) helps regulate their bowels. If these remedies are not effective, consult your doctor or pharmacist.
- Excess salivation or drooling – This often occurs at night. Use a towel on the pillow when sleeping. If this also occurs during waking hours or causes choking, speak to your doctor about other remedies.
- Weight gain – Monitor your food intake; you may notice a craving for carbohydrates (e.g., sweets, potatoes, rice, pasta), but try to avoid foods with high fat content (e.g., cakes and pastry).
- Nausea or heartburn – If this happens, take the medication with food.

Rare side effects you should report to your doctor **IMMEDIATELY** include:

- **Soreness of the mouth, gums, or throat**
- **Lethargy, weakness, fever or flu-like symptoms or other signs of infections**
- **Rapid heart beat, chest pain and shortness of breath**
- **Periods of blackouts or seizures**
- Skin rash or itching
- Unusual headache
- Severe or persistent dizziness or fainting
- Increased thirst and/or frequent urinating or loss of bladder control
- Yellow tinge in the eyes or to the skin; dark-colored urine
- Inability to have a bowel movement (more than 2–3 days)
- Worsening of repetitive behavior or obsessional symptoms

Tardive dyskinesia is an adverse effect that has been recognized in some patients who have been treated with antipsychotics, usually for many years. The risk of this adverse effect with clozapine is considered to be low, and clozapine may help in treating this problem. Tardive dyskinesia describes involuntary movements of certain muscles – usually those of the lips and tongue, and sometimes those of the hands, neck and other parts of the body.

Let your doctor know **as soon as possible** if you miss your period or suspect you may be **pregnant.**

What should you do if you forget to take a dose of your medication?

If you take your total dose of antipsychotic at bedtime and you forget to take it, DO NOT take the dose in the morning, but continue with your schedule the next day. If you take the drug several times a day, take the missed dose when you remember, then continue with your regular schedule.

Interactions with other medication

Because clozapine can change the effect of other medication, or may be affected by other medication, always check with your doctor or pharmacist before taking other drugs, including over-the-counter medication such as cold remedies. Always inform any doctor or dentist that you see that you are taking an antipsychotic medication.

Precautions

1. Do not increase or decrease your dose without consulting your doctor.
2. Take your drug with meals or with water, milk or orange juice; avoid grapefruit juice as it may interfere with the effect of the drug.
3. This drug may impair the mental and physical abilities required for driving a car or operating machinery. Avoid these activities if you feel drowsy or slowed down.
4. This drug may increase the effects of alcohol, making you more sleepy, dizzy and lightheaded.
5. Avoid exposure to extreme heat and humidity (e.g., saunas) since this drug may affect your body's ability to regulate temperature changes.
6. Antacids (e.g., Gelusil, Maalox, Amphogel, etc.) interfere with absorption of these drugs in your stomach and therefore may decrease their effect. To avoid this, take the antacid at least 2 hours before or 1 hour after taking your antipsychotic drug.
7. Excessive use of caffeinated beverages (coffee, tea, colas, etc.) can cause anxiety, agitation and restlessness and may affect the blood level of your medication.
8. Cigarette smoking can change the amount of antipsychotic that remains in your bloodstream; inform your doctor if you make any changes to your current smoking habit.
9. Do not stop your drug suddenly as this may result in withdrawal symptoms such as nausea, dizziness, sweating, headache, sleeping problems, agitation and tremor, and also result in the return of psychotic symptoms.
10. Store your medication in a clean, dry area at room temperature. Keep all medication out of the reach of children.

If you have any questions regarding this medication, do not hesitate to contact your doctor, pharmacist, or nurse.

PATIENT INFORMATION on ANTIPARKINSONIAN DRUGS

The name of your medication is ____.

Use

This medication is used to **treat muscle side effects** that some individuals experience when they are being treated with antipsychotic (neuroleptic) drugs. These muscle side effects can include:

- Muscle spasms or contractions (e.g., in the neck, eyes or tongue)
- Muscle stiffness, tremor, or a shuffling walk
- Feeling restless, unable to sit still, having a need to pace
- Muscle weakness or a slowing of movement

How quickly will the drug start working?

Antiparkinsonian drugs can reduce or stop the above side effects, usually within an hour. Sometimes they have to be given by injection for a quicker effect.

How long should you take this medication?

Most patients take antiparkinsonian drugs for 2–3 weeks, usually when first prescribed an antipsychotic drug, and while its dose is being stabilized. The doctor will then reduce the dose of this drug to see if the muscle symptoms return; if not, you may be advised to stop using this medication. **Do not increase the dose or stop the drug without consulting with your doctor.**

Some patients need to use an antiparkinsonian drug for longer time periods, because they are more sensitive to muscle side effects from the antipsychotic drug they are receiving. Others require it only from time to time, i.e., PRN (e.g., for 1 week after receiving an injection of an antipsychotic).

Side effects

Side effects occur, to some degree, with all medication. They are usually not serious and do not occur in all individuals. Most will decrease or disappear with time. If a side effect continues, speak to your doctor about appropriate treatment.

Common side effects that can occur with antiparkinsonian drugs include:

- Dry mouth – Sour candy and sugarless gum help increase saliva in your mouth; try to avoid sweet, calorie-laden beverages. Drink water and brush your teeth regularly.
- Blurred vision – This usually occurs at the start of treatment and may last 1–2 weeks. Reading under a bright light or at a distance may help; a magnifying glass can be of temporary use. If the problem continues, advise your doctor.
- Constipation – Increase bulk foods in your diet (e.g., salads, bran) and drink plenty of fluids. Some individuals find a bulk laxative (e.g., Metamucil, Fibyrax) or a stool softener (Colace, Surfak) helps regulate their bowels. If these remedies are not effective, consult your doctor or pharmacist.
- Drowsiness and lethargy – This problem goes away with time. Use of other drugs that make you drowsy will worsen the problem. Avoid driving a car or operating machinery if drowsiness persists.
- Nausea or heartburn – If this happens, take the medication with food

Less common side effects that you should report to your physician **IMMEDIATELY** include:

- Disorientation, confusion, worsening of your memory, increase in psychotic symptoms
- Inability to have a bowel movement (more than 2–3 days)
- Inability to pass urine (more than 24 hours)
- Skin rash

Let your doctor know **as soon as possible** if you miss your period or suspect you may be **pregnant**

Precautions

1. Do not increase your dose without consulting your doctor
2. Check with your doctor or pharmacist before taking other drugs, including over-the-counter medication such as cold remedies
3. This drug may impair the mental and physical abilities required for driving a car or operating machinery. Avoid these activities if you feel drowsy or slowed down.
4. This drug may increase the effects of alcohol, making you more sleepy, dizzy and lightheaded
5. Avoid exposure to extreme heat and humidity (e.g., saunas) since this drug may affect your body's ability to regulate temperature changes.
6. Store your medication in a clean, dry area at room temperature. Keep all medication out of the reach of children.

If you have any questions regarding this medication, do not hesitate to contact your doctor, pharmacist, or nurse.

PATIENT INFORMATION
on
BENZODIAZEPINE ANTIANXIETY DRUGS (ANXIOLYTICS)

The name of your medication is ______________________________.

Use

This medication is used to **treat symptoms of anxiety.** Anxiety is a universal human response to stress and is considered necessary for effective functioning and coping with daily activities. It may, however, be a symptom of many other disorders, both medical and psychiatric. There are many different types of anxiety and there are many different approaches to treating it. Anxiolytics will help relieve the symptoms of anxiety but will not alter its cause. In usually prescribed doses, they help to calm and sedate the individual; in high doses these drugs may be used to induce sleep.

How quickly will the drug start working?

Anxiolytic drugs can reduce agitation and induce calm or sedation usually within an hour. Sometimes they have to be given by injection, or dissolved under the tongue, for a quicker effect.

How long should you take this medication?

Anxiety is usually self-limiting; often when the cause of anxiety is treated or eliminated, symptoms of anxiety will decrease. Therefore, anxiolytics are usually prescribed for a limited period of time. Many individuals take the medication only when needed (during periods of excessive stress) rather than on a daily basis. Tolerance or loss of effectiveness can occur in some individuals if they are used continuously beyond 4 months. If you have been taking the medication for a continuous period of time, the physician may try to reduce the dose of this drug slowly to see if the anxiety symptoms return; if not, the dosage may be further reduced and you may be advised to stop using this medication. **Do not increase the dose or stop the drug without consulting with your doctor.** Some patients need to use an anxiolytic drug for longer time periods, because of the type of anxiety they may be experiencing. Others require it only from time to time, i.e., as needed.

Side effects

Side effects occur, to some degree, with all medication. They are usually not serious and do not occur in all individuals. Most will decrease or disappear with time. If a side effect continues, speak to your doctor about appropriate treatment.

Common side effects that can occur with anxiolytic drugs include:

- Drowsiness and lethargy – This problem goes away with time, or when the dose is reduced. Use of other drugs that make you drowsy will worsen the problem. Avoid driving a car or operating machinery if drowsiness persists.
- Muscle incoordination, weakness or dizziness – Inform your doctor; an adjustment in your dosage may be needed.
- Forgetfulness, memory lapses – Inform your doctor.
- Slurred speech – An adjustment in your dosage may be needed.
- Nausea or heartburn – If this happens, take the medication with food.

Less common side effects that you should report to your physician **IMMEDIATELY** include:

- Disorientation, confusion, worsening of memory, blackouts or amnesia
- Nervousness, excitement or any behavior changes
- Incoordination leading to falls
- Skin rash

Let your doctor know **as soon as possible** if you miss your period or suspect you may be **pregnant**

Precautions

1. Do not increase your dose without consulting your doctor
2. Take your medication with meals or with water, milk, orange or apple juice. Avoid grapefruit juice as it may interfere with the effects of the drug.
3. Check with your doctor or pharmacist before taking other drugs, including over-the-counter medication such as cold remedies
4. This drug may impair the mental and physical abilities required for driving a car or operating machinery. Avoid these activities if you feel drowsy or slowed down.
5. This drug may increase the effects of alcohol, making you more sleepy, dizzy and lightheaded
6. Do not stop taking the drug suddenly, especially if you have been on the medication for a number of months or have been taking high doses. Anxiolytics need to be withdrawn gradually to prevent withdrawal reactions.
7. Avoid excessive consumption of caffeinated beverages (i.e., more than 4 cups of coffee, 6 cups of tea or cola) as it may counteract the beneficial effects of the anxiolytic.
8. Store your medication in a clean, dry area at room temperature. Keep all medication out of the reach of children.

If you have any questions regarding this medication, do not hesitate to contact your doctor, pharmacist, or nurse.

PATIENT INFORMATION on BUSPIRONE

Buspirone is an anti-anxiety drug (anxiolytic).

Use

Buspirone is used to **treat symptoms of chronic anxiety.** Anxiety is a universal human response to stress and is considered necessary for effective functioning and coping with daily activities. It may, however, be a symptom of many other disorders, both medical and psychiatric. There are many different types of anxiety and there are many different approaches to treating it.

Though not approved for these indications, buspirone has also been found effective in other conditions, including posttraumatic stress disorder, social phobia, body dysmorphic disorder, agitation, irritability, aggression, and antisocial behavior, and as an aid in smoking cessation and alcohol withdrawal. It has been used alone or in combination with antidepressants in the treatment of depression and obsessive compulsive disorder.

How quickly will the drug start working?

Buspirone causes a gradual improvement in symptoms of anxiety and can reduce agitation and induce calm usually within 1 to 2 weeks.

Improvement in symptoms of other disorders, for which buspirone may be prescribed, occur gradually over several weeks.

How long should you take this medication?

Anxiety is usually self-limiting; often when the cause of anxiety is treated or eliminated, symptoms of anxiety will decrease. Therefore, anxiolytics are usually prescribed for a limited period of time. To maintain effectiveness, buspirone cannot be taken only when needed (during periods of excessive stress), but needs to be taken on a daily basis. The physician may try to reduce the dose of this drug to see if the anxiety symptoms return; if not, the dosage may be further reduced and you may be advised to stop using this medication. **Do not increase the dose or stop the drug without consulting with your doctor.** Some patients need to use an anxiolytic drug for longer time periods, because of the type of anxiety they may be experiencing.

Long-term treatment is generally recommended for certain other indications such as social phobia, body dysmorphic disorder or antisocial behavior.

Side effects

Side effects occur, to some degree, with all medication. They are usually not serious and do not occur in all individuals. Most will decrease or disappear with time. If a side effect continues, speak to your doctor about appropriate treatment.

Common side effects that can occur with buspirone include:
- Drowsiness – This problem goes away with time, or when the dose is reduced. Avoid driving a car or operating machinery if drowsiness persists.
- Headache – tends to be temporary and can be managed by taking analgesics (e.g., aspirin, acetaminophen) when required.
- Nausea or heartburn – If this happens, take the medication with food.
- Dizziness, lightheadedness – sit or lie down; if symptoms persist, contact your doctor.
- Energized/agitated feeling – some individuals may feel nervous for a few days after starting this medication. Report this to your doctor.
- Tingling or numbing in fingers or toes – report this to your doctor.

Less common side effects that you should report to your physician **IMMEDIATELY** include:
- Severe agitation, excitement or any changes in behavior.

Let your doctor know **as soon as possible** if you miss your period or suspect you may be **pregnant**

Precautions

1. Do not increase your dose without consulting your doctor
2. Take your medication with meals or with water, milk, orange or apple juice. Avoid grapefruit juice as it may interfere with the effects of the drug.
3. Avoid excessive consumption of caffeinated beverages (i.e., more than 4 cups of coffee, 6 cups of tea or cola) as it may counteract the beneficial effects of the anxiolytic.
4. Check with your doctor or pharmacist before taking other drugs, including over-the-counter medication or herbal remedies.
5. Store your medication in a clean, dry area at room temperature. Keep all medication out of the reach of children.

If you have any questions regarding this medication, do not hesitate to contact your doctor, pharmacist, or nurse.

PATIENT INFORMATION
on
HYPNOTICS/SEDATIVES

The name of your medication is ____.

Use

This medication is used to **treat sleep problems,** such as the inability to fall asleep or to remain asleep for a reasonable number of hours or waking up often during the night. Sleeping problems occur in most individuals from time to time. If, however, sleeping problems persist, this may be a symptom of some other disorder, either medical and psychiatric.

A person may have difficulty in falling asleep because of stress or anxiety felt during the day, pain, physical discomfort or changes in daily routine (e.g., jet lag, changes in work shifts, etc.) Any disease that causes pain (e.g., ulcers) or breathing difficulties (e.g., asthma or a cold) can interfere with continuous sleep. Stimulant drugs, including caffeine, may also contribute to problems falling asleep; other medications may change sleep patterns when they are stopped (e.g., antidepressants, antipsychotics). Sleep will improve when these causes have been identified, corrected, or treated.

Problems remaining asleep may be due to age, as older people tend to sleep less at night. Certain disorders, including depression, may also affect sleep.

Hypnotic/sedatives are similar to antianxiety drugs, but tend to cause more drowsiness and incoordination; therefore, sometimes antianxiety drugs are given to treat sleep problems.

How quickly will the drug start working?

Hypnotics/sedatives can induce calm or sedation usually within an hour. As some drugs act quickly, take the medication just prior to going to bed and relax in bed until the drug takes effect.

How long should you take this medication?

Sleep problems are usually self-limiting; often when the cause of sleep difficulties is treated or eliminated, sleep will improve. Therefore, hypnotic/sedatives are usually prescribed for a limited period of time. Many individuals take the medication only when needed (during periods of insomnia) rather than on a daily basis. It is suggested that once you have slept well for 2 or 3 consecutive nights, try to get to sleep without taking the sedative/hypnotic. Tolerance or loss of effectiveness can occur in some individuals if they are used continuously beyond four months. Individuals taking hypnotics for long periods of time have a risk of developing dependence – they may have difficulty stopping the medication and may experience withdrawal symptoms.

If you have been taking the medication for a continuous period of time, the physician may try to reduce the dose of this drug slowly to see if sleeping problems persist; if not, the dosage may be further reduced and you may be advised to stop using this medication. **Do not increase the dose or stop the drug without consulting with your doctor.**

Some patients need to use a sedative/hypnotic drug for longer time periods, because of the type of problems they may be experiencing. Others require it only from time to time, i.e., PRN.

Side effects

Side effects occur, to some degree, with all medication. They are usually not serious and do not occur in all individuals. Most will decrease or disappear with time. If a side effect continues, speak to your doctor about appropriate treatment.

Common side effects that can occur with sedative/hypnotics drugs include:

- Morning hangover, drowsiness and lethargy – This problem may decrease with time; inform your doctor. Use of other drugs that make you drowsy will worsen the problem. Avoid driving a car or operating machinery if drowsiness persists.
- Muscle incoordination, weakness, lightheadedness or dizziness – Inform your doctor; an adjustment in your dosage may be needed.
- Forgetfulness, memory lapses – Inform your doctor.
- Slurred speech – An adjustment in your dosage may be needed.
- Nausea or heartburn – If this happens, take the medication with food.
- Bitter taste – Can occur with certain drugs (e.g., zopiclone). Avoid milk in the morning to lessen this effect.

Less common side effects that you should report to your physician **IMMEDIATELY** include:

- Disorientation, confusion, worsening of your memory, periods of blackouts, or amnesia
- Nervousness, excitement, agitation, hallucinations or any behavior changes
- Worsening of depression, suicidal thoughts
- Incoordination leading to falls
- Skin rash

Let your doctor know **as soon as possible** if you miss your period or suspect you may be **pregnant.**

Precautions

1. Do not increase your dose without consulting your doctor
2. Check with your doctor or pharmacist before taking other drugs, including over-the-counter medication such as cold remedies
3. Speak to your doctor if you experience sleeping problems after starting any new medication (e.g., for a medical condition)
4. This drug may impair the mental and physical abilities required for driving a car or operating machinery. Avoid these activities if you feel drowsy or slowed down.
5. This drug may increase the effects of alcohol, making you more sleepy, dizzy and lightheaded
6. Take your medication about half an hour before bedtime; do not smoke in bed afterwards.
7. Do not stop taking the drug suddenly, especially if you have been on the medication for a number of months or have been taking high doses. Hypnotics/sedatives need to be withdrawn gradually to prevent withdrawal reactions.
8. Avoid excessive consumption of caffeinated beverages (i.e., more than 4 cups of coffee, 6 cups of tea or cola) as it may counteract the beneficial effects of the anxiolytic.
9. Store your medication in a clean, dry area at room temperature. Keep all medication out of the reach of children.

Some nondrug methods to help you sleep include:

1. Avoid caffeine-containing beverages or foods (e.g., chocolate) after 6 pm and avoid heavy meals several hours before bedtime. A warm glass of milk is effective for some people.
2. Napping and sleeping during the day will make restful sleep at night difficult. Keep active during the day and exercise regularly.
3. Engage in relaxing activities prior to bedtime such a reading, listening to music or taking a warm bath. Strenuous exercise (e.g., jogging) immediately before bedtime may make it difficult to get to sleep.
4. Establish a routine or normal pattern of sleeping and waking.
5. Use the bed and bedroom only for sleep and sexual activity.
6. Minimize external stimuli which might disturb sleep. If necessary, use dark shades over windows or wear ear plugs.
7. Once in bed, make sure you are comfortable (i.e., not too hot or cold); use a firm mattress.
8. Relaxation techniques (e.g., muscle relaxation exercises, yoga) may be helpful in decreasing anxiety and promoting sleep
9. If you have problems getting to sleep, rather than toss and turn in bed, have some warm milk, read a book, listen to music, or try relaxation techniques until you again begin to feel tired.
10. Don't worry about the amount of sleep you are getting as the amount will vary from day to day. The more you worry the more anxious you will get and this may make it harder for you to fall asleep.

If you have any questions regarding this medication, do not hesitate to contact your doctor, pharmacist, or nurse.

PATIENT INFORMATION
on
LITHIUM

Lithium is classified as a mood stabilizer. It is a simple element, found in nature in some mineral waters, and is also present in small amounts in the human body.

Uses

Lithium is used primarily in the treatment of acute mania and in the long-term control or prophylaxis of Manic Depressive Illness (Bipolar Disorder).

Though not approved for these indications, lithium has also been found to augment the effects of antidepressants in depression and obsessive compulsive disorder, and is useful in the treatment of cluster headaches, as well as chronic aggression or impulsivity.

How does the doctor decide what dose (how many milligrams) to prescribe?

The dose of lithium is different for every patient and is based on how much lithium is in the blood, as well as the response to treatment. The doctor will measure the lithium level in the blood on a regular basis during the first few months. The lithium level that is usually found to be effective for most patients is between 0.6 and 1.2 mmol/L (mEq/L).

You may initially take your medication several times a day (2 or 3); after several weeks, the doctor may decide to prescribe the drug once daily. It is important to drink 8–12 cups of fluid daily when on lithium (e.g., water, juice, milk, broth, etc.).

On the morning of your lithium blood test, take the morning dose of lithium **after** the test to avoid inaccurate results.

How quickly will the drug start working?

Control of manic symptoms may require up to 14 days of treatment. Because lithium takes time to work, **do not decrease or increase the dose or stop the medication** without discussing this with your doctor.

Improvement in symptoms of depression, obsessive compulsive disorder, cluster headaches, as well as aggression/impulsivity also occur gradually.

DO NOT STOP taking your medication if you are feeling better, without first discussing this with your doctor.

How long should you take this medication?

Following the first episode of mania it is recommended that lithium be continued for a minimum of one year; this decreases the chance of being ill again. The doctor may then decrease the drug slowly and monitor for any symptoms; if none occur, the drug can gradually be stopped.

For individuals who have had several episodes of mania or depression, lithium should be continued indefinitely.

Long-term treatment is generally recommended for recurring depression, obsessive-compulsive disorder, cluster headaches or aggression/impulsivity.

DO NOT STOP taking your medication if you are feeling better, without first discussing this with your doctor.

Side effects

Side effects occur, to some degree, with all medication. They are usually not serious and do not occur in all individuals. They may sometimes occur before beneficial effects of the medication are noticed. If a side effect continues, speak to your doctor about appropriate treatment.

Common side effects that should be reported to your doctor at the next appointment include:

- Lethargy, difficulty concentrating – This problem usually goes away with time. Use of other drugs that make you drowsy will worsen the problem. Avoid driving a car or operating machinery if drowsiness persists.
- Nausea or heartburn – If this happens, take the medication with food. If vomiting or diarrhea occur and persist for more than 24 hours, call your doctor.
- Muscle tremor, weakness, shakiness, stiffness – Speak to your doctor as this may require an adjustment in your dosage.
- Changes in sex drive or sexual performance – Discuss this with your doctor.
- Weight changes – Monitor your food intake; avoid foods with high fat content (e.g., cakes and pastry).
- Increased thirst and increase in frequency of urination – Discuss this with your doctor.
- Skin changes, e.g., dry skin, acne, rashes.

Side effects you should report IMMEDIATELY, as they may indicate the amount of lithium in the body is higher than it should be, include:

- Loss of balance
- Slurred speech
- Visual disturbances (e.g., double-vision)
- Nausea, vomiting, stomach ache
- Watery stools, diarrhea (more than twice a day)
- Abnormal general weakness or drowsiness

- Marked trembling (e.g., shaking that interferes with holding a cup), muscle twitches, jaw shaking

IF THESE OCCUR CALL YOUR DOCTOR RIGHT AWAY. If you cannot reach your doctor, stop taking the lithium until you get in touch with him. Drink plenty of fluids and snack on salty foods (e.g., chips, crackers). If symptoms continue to get worse, or if they do not clear within 12 hours, go to the Emergency Department of the nearest hospital. A clinical check-up and a blood test will show the cause of the problem.

Rare side effects you should report to your doctor **IMMEDIATELY** include:
- Soreness of the mouth, gums, or throat
- Skin rash or itching, swelling of the face
- Nausea, vomiting, loss of appetite, lethargy, weakness, fever, or flu-like symptoms
- Swelling of the neck (goitre)
- Abnormally frequent urination and increased thirst (e.g., having to get up in the night several times to pass urine)

Let your doctor know **as soon as possible** if you miss your period or suspect you may be **pregnant**.

What should you do if you forget to take a dose of your medication?

If you take your total dose of lithium in the morning and you forget to take it for more than 6 hours, skip the missed dose and continue with your schedule the next day. **DO NOT DOUBLE THE DOSE**. If you take the drug several times a day, take the missed dose when you remember, then continue with your regular schedule.

Interactions with other medication

Because lithium can change the effect of other medication, or may be affected by other medication, always check with your doctor or pharmacist before taking other drugs, including over-the-counter medication such as cold remedies. Always inform any doctor or dentist that you see that you are taking lithium.

Precautions

1. Do not increase or decrease your dose without consulting your doctor.
2. This drug may impair the mental and physical abilities and reaction time required for driving a car or operating other machinery. Avoid these activities if you feel drowsy or slowed down.
3. Do not stop your drug suddenly as this may result in withdrawal symptoms such as anxiety, irritability and emotional lability.
4. Report any changes in mood or behavior to your physician.
5. It is important to drink 8–12 cups of fluids daily (e.g., water, juice, milk, broth, etc.)
6. Do not change your salt intake during your treatment, without first speaking to your doctor (e.g., avoid no-salt or low-salt diets).
7. If you have the flu, especially if vomiting or diarrhea occur, check with your doctor regarding your lithium dose.
8. Use extra care in hot weather and during activities that cause you to sweat heavily (e.g., hot baths, saunas, exercising). The loss of too much water and salt from your body may lead to changes in the level of lithium in your body.
9. Tablets or capsules of lithium should be swallowed whole; do not crush them.
10. Store your medication in a clean, dry area at room temperature. Keep all medication out of the reach of children.

If you have any questions regarding this medication, do not hesitate to contact your doctor, pharmacist, or nurse.

PATIENT INFORMATION
on
ANTICONVULSANT MOOD STABILIZERS

The name of your medication is ____.

Uses

Anticonvulsants can be used in the treatment of acute mania and in the long-term control or prophylaxis of Manic Depressive Illness (Bipolar Disorder).

They are also used in the treatment of seizure disorders as well as certain pain syndromes (e.g., trigeminal neuralgia – carbamazepine; migraines – valproate).

Though not approved for these indications, these drugs have has also been found to be useful in the treatment of several other conditions, including: augmentation of antidepressants in the treatment of depression, augmentation of antipsychotics in the treatment of schizophrenia, withdrawal reactions from alcohol or sedative/hypnotics, and in behavior disturbances, such as chronic aggression or impulsivity.

How does the doctor decide what dose (how many milligrams) to prescribe?

The dose of the medication is different for every patient and is based on the amount of drug in the blood (for carbamazepine and valproate) as well as the response to treatment. You may initially take your medication several times a day (2 or 3); after several weeks, the doctor may decide to prescribe the drug once daily.

How often will you need to have blood levels done with carbamazapine and valproate?

The doctor will measure the drug level in the blood on a regular basis during the first few months until the dose is stable. Thereafter, drug levels will be done at least once a year or whenever there is a change in drug therapy.

What do the blood levels mean?

The carbamazepine level that is usually found to be effective for most patients is between 17 and 50 µmol/L (4–12 µg/ml). The valproate level that is usually found to be effective for most patients is between 350 and 700 µmol/L (50–100 µg/ml).

On the morning of your blood test, take the morning dose of your medication **after** the test to avoid inaccurate results.

Blood levels do not need to be done with either lamotrigine or gabapentin.

How quickly will the drug start working?

Control of manic symptoms or stabilization of mood may require up to 14 days of treatment. Because these medications need time to work, **do not decrease or increase the dose or stop the medication** without discussing this with your doctor.

Improvement in seizures, pain symptoms, as well as aggression/impulsivity also occur gradually.

How long should you take this medication?

Following the first episode of mania it is recommended that these drugs be continued for a minimum of one year; this decreases the chance of being ill again. The doctor may then decrease the drug slowly and monitor for any symptoms; if none occur, the drug can gradually be stopped. For individuals who have had several episodes of mania or depression, medication may need to be continued indefinitely.

Long-term treatment is generally recommended for recurring depression, seizure disorder and aggression/impulsivity.

Side effects

Side effects occur, to some degree, with all medication. They are usually not serious and do not occur in all individuals. They may sometimes occur before beneficial effects of the medication are noticed. If a side effect continues, speak to your doctor about appropriate treatment.

Common side effects that should be reported to your doctor at the next appointment include:

- Drowsiness and lethargy, difficulty concentrating – This problem goes away with time. Use of other drugs that make you drowsy will worsen the problem. Avoid driving a car or operating machinery if drowsiness persists.
- Dizziness – Get up from a lying or sitting position slowly; dangle your legs over the edge of the bed for a few minutes before getting up. Sit or lie down if dizziness persists or if you feel faint – then call the doctor.
- Ataxia or unsteadiness – Discuss this with your doctor as this may require an adjustment in your dosage.
- Blurred vision – This usually occurs at the start of treatment and tends to be temporary. Reading under a bright light or at a distance may help; a magnifying glass can be of temporary use. If the problem continues, advise your doctor.
- Dry mouth – Sour candy and sugarless gum help increase saliva in your mouth;

try to avoid sweet, calorie-laden beverages. Drink water and brush your teeth regularly.

- Nausea or heartburn – If this happens, take the medication with food. If vomiting or diarrhea occur and persist for more than 24 hours, call your doctor.
- Muscle tremor – Speak to your doctor as this may require an adjustment in your dosage.
- Changes in hair texture, hair loss (valproate).
- Changes in the menstrual cycle (valproate).
- Changes in sex drive or sexual performance – Discuss this with your doctor.
- Weight changes – Monitor your food intake; avoid foods with high fat content (e.g., cakes and pastry).

Rare side effects you should report to your doctor **IMMEDIATELY** include:

- Soreness of the mouth, gums, or throat, mouth lesions
- Skin rash or itching, swelling of the face (especially with carbamazepine and lamotrigine)
- Acute abdominal pain, nausea, vomiting, loss of appetite
- Lethargy, weakness, fever, or flu-like symptom
- Confusion or disorientation
- Easy bruising, bleeding, appearance of splotchy purplish darkening of the skin
- Yellowing of the skin or eyes, darkening of urine
- Unusual eye movements
- Severe dizziness or falls

Let your doctor know **as soon as possible** if you miss your period or suspect you may be **pregnant**.

What should you do if you forget to take a dose of your medication?

If you take your total dose of medication in the morning and you forget to take it for more than 6 hours, skip the missed dose and continue with your schedule the next day. **DO NOT DOUBLE THE DOSE**. If you take the drug several times a day, take the missed dose when you remember, then continue with your regular schedule.

Interactions with other medication

Because these drugs can change the effect of other medication, or may be affected by other medication, always check with your doctor or pharmacist before taking other drugs, including over-the-counter medication such as cold remedies. Always inform any doctor or dentist that you see that you are taking this drug.

Precautions

1. Do not increase or decrease your dose without consulting your doctor.
2. Avoid drinking grapefruit juice while on carbamazepine as it can affect the level of carbamazepine in your body.
3. If your are on liquid carbamazepine, do not mix it with any other liquid medication. The liquid form of valproic acid should not be mixed with carbonated beverages, such as soda pop. This may cause an unpleasant taste or mouth irritation.
4. Unless you are prescribed a chewable tablet, capsules or tablets should be swallowed whole; do not break or crush them.
5. These drugs may impair the mental and physical abilities and reaction time required for driving a car or operating other machinery. Avoid these activities if you feel drowsy or slowed down.
6. Do not stop your drug suddenly as this may result in withdrawal symptoms such as anxiety, irritability and emotional lability.
7. To treat occasional pain, avoid the use of ASA (aspirin and related products) if you are taking divalproex or valproic acid, as it can affect the blood level of this drug; acetaminophen (Tylenol) or ibuprofen (Motrin, Advil) are safer alternatives.
8. Report any changes in mood or behavior to your physician.
9. Store your medication in a clean, dry area at room temperature. Keep all medication out of the reach of children.

If you have any questions regarding this medication, do not hesitate to contact your doctor, pharmacist, or nurse.

PATIENT INFORMATION
on
L-TRYPTOPHAN

L-tryptophan is an amino acid, a natural body chemical.

Uses

L-tryptophan is used primarily as an add-on therapy in the treatment of acute mania or depression, and in the long-term control or prophylaxis of Manic Depressive Illness (Bipolar Disorder).

Though not approved for these indications, L-tryptophan has also been found to be useful as a sedative in insomnia and in behavior disturbances, such as chronic aggression or antisocial behavior.

How quickly will the drug start working?

Control of manic symptoms may require up to 14 days of treatment. Because L-tryptophan takes time to work, **do not decrease or increase the dose or stop the medication** without discussing this with your doctor.

Improvement in sleep disorders tends to occur relatively quickly (with the first dose). Benefits in behavior disturbances occur gradually.

How long should you take this medication?

L-tryptophan is often prescribed to increase the effectiveness of an antidepressant, an antipsychotic or another mood stabilizer. Long-term treatment is generally recommended for recurring depression or mood disorder.

As sleep problems are usually self-limiting, many individbuals take L-tryptophan only when needed (during periods of insomnia). Long-term treatment is generally recommended for treatment of behavior disturbances.

Side effects

Side effects occur, to some degree, with all medication. They are usually not serious and do not occur in all individuals. They may sometimes occur before beneficial effects of the medication are noticed. If a side effect continues, speak to your doctor about appropriate treatment.

Common side effects that should be reported to your doctor at the next appointment include:

- Drowsiness and lethargy, difficulty concentrating – This problem goes away with time. Use of other drugs that make you drowsy will worsen the problem. Avoid driving a car or operating machinery if drowsiness persists.
- Ataxia or unsteadiness, incoordination – Discuss this with your doctor as this may require an adjustment in your dosage.
- Nausea or heartburn – If this happens, take the medication with food.
- Dry mouth – Sour candy and sugarless gum help increase saliva in your mouth; try to avoid sweet, calorie-laden beverages. Drink water and brush your teeth regularly.

Rare side effects you should report to your doctor **IMMEDIATELY** include:

- Muscle twitches, tremor, incoordination, shivering, confusion
- Soreness of the mouth, gums, or throat, mouth lesions
- Skin rash or itching, swelling of the face
- Vomiting, abdominal pain
- Lethargy, weakness, fever or flu-like symptoms
- Yellowing of the skin or eyes, darkening of urine
- Severe dizziness
- Switch in mood to an unusual state of happiness, excitement, irritability

Let your doctor know **as soon as possible** if you miss your period or suspect you may be **pregnant**.

What should you do if you forget to take a dose of your medication?

If you take your total dose of L-tryptophan in the evening and you forget to take it that evening, skip the missed dose and continue with your schedule the next day. **DO NOT DOUBLE THE DOSE**. If you take the drug several times a day, take the missed dose when you remember, then continue with your regular schedule.

Interactions with other medication

Because L-tryptophan can change the effect of other medication, or may be affected by other medication, always check with your doctor or pharmacist before taking other drugs, including over-the-counter or herbal medication. Always inform any doctor or dentist you see that you are taking this drug.

Precautions

1. Do not increase or decrease your dose without consulting your doctor.

2. This drug may impair the mental and physical abilities and reaction time required for driving a car or operating other machinery. Avoid these activities if you feel drowsy or slowed down.
3. Inform your doctor before starting any protein-reduced diets as these can interfere with the action of this medication.
4. Report any changes in mood or behavior to your physician.
5. Store your medication in a clean, dry area at room temperature. Keep all medication out of the reach of children.

If you have any questions regarding this medication, do not hesitate to contact your doctor, pharmacist, or nurse.

PATIENT INFORMATION on PSYCHOSTIMULANTS

The name of your medication is ____.

Use

Psychostimulants are primarily used in the treatment of Attention Deficit Hyperactivity Disorder (ADHD) in children and adults. These drugs are also approved for use in Parkinson's Disease and Narcolepsy (a sleeping disorder).

Though they are currently not approved for this indication, psychostimulants have been found useful in the treatment of refractory depression.

How quickly will the drug start working?

Some response to psychostimulants is usually noted within the first week of treatment of ADHD and tends to increase over the next 3 weeks.

How does the doctor decide on the dosage?

Psychostimulants come in various preparations including short-acting and slow-release (i.e., spansules or extended-release) forms. The dose is based on the body weight and is usually given several times a day. Take the drug exactly as prescribed; **do not increase or decrease the dose without speaking to your doctor.**

How long should you take this medication?

Psychostimulants are usually prescribed for a period of several years. Some clinicians may decide to prescribe "drug holidays" to individuals on this medication, i.e., the drug is not taken at certain times (e.g., week-ends, vacations, etc.).

Side effects

Side effects occur, to some degree, with all medication. They are usually not serious and do not occur in all individuals. They may sometimes occur before beneficial effects of the medication are noticed. If a side effect continues, speak to your doctor about appropriate treatment.

Common side effects that should be reported to your doctor at the next appointment include:

- Energizing/agitated feeling, excitability – Some individuals may feel nervous or have difficulty sleeping for a few days after starting this medication. If you are taking the medication in the evening, the physician may decide to prescribe it earlier in the day.
- Increased heart rate and blood pressure – Speak to your doctor.
- Headache – This tends to be temporary and can be managed by taking analgesics (aspirin, acetaminophen) when required. Blood pressure should be checked.
- Nausea or heartburn – If this happens, take the medication with food or milk.
- Dry mouth – Sour candy and sugarless gum help increase saliva in your mouth; try to avoid sweet, calorie-laden beverages. Drink water and brush your teeth regularly.
- Loss of appetite, weight loss – Taking the medication after meals, eating smaller meals more frequently or drinking high calorie drinks may help.
- Blurred vision – This usually occurs at the start of treatment and may last 1–2 weeks. Reading under a bright light or at a distance may help; a magnifying glass can be of temporary use. If the problem continues, advise your doctor.
- Mild hair loss – Inform your doctor.
- Respiratory symptoms including sinusitis, sore throat or coughing.

Rare side effects you should report to your doctor **IMMEDIATELY** include:

- Muscle twitches, tics or movement problems
- Fast or irregular heart beat
- Persistent throbbing headache
- Soreness of the mouth, gums, or throat
- Skin rash or itching, swelling of the face
- Any unusual bruising or bleeding, appearance of splotchy purplish darkening of the skin
- Nausea, vomiting, loss of appetite, lethargy, weakness, fever, or flu-like symptoms
- Yellow tinge in the eyes or to the skin; dark-colored urine
- Severe agitation or restlessness
- **A switch in mood to an unusual state of happiness or irritability; fluctuations in mood**

Let your doctor know **as soon as possible** if you miss your period or suspect you may be **pregnant**.

What should you do if you forget to take a dose of your medication?

If you take the psychostimulant 2–3 times a day and forget to take a dose by more than 4 hours, skip the missed dose and continue with your regular schedule. **DO NOT DOUBLE THE DOSE.**

Interactions with other medication

Because psychostimulants can change the effect of other medication, or may be affected by other medication, always check with your doctor or pharmacist before taking other drugs, including over-the-counter medication such as cold remedies. Always inform any doctor or dentist that you see that you are taking a psychostimulant drug.

Precautions

1. Do not increase or decrease your dose without consulting your doctor.
2. Do not chew or crush the tablets or capsules.
3. Use caution while driving or performing tasks requiring alertness as these drugs can mask symptoms of fatigue and impair concentration.
4. Report to your doctor any changes in sleeping or eating habits or changes in mood or behavior.
5. Do not stop your drug suddenly as this may result in withdrawal symptoms such as insomnia and changes in mood and behavior.
6. This drug may interact with medication prescribed by your dentist, so let him/her know the name of the drug you are taking.
7. Store your medication in a clean, dry area at room temperature. Keep all medication out of the reach of children.

If you have any questions regarding this medication, do not hesitate to contact your doctor, pharmacist, or nurse.

PATIENT INFORMATION
on
COGNITION ENHANCERS

The name of your medication is ____.

Use

Cognition enhancers are primarily used in the **symptomatic treatment of mild to moderate Alzheimer's dementia.**

How quickly will the drug start working?

Improvement in concentration and attention is noted over a period of several weeks. Because these drugs take time to work **do not decrease or increase the dose** without discussing this with the doctor.

How does the doctor decide on the dosage?

The drug is started at a low dose to minimize the chance of side effects. The dose can be increased after several weeks if minimal improvement is seen. The dose of the drug tacrine is determined by the results of tests of liver function, which the physician performs on a regular basis.

How long should you take this medication?

Cognition enhancers are usually prescribed for a period of several years.

Side effects

Side effects occur, to some degree, with all medication. They are usually not serious and do not occur in all individuals. They may sometimes occur before beneficial effects of the medication are noticed. If a side effect continues, speak to your doctor about appropriate treatment.

Common side effects that should be reported to your doctor at the next appointment include:

- Energizing/agitated feeling, excitability – Some individuals may feel nervous or have difficulty sleeping for a few days after starting this medication. If you are taking the medication in the evening, the physician may decide to prescribe it earlier in the day.
- Headache – This tends to be temporary and can be managed by taking analgesics (aspirin, acetaminophen) when required.
- Nausea, vomiting, stomach pains, heartburn – If this happens, take the medication with food or milk.
- Diarrhea or constipation, flatulence.
- Loss of appetite, weight loss – Taking the medication after meals, eating smaller meals more frequently or drinking high calorie drinks may help.
- Weakness, fatigue
- Muscle aches or cramps – Can be managed by taking analgesics when required.
- Nasal congestion.
- Hot flushes.

Rare side effects you should report to your doctor **IMMEDIATELY** include:

- Yellow tinge in the eyes or to the skin; dark-colored urine
- Soreness of the mouth, gums, or throat
- Skin rash or itching, swelling of the face
- Nausea, vomiting, loss of appetite, lethargy, weakness, fever, or flu-like symptoms
- Severe agitation or restless

What should you do if you forget to take a dose of your medication?

If you take your total dose of the drug in the morning and you forget to take it for more than 6 hours, skip the missed dose and continue with your schedule the next day. **DO NOT DOUBLE THE DOSE**. If you take the drug several times a day, take the missed dose when you remember, then continue with your regular schedule.

Interactions with other medication

Because these drugs can change the effect of other medication, or may be affected by other medication, always check with your doctor or pharmacist before taking other drugs, including over-the-counter medication such as cold remedies. Always inform any doctor or dentist that you see that you are taking a cognition enhancer.

Precautions

1. Do not increase or decrease your dose without consulting your doctor
2. Report to your doctor any changes in sleeping or eating habits or changes in mood or behavior.
3. Do not stop your drug suddenly as this may result in changes in behavior and/or concentration. If rivastigmine was stopped for more than 3 days, DO NOT restart without contacting your doctor.

4. This drug may interact with medication prescribed by your dentist, so let him/her know the name of the drug you are taking.
5. Do not take any other medication (including over-the-counter and herbal products) without consulting with your doctor or pharmacist.
6. Store your medication in a clean, dry area at room temperature. Keep all medication out of the reach of children.

If you have any questions regarding this medication, do not hesitate to contact your doctor, pharmacist, or nurse.

Practical recommendations for caregivers to decrease agitation and improve communication with patients with dementia

1. Decrease environmental stimuli and modify the environment to maintain safety.
2. Maintain physical comfort.
3. Slow down your pace and simplify your actions (i.e., one demand at a time).
4. Use simple direct statements; limit choices. Speak clearly and slowly and allow time for response.
5. Match verbal and nonverbal signals; maintain eye contact and relaxed posture.
6. Identify situations/actions that result in agitation; modify these if possible.

PATIENT INFORMATION
on
SEX-DRIVE DEPRESSANTS

The name of your medication is ______________________________.

Use

These drugs are primarily used in the **reduction of sexual arousal and libido.**

How quickly will the drug start working?

These drugs interfere with the formation of the hormone testosterone in the body; their effect on sexual arousal and libido is noted over a period of several weeks. Because these drugs take time to work **do not decrease or increase the dose** without discussing this with the doctor.

How does the doctor decide on the dosage?

These drugs are available in different forms, including tablets and long-acting injections. For oral tablets, the dose of the drug is increased gradually until a good response is noted. A testosterone test, or your own report of the effects, can determine the correct dosage. The dose of the injection may also be related to whether the drug will be given every month or every 3 months.

How long should you take this medication?

Sex-drive depressants are usually prescribed for a period of several years.

Side effects

Side effects occur, to some degree, with all medication. They are usually not serious and do not occur in all individuals. They may sometimes occur before beneficial effects of the medication are noticed. If a side effect continues, speak to your doctor about appropriate treatment.

Common side effects that should be reported to your doctor at the next appointment include:
- Sweating, hot flashes
- Impotence
- Muscle aches or spasms – can be managed by taking analgesics when required.
- Breast swelling
- Decrease in body hair
- Lethargy, depressed mood
- Nervousness, insomnia

Rare side effects you should report to your doctor **IMMEDIATELY** include:
- Yellow tinge in the eyes or to the skin; dark-colored urine
- Soreness of the mouth, gums, or throat
- Skin rash or itching, swelling of the face
- Nausea, vomiting, loss of appetite, lethargy, weakness, fever, or flu-like symptoms
- Changes in mental or motor ability
- Swelling or pain in the legs

What should you do if you forget to take a dose of your medication?

If you take your total dose of the drug in the morning and you forget to take it for more than 6 hours, skip the missed dose and continue with your schedule the next day. **DO NOT DOUBLE THE DOSE**. If you miss your injection, contact your doctor and try to get an injection as soon as possible.

Interactions with other medication

Because these drugs can change the effect of other medication, or may be affected by other medication, always check with your doctor or pharmacist before taking other drugs, including over-the-counter medication such as cold remedies. Always inform any doctor or dentist that you see that you are taking this medication.

Precautions

1. Do not increase or decrease your dose without consulting your doctor.
2. Report to your doctor any changes in sleeping or eating habits or changes in mood or behavior.
3. Store your medication in a clean, dry area at room temperature. Keep all medication out of the reach of children.

If you have any questions regarding this medication, do not hesitate to contact your doctor, pharmacist, or nurse.

PATIENT INFORMATION on DISULFIRAM

Use

Disulfiram is primarily used as a **deterrent to alcohol use/abuse.**

How quickly will the drug start working?

Disulfiram inhibits the breakdown of alcohol in the body, resulting in a build-up of a chemical called acetaldehyde; this results in an unpleasant reaction when alcohol is consumed. The reaction can occur 10–20 minutes after drinking alcohol and may last up to 2 hours.

The reaction consists of: flushing, choking, nausea, vomiting, increased heart rate and decreased blood pressure (dizziness).

How long should you take this medication?

Disulfiram is usually prescribed for a set period of time to help the individual stop the use of alcohol. **Do not decrease or increase the dose** without discussing this with the doctor.

Side effects

Side effects occur, to some degree, with all medication. They are usually not serious and do not occur in all individuals. They may sometimes occur before beneficial effects of the medication are noticed. If a side effect continues, speak to your doctor about appropriate treatment.

Common side effects that should be reported to your doctor at the next appointment include:

- Drowsiness, lethargy, depression – This problem goes away with time. Use of other drugs that make you drowsy will worsen the problem. Avoid driving a car or operating machinery if drowsiness persists.
- Energizing/agitated feeling – Some individuals may feel nervous or have difficulty sleeping for a few days after starting this medication.
- Headache – Temporary use of analgesics (e.g., acetaminophen, ASA).
- Skin rash – Contact your doctor.
- Garlic-like taste

Rare side effects you should report to your doctor **IMMEDIATELY** include:

- Yellow tinge in the eyes or to the skin; dark-colored urine
- Soreness of the mouth, gums, or throat
- Skin rash or itching, swelling of the face
- Nausea, vomiting, loss of appetite, lethargy, weakness, fever, or flu-like symptoms

What should you do if you forget to take a dose of your medication?

If you take your total dose of the drug in the morning and you forget to take it for more than 6 hours, skip the missed dose and continue with your schedule the next day. **DO NOT DOUBLE THE DOSE**.

Interactions with other medication

Because disulfiram can change the effect of other medication, or may be affected by other medication, always check with your doctor or pharmacist before taking other drugs, including over-the-counter medication such as cold remedies. Always inform any doctor or dentist that you see that you are taking this medication.

Precautions

1. Do not increase or decrease your dose without consulting your do
2. Report to your doctor any changes in sleeping or eating habits or changes in mood or behavior.
3. Avoid all products (food and drugs) containing alcohol, including tonics, cough syrups, mouth washes and alcohol-based sauces. A delay in the reaction may be as long as 24 hours.
4. Exposure to alcohol-containing rubs or solvents (e.g., after-shave) may trigger a reaction.
5. Carry an identification card stating the name of the drug you are taking.
6. Store your medication in a clean, dry area at room temperature. Keep all medication out of the reach of children.

If you have any questions regarding this medication, do not hesitate to contact your doctor, pharmacist, or nurse.

PATIENT INFORMATION
on
NALTREXONE

Use

Naltrexone is primarily used as an aid in the treatment of alcohol dependence or addiction to opiates. Though not approved for this indication, naltrexone has also been used in the treatment of behavior and impulse-control disorders and obsessive-compulsive disorder.

How quickly will the drug start working?

Naltrexone blocks the "craving" for alcohol and opiates. It does not suppress withdrawal symptoms that can occur in opiate user and should not be used in anyone using narcotics in the previous 10 days; these individuals must undergo detoxification programs before starting naltrexone. Naltrexone is started at a low dose and increased gradually based on effectiveness. Onset of response is quick (within the hour).

How long should you take this medication?

Naltrexone is usually prescribed for a set period of time to help the individual discontinue the use of alcohol or opiates. Naltrexone is used for a prolonged period of time in the treatment of behavior and impulse- control problems and obsessive-compulsive disorder. **Do not decrease or increase the dose** without discussing this with the doctor.

Side effects

Side effects occur, to some degree, with all medication. They are usually not serious and do not occur in all individuals. They may sometimes occur before beneficial effects of the medication are noticed. If a side effect continues, speak to your doctor about appropriate treatment.

Common side effects that should be reported to your doctor at the next appointment include:

- Lethargy, confusion, depression – This problem goes away with time. Use of other drugs that make you drowsy will worsen the problem. Avoid driving a car or operating machinery if drowsiness persists.
- Nervousness, anxiety, insomnia – Some individuals may feel nervous or have difficulty sleeping for a few days after starting this medication.
- Headache – Temporary use of analgesics (e.g., acetaminophen, ASA).
- Joint and muscle pain – Temporary use of analgesics
- Abdominal pain, cramps, nausea and vomiting – If this happens take the medication with food or milk.
- Weight loss.

Rare side effects you should report to your doctor **IMMEDIATELY** include:

- Yellow tinge in the eyes or to the skin; dark-colored urine
- Soreness of the mouth, gums, or throat
- Skin rash or itching, swelling of the face
- Nausea, vomiting, loss of appetite, lethargy, weakness, fever, or flu-like symptoms

What should you do if you forget to take a dose of your medication?

If you take your total dose of the drug in the morning and you forget to take it for more than 6 hours, skip the missed dose and continue with your schedule the next day. **DO NOT DOUBLE THE DOSE.** If you take the drug several times a day, take the missed dose when you remember, then continue with your regular schedule.

Interactions with other medication

Because naltrexone can change the effect of other medication, or may be affected by other medication, always check with your doctor or pharmacist before taking other drugs, including over-the-counter medication such as cold remedies. Always inform any doctor or dentist that you see that you are taking this medication.

Precautions

1. Do not increase or decrease your dose without consulting your do
2. Report to your doctor any changes in sleeping or eating habits or changes in mood or behavior.
3. Carry an identification card stating the name of the drug you are taking.
4. Store your medication in a clean, dry area at room temperature. Keep all medication out of the reach of children.

If you have any questions regarding this medication, do not hesitate to contact your doctor, pharmacist, or nurse.

PATIENT INFORMATION on METHADONE

Use

Methadone is primarily used as a substitute drug in the treatment of narcotic (opiate) dependent patients who desire maintenance therapy. It suppresses withdrawal symptoms of other narcotic analgesics as well as the craving for narcotics.

How quickly will the drug start working?

Methadone blocks the "craving" and withdrawal reactions from narcotics/opiates immediately. Methadone is started at a low dose and increased gradually, based on effectiveness, to a maintenance dose. It is then prescribed once daily.

Why is methadone given on a daily basis?

Methadone is a narcotic and its dispensing and usage is governed by Federal regulations. It is prepared as a liquid, mixed with orange juice. Most patients receive their methadone, on a daily basis, from the Pharmacy and are required to drink the contents of the bottle in the presence of the pharmacist.

Some patients (who are stable on their medication) are permitted to carry several days' supply of methadone.

How long should you take this medication?

The length of time methadone is prescribed varies among individuals and depends on a number of factors, including their progress in therapy; most patients receive methadone for several months, while others may require it for several years. Any decreases in dose should be done very gradually under the direction of the physician. It has been demonstrated that methadone is beneficial in helping patients avoid illicit narcotic use and helps them attain social stability.

Side effects

Side effects occur, to some degree, with all medication. They are usually not serious and do not occur in all individuals. They may sometimes occur before beneficial effects of the medication are noticed. If a side effect continues, speak to your doctor about appropriate treatment.

Common side effects that should be reported to your doctor at the next appointment include:

- Lethargy, confusion, depression – This problem goes away with time. Use of other drugs that make you drowsy will worsen the problem. Avoid driving a car or operating machinery if drowsiness persists.
- Energized feeling, insomnia – Some individuals may feel nervous or have difficulty sleeping for a few days after starting this medication.
- Dizziness, lightheadedness, weakness – This should go away with time.
- Joint and muscle pain – Temporary use of analgesics may help.
- Nausea and vomiting – If this happens take the medication after eating.
- Loss of appetite, weight loss – Taking the medication after meals, eating smaller meals more frequently or drinking high calorie drinks may help.
- Changes in sex drive or sexual performance – Though rare, should this problem occur, discuss it with your doctor.
- Sweating, flushing – You may sweat more than usual; frequent showering, use of deodorants and talcum powder may help.
- Constipation – Increase bulk foods in your diet (e.g., salads, bran) and drink plenty of fluids. Some individuals find a bulk laxative (e.g., Metamucil, Fibyrax) or a stool softener (Colace, Surfak) helps regulate their bowels. If these remedies are not effective, consult your doctor or pharmacist.

Rare side effects you should report to your doctor **IMMEDIATELY** include:

- Yellow tinge in the eyes or to the skin; dark-colored urine
- Soreness of the mouth, gums, or throat
- Skin rash or itching, swelling of the face
- Nausea, vomiting, loss of appetite, lethargy, weakness, fever, or flu-like symptoms

What should you do if you forget to take a dose of your medication?

It is important to take this medication at approximately the same time, on a daily basis. Missing a dose can result in a withdrawal reaction, consisting of restlessness, insomnia, nausea, vomiting, headache, increased perspiration, congestion, "gooseflesh," abdominal cramps, muscle and bone pain.

Interactions with other medication

Because methadone can change the effect of other medication, or may be affected by other medication, always check with your doctor or pharmacist before taking other drugs, including over-the-counter medication such as cold remedies. Always inform any doctor or dentist that you see that you are taking this medication.

Precautions

1. Do not share this medication with anyone. If you receive "carries" of methadone, store them out of the reach of children (preferably in a lockable compartment in the refrigerator); methadone can be poisonous to individuals who do not take opiates.
2. Report to your doctor any changes in sleeping or eating habits or changes in mood or behavior.
3. Carry an identification card stating the name of the drug you are taking.

If you have any questions regarding this medication, do not hesitate to contact your doctor, pharmacist, or nurse.

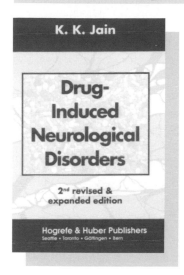

A uniquely beautiful textbook, with a uniquely practical orientation.

visit **www.hhpub.com** to see a sample chapter, or order an inspection copy

One of the most popular and highly regarded behavioral science and psychology textbooks, the new, third edition of this well-established resource has been fully updated and revised in response to changes in the health care delivery system and the increased importance of psychology and behavioral science in medical training and practice. Competitively priced compared to many, much less comprehensive, question-and-answer-type course review works, the main features of Danny Wedding's *Behavior and Medicine* are its:

- **Practical, clinical emphasis, focusing on the behavioral aspects of health care delivery vital in training and practice**
- **Comprehensive, trustworthy, and up to date coverage**
- **Contributions from leading educators at major medical faculties**
- **Numerous case examples, tables, charts, and boxes for quick access to information**
- **Learning and exam aids, such as sample USMLE review questions after each section**
- **Use of hundreds of thought-provoking works of art and poetry to illuminate the main points**
- **New chapters on alternative medicine, disability, and cancer, as well as on psychopathology and the ways in which mental illness presents in primary care settings**

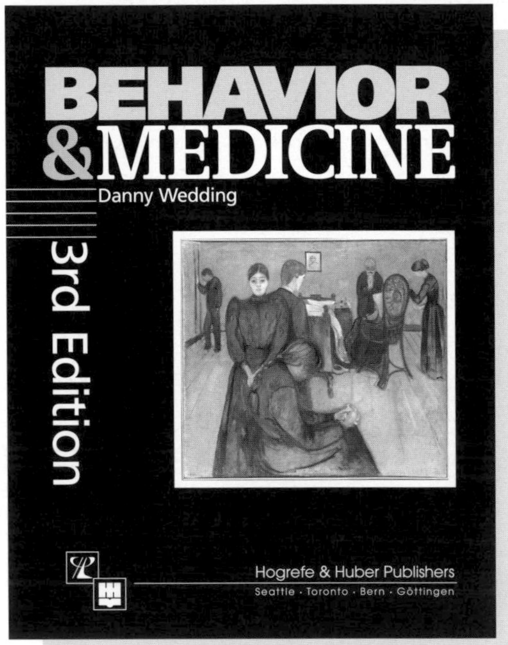

US $34.95
ISBN: 0-88937-238-1
softcover, 504 pages

Table of Contents

A comprehensive and up-to-date text, with a practical, clinical emphasis and a structure that mirrors the way psychology and behavioral science are approached in the medical school classroom.

Order via www.hhpub.com or call (800) 228-3749

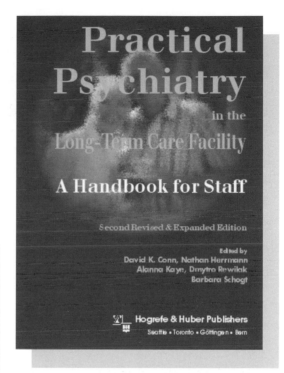

Hogrefe & Huber Publishers
USA • Canada • Germany • Switzerland

Serving the medical and social science communities for more than three generations

Order online at www.hhpub.com

ORDER FORM

Clinical Handbook of Psychotropic Drugs 12th Edition

Price	Quantity	Total
Book edition, ISBN 0-88937-258-6, US $49.95	____	______
Subscription ed., ISBN 0-88937-259-4, US $94.95	____	______
Postage & Handling (add $4.60 for first item and $1.00 for each additional item)		______
Washington State residents, please add 8.8% sales tax Canadians, please add 7% GST		______
Total		______

- Professor examination copies available
- Discounts apply with bulk orders of 10 copies or more
- Enquire for details

❑ Check in the amount of______________ enclosed

❑ Charge my: Visa____ Mastercard____ Amex____

Cardholder name ______________________________

Card #: ______________________________

Signature: ______________________________

Expiry Date: ____________

❑ Put me on your mailing list ❑ Send catalogue

❑ Please send me future editions with the appropriate invoice.

Make check payable to and send order to:
HOGREFE & HUBER Publishers or call

(800) 228-3749

Name: ______________________________

Address: ______________________________

____

____

____

Tel.: ______________________________

Fax: ______________________________

E-mail: ______________________________

Hogrefe & Huber Publishers
USA • Canada • Germany • Switzerland

Serving the medical and social science communities for more than three generations

Order online at www.hhpub.com

ORDER FORM

Clinical Handbook of Psychotropic Drugs 12th Edition

Price / Quantity / Total
Book edition, ISBN 0-88937-258-6, US $49.95
Subscription ed., ISBN 0-88937-259-4, US $94.95
Postage & Handling (add $4.60 for first item and $1.00 for each additional item)
Washington State residents, please add 8.8% sales tax
Canadians, please add 7% GST
Total

- Professor examination copies available
- Discounts apply with bulk orders of 10 copies or more
- Enquire for details

❑ Check in the amount of______________ enclosed
❑ Charge my: Visa____ Mastercard____ Amex____
Cardholder name ______________________________
Card #: ______________________________
Signature: ______________________________
Expiry Date: ____________
❑ Put me on your mailing list ❑ Send catalogue
❑ Please send me future editions with the appropriate invoice.
Make check payable to and send order to:
HOGREFE & HUBER Publishers or call
(800) 228-3749
Name:
Address:
Tel.:
Fax:
E-mail:

Hogrefe & Huber Publishers
USA • Canada • Germany • Switzerland

Serving the medical and social science communities for more than three generations

ORDER FORM

Clinical Handbook of Psychotropic Drugs 12th Edition

Price / Quantity / Total
Book edition, ISBN 0-88937-258-6, US $49.95
Subscription ed., ISBN 0-88937-259-4, US $94.95
Postage & Handling (add $4.60 for first item and $1.00 for each additional item)
Washington State residents, please add 8.8% sales tax
Canadians, please add 7% GST
Total

- Professor examination copies available
- Discounts apply with bulk orders of 10 copies or more
- Enquire for details

❑ Check in the amount of______________ enclosed
❑ Charge my: Visa____ Mastercard____ Amex____
Cardholder name ______________________________
Card #: ______________________________
Signature: ______________________________
Expiry Date: ____________
❑ Put me on your mailing list ❑ Send catalogue
❑ Please send me future editions with the appropriate invoice.
Make check payable to and send order to:
HOGREFE & HUBER Publishers or call
(800) 228-3749
Name:
Address:
Tel.:
Fax:
E-mail:

Hogrefe & Huber Publishers
Customer Service Department
P.O. Box 2487
Kirkland, WA 98083

Please return the order cards to one of our offices listed below, whichever is most convenient to you:

❑ – USA
Hogrefe & Huber Publishers
P.O. Box 2487
Kirkland, WA 98083
Phone (800) 228-3749
Fax (425) 823-8324

❑ – CANADA
Hogrefe & Huber Publishers
Suite 514, 1543 Bayview Ave
Toronto, Ontario M4G 3B5
Phone (425) 820-1500
Fax (425) 823-8324

❑ – GERMANY
Hogrefe & Huber Publishers
Rohnsweg 25
D-37085 Göttingen
Phone +49 551 49609-0
Fax +49 551 49609-88

❑ – SWITZERLAND
Verlag Hans Huber
Länggass-Strasse 76
CH-3000 Bern 9
Phone +41 31 300-4500
Fax +41 31 300-4590

Or order at our website: www.hhpub.com

Hogrefe & Huber Publishers
Customer Service Department
P.O. Box 2487
Kirkland, WA 98083